Participation in Health and Welfare Services

T0187852

Today, healthy ageing and active, meaningful lives are core values and aims for international and national health policies. Health services are challenged to ensure that the recipients of their services are active participants in their own care and beyond. Participation allows patients to become less dependent on healthcare providers, increasing their control over their own treatment and health. Increasingly, the idea of 'participation' is shifting, from participation in services to participation in mainstream society.

This book examines the concept of participation, as well as the different meanings it takes on in the context of health and welfare services. It asks how services can enable and stimulate participation outside of those services. The contributions in this volume particularly focus on participation as engagement in daily life and 'everyday life' in order to develop the field of participation beyond the sphere of health and social care services. This book will appeal to researchers in the fields of health and social care, social services, occupational therapy and the sociology of health and illness. It will be of interest to practitioners of health and welfare services.

Arne H. Eide, Norwegian University for Science and Technology and SINTEF Technology and Society, Norway.

Staffan Josephsson, Norwegian University for Science and Technology and Karolinska Institutet, Sweden.

Kjersti Vik, Norwegian University for Science and Technology.

Routledge Studies in Health and Social Welfare

For a full list of titles in this series, please visit www.routledge.com

Participation in Health and Welfare Services

Professional Concepts
and Lived Experience

**Edited by Arne H. Eide,
Staffan Josephsson and Kjersti Vik**

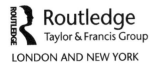

Routledge
Taylor & Francis Group

LONDON AND NEW YORK

First published 2017 by Routledge

2 Park Square, Milton Park, Abingdon, Oxfordshire OX14 4RN
52 Vanderbilt Avenue, New York, NY 10017

Routledge is an imprint of the Taylor & Francis Group, an informa business

First issued in paperback 2019

Copyright © 2017 selection and editorial matter, Arne H. Eide, Staffan Josephsson, Kjersti Vik; individual chapters, the contributors

The right of Arne H. Eide, Staffan Josephsson and Kjersti Vik to be identified as the authors of the editorial material, and of the authors for their individual chapters, has been asserted in accordance with sections 77 and 78 of the Copyright, Designs and Patents Act 1988.

All rights reserved. No part of this book may be reprinted or reproduced or utilised in any form or by any electronic, mechanical, or other means, now known or hereafter invented, including photocopying and recording, or in any information storage or retrieval system, without permission in writing from the publishers.

Notice:
Product or corporate names may be trademarks or registered trademarks, and are used only for identification and explanation without intent to infringe.

British Library Cataloguing-in-Publication Data
A catalogue record for this book is available from the British Library

Library of Congress Cataloging-in-Publication Data
A catalog record for this book has been requested

ISBN: 978-1-138-64485-4 (hbk)
ISBN: 978-0-367-23641-0 (pbk)

Typeset in Times New Roman
by Apex CoVantage, LLC

This book is dedicated to Dr. David Gray, who is co-author in one of the chapters and who unfortunately passed away before the book was finalised. From his base at Washington University in St. Louis, USA, David was a pioneer in participation research and a great inspiration to many of us. His influence on this book, as well as in the area of participation, is priceless.

Contents

Contributors

Sissel Alsaker, PhD, is Associate Professor at the Norwegian University of Science and Technology, Faculty of Health and Social Sciences, Program of Mental Health Work. She is engaged in research that is contributing to new knowledge in the interdisciplinary field of mental health work. The knowledge base is in the field of social and occupational science, studying everyday life in the cultural contexts where humans live and act. More broadly, Alsaker studies how humans can be enabled to change and adjust their social practices and enhance their participation in their cultural contexts.

Peter Beresford, OBE, is Professor of Citizen Participation at the University of Essex and Emeritus Professor of Social Policy at Brunel University London. He is Co-Chair of Shaping Our Lives, the UK independent disabled people's and service users' organisation, network and think tank. He is a long-term user of mental health services and has a longstanding background of involvement in issues of participation as a writer, researcher, activist and teacher. His latest book is *All Our Welfare: Towards Participatory Social Policy* (Policy Press, 2016).

Ebba Langum Bredland is an Associate Professor at the Department of Health and Social Science at the Norwegian University of Science and Technology. Bredland has had a part-time position in the clinical field since 2008. She has experienced challenges, both physically and psychosocially, among elderly patients, which has strongly influenced her research interest. Bredland has competence and experience integrating interdisciplinary perspectives into health promotion in the community. Her present research is about older people's everyday life, inclusion and participation. She participates in national and international research networks.

Jessica Dashner, OTD OTR/L, is an Instructor in Occupational Therapy (OT) and Neurology at Washington University School of Medicine. In 2002, she received a Clinical Doctorate in OT from Washington University. For over 10 years she worked as a Research Associate in the Disability & Community Participation Research Laboratory with Dr. David Gray at Washington University. Her research interests include developing and testing interventions to improve participation of individuals with sensory and mobility impairments. Dr. Dashner teaches the Environmental Factors Facilitating Performance and Participation I & II and the Health Promotion, Participation and Wellness for Persons with Chronic Disease classes at Washington University.

Virginia Dickie retired in 2012 from the University of North Carolina Chapel Hill, where she was an Associate Professor and Director of the Division of Occupational Science and Occupational Therapy. Following her retirement, she held a part-time appointment as a visiting researcher at Luleå Uåniversity of Technology in Lule, Sweden, for a year and a half. She is an occupational therapist (MS, University of Wisconsin, Madison; MS, Wayne State University) and anthropologist (PhD, Wayne State University) whose research has focused on the occupations of making quilts and of being a self-employed crafter, selling in small-scale local markets. This research led to her collaboration in the development of a transactional perspective on occupation.

Grainne Donellan is an Occupational Therapist within the Primary Care Services based in North Dublin, Ireland. She completed her research thesis at the Department of Occupational Therapy, University of Limerick, Ireland. Her research explored mental health service users' perspectives on social inclusion and participation.

Arne H. Eide is Chief Scientist at SINTEF Technology and Society, Norway; Professor at the Norwegian University of Science and Technology (NTNU); and Guest Professor at Stellenbosch University, South Africa. He has been the lead researcher on activity and participation at Sør-Trøndelag University College/NTNU for the last 10 years and has long experience with participatory research on disability, both in Norway and in low-income contexts.

Toril Anne Elstad is Associate Professor at the Program for Master and Diploma Course in Mental Health Work, Faculty of Health and Social Sciences, Norwegian University of Science and Technology, Trondheim. She has a clinical background as a mental health nurse, and her research interests are in the areas of participation and social inclusion related to mental health and mental health services research. Her PhD thesis is an ethnographic study within a community mental health service.

David B. Gray, PhD, was a Professor in the Occupational Therapy program at Washington University School of Medicine in St. Louis, Missouri, for 20 years. Throughout his time at Washington University, his work encompassed a community-based approach. His research focus was participation of people with disabilities in the environment. He developed outcome measures with participation at the core as well as tested interventions (such as exercise, enhanced personal assistance services and assistive technology) to improve community participation for people with disabilities. His measures of community participation and environmental facilitators and barriers have been internationally recognized. He authored and co-authored numerous publications related to disability, participation and environment.

Jade Gross, OTD, OTR/L, CSLT, is a full-time Occupational Therapist working in an outpatient clinic and a part-time Professor of Occupational Therapy at Georgia State University. Gross received her bachelor's degree in psychology at the University of Kansas and doctorate degree in occupational therapy at Washington University School of Medicine's program in occupational therapy. Jade's career interests are in rehabilitation of the upper extremity, lymphedema and breast cancer rehabilitation, and helping to ensure equal access to quality healthcare for all consumers.

Kirsti Haracz, PhD, MSc, BAppSC OT, is a Lecturer in Occupational Therapy at the University of Newcastle (Australia). Haracz worked in mental health settings in Australia and England before commencing her academic career in 2006. The field of mental health recovery remains central to Haracz's work in her teaching and research.

Helena Hemmingsson, PhD, holds a position as Professor in Occupational Therapy at the Department of Social and Welfare Studies, Linköping University, Sweden. Her research has a focus on disability in everyday life with a major research line in school participation and the transition to working life for young people with disabilities. In addition, several research projects focus on enabling technology and digital equality. Her research group cooperates internationally with researchers in Europe, the USA and Australia.

Clare Hocking has worked at the Auckland University of Technology for more than 25 years. She is an Associate Professor at the University of Plymouth in the UK and Chiang Mai University in Thailand. Hocking serves as the Executive Editor of the *Journal of Occupational Science*, co-authored the third edition of Wilcock's *Occupational Perspective of Health* (2015) and co-edited *Occupational Science: Society, Inclusion, Participation* (2012). The author of 100 refereed articles and 25 book chapters, her major focus is occupational justice and human rights. As the current Chair of the World Federation of Occupational Therapists (WFOT) Advisory Group on Human Rights, she co-ordinated input to the Revised Minimum Standards for the Education of Occupational Therapists (2016).

Holly Hollingsworth, PhD, is an Associate Research Professor (Retired) at the Program in Occupational Therapy in the Washington University School of Medicine. He has a BA in Mathematics, San Francisco State University; and a MA in Mathematical Statistics and a PhD in Applied Statistics and Measurement, University of Illinois, Champaign-Urbana. His research interests are in social participation in the community of people with mobility impairments. He has authored and co-authored several articles in this area.

Sissel Horghagen is Associate Professor at the Norwegian University of Science and Technology. She is the Program Director of the Occupational Therapy Education and responsible for a master course in Occupational Science. Horghagen is a co-editor of the Norwegian journal *Ergoterapeuten*, and has co-authored two Norwegian books about occupational therapy. Her major focus is the transformative potential of cultural and creative activities for people in vulnerable life situations, transition from education to work for people with disabilities, and health promotion.

Klara Jakobsen is an Occupational Therapist and a Professor in Health Science in the Faculty of Health and Social Sciences, Occupational Therapy, at the Norwegian University of Science and Technology. Her research focus explores current challenges and health-promoting solutions when vulnerable or disadvantaged groups are to be assisted to work participation.

Gundi Schrötter Johannsen is a Senior Lecturer at the University College South, Denmark. She has a background as a social educator in the field of mental health services, and a candidate degree from the Danish University of Social Education. Her theoretical interests are grounded anthropology, sociology and social psychology.

Staffan Josephsson is Professor at Karolinska Institutet, Sweden, and at the Norwegian University of Science and Technology (NTNU). He has been a researcher on activity in relation to creativity, involvement and participation for people with chronic disabilities for more than two decades, the last 10 of these with an affiliation also at Sør-Trøndelag University College/NTNU.

Ulla Kroksmark, MA, is a registered Occupational Therapist and Researcher at the Institute of Neurology and Physiology/Ophthalmology, Sahlgrenska Academy, University of Gothenburg, Sweden. She has taught at the bachelor program in occupational therapy and health promotion at the University in Lund, Gothenburg and Umeå. Her main research areas are living habits in everyday life and participation and health promotion.

Terry Krupa is a Professor and Associate Director (Research and Post-Professional Programs) in the School of Rehabilitation Therapy at Queen's University in Kingston, Ontario. Her practice and scholarly work has focused primarily on the development and research of approaches directed to improving the health, well-being and full community participation of people with mental illness.

Lisbeth Kvam is a sociologist, MS, and is currently working as Associate Professor/PhD at The Faculty of Health and Social Science, at the Norwegian University of Science and Technology. In her doctoral work, she investigated the concept of participation in major life areas among men and women in vocational rehabilitation. She has experience from working in the Norwegian Labour and Welfare Administration. Her main research interests include participatory and inclusive research, vocational rehabilitation, and participation and work inclusion for persons with intellectual disability.

Annelie Schedin Leiulfsrud is Occupational Therapy Specialist, St. Olav's University Hospital, Trondheim. Schedin Leiulfsrud has a background in clinical rehabilitation of persons with a spinal cord injury (SCI) since the late 1980s in Sweden and in Norway. She played an important role in establishing the

Norwegian SCI Registry. She has collaborated with researchers working within the International Classification of Functioning, Disability and Health (ICF) framework in several international SCI projects on social participation, employment and living conditions. Her doctoral thesis from 2016 is entitled 'Exploring Persons with a Spinal Cord Injury's Participation in Society'.

Margareta Lilja, PhD, holds a position as Professor in Occupational Therapy at the Department of Health Science, Luleå University of Technology, Sweden. Her research is mostly focused on older adults' needs and interests in relation to his/her occupational performance, environment and participation in society. Of particular interest is technology as a resource in community-based rehabilitation. She is also involved in several research networks, both national and international.

Rosemary Lysaght is an Associate Director (Occupational Therapy) of the School of Rehabilitation Therapy at Queen's University in Kingston, Ontario, and Associate Professor. Her professional expertise is in the areas of work rehabilitation, assistive technologies, and program administration and evaluation. Her primary research focuses are work participation and social inclusion of people in marginalized groups.

Eva Magnus, PhD, is an Associate Professor at the Norwegian University of Technology and Science, Department of Health Science. She teaches at the bachelor level in occupational therapy and master level in occupational and movement science. Her main research areas are disability studies, with a focus on disabled students and transitioning from education to employment, everyday life and participation and health promotion.

Deirdre Mahon works as a Specialist Occupational Therapist in the field of Neurological Rehabilitation and is currently based at London's Imperial College Healthcare Trust. Since graduating from the University of Limerick in 2009, she has worked in Ireland, Australia and the UK.

Elizabeth McKay is Reader at Brunel University and an educator and qualitative researcher. Her research topics includes mental health service users' experiences, professional education, transition into the professional workplace, and palliative care stakeholders' views on hospice at home.

Turid Midjo is Associate Professor/PhD at The Faculty of Health and Social Science, Norwegian University of Science and Technology. Her main research fields today are on child welfare and learning disabilities with a special interest in institutional talk, participation and transition processes. She has published several reports and different types of articles.

Nils Erik Ness is Associate Professor at the Norwegian University of Science and Technology, Faculty of Health and Social Sciences, Occupational Therapy and President of the Norwegian Occupational Therapy Association. Together with other user and professional associations, Ness has been politically active in developing primary healthcare to ensure inclusion and participation, especially within the areas of re-ablement and assistive technology.

Kersti Nordell is a PhD in Human Geography. She is a former teacher and researcher at the University of Gothenburg, Sweden, with a focus on the opportunities to use the time-geographic approach in areas of disability and health. Now she is self-employed with consulting assignments connected to her former research, among them developing The Aday System based on the time-geographic method, together with Ulla Kroksmark.

Heidi Pedersen has worked as a social worker in the Norwegian Labour and Welfare Administration and as a researcher at the Norwegian University of Science and Technology (NTNU) Social Research, and she is now a PhD student at The Department of Health Science (NTNU). In her doctoral thesis, she studies user experiences with adaptive technology, users' needs in the dissemination of adaptive technology, and how adaptive technology can contribute to activity and participation on users' own terms. An important field of interest has been how different forms of organization are significant for social work practice and service delivery. The topic has been studied on the basis of application of employability assessments in the Norwegian Labour and Welfare Administration. Professional understanding and user involvement have been key topics for exploration.

Skender Redzovic is Associate Professor and Head of the Department of Applied Social Science at the Norwegian University of Science and Technology. He is responsible for the direction and management of research and development projects within multiple research areas. His completed PhD degree in organizational psychology is an explorative study of the relationship between organizational norms and subjective well-being at work. His primary areas of teaching and research include organizational culture, occupation and participation, innovation and entrepreneurship within health and social sciences, as well as mental health. Redzovic has been a visiting researcher at the University of California, Berkeley.

Susan Ryan, PhD, MSc, BAppSc OT, is currently a Professor Emerita at University College Cork, Ireland; a Conjoint Professor at The University of Newcastle, Australia; and an Adjunct Professor at Charles Sturt University, Australia. Ryan has headed occupational therapy programs in Cork, Ireland; Newcastle, Australia; and a suite of Master's Programs in London, England. Her research expertise and experience lies in the educational development of thinking and reasoning in therapy at the undergraduate and graduate levels. Susan applies this knowledge to program and module design and research grant applications to develop online e-learning materials to enhance students' professional abilities.

Sarah Sheldon, BOccThy, Hons, graduated from Occupational Therapy at the University of Newcastle (Australia) in 2010. Sheldon has since worked for a short time in Sydney before relocating to the United Kingdom. She is currently working as Occupational Therapist at Headley Court. Sheldon is involved in treating a complex physical and psychosocial case mix.

Sylvia Söderström, PhD, holds a position as an Associate Professor at the Department of Health and Social Science at the Norwegian University of Science and Technology. Her research field is within Disability Studies with a special focus on disability and technology within a Science, Technology and Society (STS) studies perspective. Her research is concerned with young disabled people's everyday life, inclusion and participation, as well as identity negotiations, categorisation and intersectionality. She participates in national and international research networks and collaborates with researchers nationally, in Sweden, in the UK and in Nepal.

Kjersti Vik is Professor at the Department of Occupational Therapy, Faculty of Medicine and Health Sciences, Norwegian University of Science and Technology (NTNU). Her main research field is on older adults and participation, with a special focus on community healthcare and rehabilitation. Vik has published several textbooks about older adults and rehabilitation. She is the leader of the research group Activity and Participation at NTNU. Professor Vik's research group is leading in its field in Norway and has extensive collaboration with research institutions internationally.

Aud Elisabeth Witsø is a Disability Nurse and currently works as Associate Professor/PhD at The Faculty of Health and Social Science, at the Norwegian University of Science and Technology. Her doctoral work explored the concept of participation in older adults in the context of living in place and receiving home-based services. She has academic and clinical experience of working in the fields of aging, intellectual disability, disability and educational research. Her particular research interests include participatory and inclusive research, the improvement and innovation of activity, participation and services for older adults and persons with intellectual disability.

1 Introduction and rationale

*Arne H. Eide, Staffan Josephsson,
Kjersti Vik and Nils Erik Ness*

The relevance for service delivery

Current and future health and welfare services in developed countries face enormous challenges due to demographic changes, increasing chronic health problems, medical and technological progress, marginalisation, unemployment and poverty. In tandem with this, there is an ambition to address criticism of paternalistic tendencies in service delivery, and to make room for more active agency and involvement of individuals and groups in matters concerning life and health. A growing elderly population and subsequent growth in chronic diseases imply that a substantial proportion of the population will be permanently or long-term dependent on health, care or rehabilitation services (WHO 2004). Likewise, a substantial number of people who depend on welfare services are at risk of exclusion in various forms (Salonen in Matthies and Uggerhøj 2014). Healthy ageing (WHO 2002), social inclusion, active citizens, empowerment and participation (EU 2007a; Newman and Tonkens 2011) have become core values and aims of the welfare state, as well as in international and national health and welfare policies. The drive for participation and inclusion in society are central in equality and diversity policies, for instance, regarding individuals with disability (UN 2006) and immigrants (EU 2005).

Exclusion and marginalisation have become major concerns for policymakers, both in Europe and globally. Services are challenged, not only in their capacity to do more of the same, but also in terms of facing strong pressure to develop a new fundament for the services with active, participating users (EC 2007b). This is driving a qualitative change in objectives, professional practice, the role of patients/users, and the balance of power between patients/users and providers. An additional driver in this development is technological innovation, which is increasingly altering communication between patients and medical personnel, as well as patients' control over their own health and patterns of service use. In years to come, this will strongly contribute to change in existing practice.

While service users clearly comprise a large heterogeneous group, people with chronic health problems and dependency on welfare services are vulnerable to exclusion and marginalisation, which are often the reasons for service needs in the first place. The broad notion of vulnerability (Flaskerud and Winslow 1998, p. 69) thus defines the groups that are of main interest to the authors of this book. Matthies (2014) suggests participation and marginalisation as twin concepts, forming the two ends of a continuum. We feel that this greatly contributes to our understanding of participation.

The turn to participation as feature and fundament within healthcare and social service is not without complications. Participation is a multidimensional concept with different uses and meanings (Cornwall 2008). Therefore, when this term is increasingly used in legislation, policy documents, clinical guidelines and among activists within disability and user organisations, the need for reflection and discussion relating to participation as a concept and its use becomes pertinent. A precise, conscious and reflected use of participation in the health and welfare services discourse is necessary in order to understand the impact and potential of an emerging conceptual development, to tackle its complexity and multidimensionality, and to avoid conceptual deflation. There is a growing awareness in the literature that participation as involvement in everyday life situations might differ in important respects from participation as used in discourses within health and welfare practice. Inherent in this distinction is also the divide between participation as a professional concept and as an everyday phenomenon within peoples' lives. It is an ambition of this book to make both levels of understanding of participation, i.e. the professional and the popular – belonging to peoples' everyday life – and their relationship visible. Knowledge of how these two understandings can communicate and work together is important for health and welfare services in order for them to enable and stimulate participation in mainstream society.

Even if participation as an ideal for health and welfare services has been around for decades and has influenced professional practice, it is also true that, at least in healthcare, involvement of users has been limited, and the complexity of participation and its facilitators and barriers need further attention (Collins et al. 2007). This book takes on these challenges by describing and discussing participation as a phenomenon and as a conceptual frame of reference for research on the user/ patient–provider interface, and how this is intertwined with daily and social life, with examples from practice.

Whilst the purpose of this book is to highlight participation both as an aspect of and as an outcome of service delivery, it is not intended as a reader on user involvement, but rather draws on the rich literature on participation in health and welfare services. With this in mind, there are several concepts associated with participation as it has been defined and practised that are important for this book, not least for clarifying the particular position of the contribution we intend to make. First, *user involvement* mainly refers to users as 'experts by experience', recognising that involving users in important decisions about the way services are delivered leads to those services being more likely to meet the needs of people who come into contact with them. Second, the term *co-production* was originally coined in the late 1970s, implying that services should be delivered in an equal and reciprocal relationship between providers and users to enable services to improve their role as change agents (http://www.nesta. org.uk/). *Shared decision-making* refers particularly to the relationship between patient and health worker in deciding on the treatment course and ensuring that medical care better aligns with patients' preferences and values (Lee and Emanuel 2013). Finally, here, *engagement in service delivery* may be understood as a challenge to the traditional concept of professionalism, involving rethinking consumer control and the distribution of power, and calling on human-service professionals to work for social change.

Research has confirmed the benefits of patient involvement, for instance, in rehabilitation (e.g. Petersen, Hounsgaard and Nielsen 2008; Rickard and Clarke 2015) and in care services (e.g. Hurley et al. 2014). A systematic review of public involvement in healthcare policy did, on the other hand, conclude that evidence of impact on health outcome is scarce (Conklin, Morris and Nolte 2012). Clearly, the development of various forms of user involvement is not only relevant, but also important as a vehicle for increased control over one's own life, including the form and content of service delivery. This is seen as a positive value in itself, contributing to improved health and well-being through increased participation in daily and social life.

While participation is not a new concept in health and welfare services, the International Classification of Functioning, Disability and Health (ICF) (WHO 2001) has contributed strongly to the emerging importance of participation, at least in healthcare. Participation as a dimension of ICF has become an important point of reference for the discourse on participation, and it has gained prominence in rehabilitation and health-service contexts as an outcome variable, therapeutic goal and research topic. One of the major contributions of ICF is the attempt to develop a common terminology, or common language, among all parties involved in health, i.e. different professional levels, researchers, as well as patients and users of services, with participation as a key concept. The ICF model is far from being a fully fledged theory on participation, and is basically built on a consensus among key stakeholders, including important input from the user/disability movement. Systematic reviews have shown that so far, ICF, and the ICF model to a limited extent, has been used in participation research (Cerniauskaite et al. 2011) and among people with chronic conditions (Alford et al. 2016); we argue, however, that the model represents an important step forward in the attempt to merge the medical and the social model of health into an interactional model (Shakespeare 2006). It is therefore also potentially useful in connecting different types of research on participation. As we move forward, research on participation can contribute to refining and revising the model, and thus enhance our understanding of health, participation and other components in the model.

One of the innovations within the ICF framework is the ambition to match healthcare with the everyday world of people in need of its services. In the framework, this is expressed as 'engagement in everyday life and involvement in life situations'. From this ambition follows a need to give voice to the people using health and social care, and to include perspectives from the user in the definitions and conceptual frameworks of participation. There are, however, several issues in need of attention when tuning the concept of participation to embrace not only service-driven but also user-driven knowledge, and an everyday perspective as part of its fundament. First, the concept of participation may have other connotations and meanings as an everyday word used in various cultures and situations. Second, everyday life itself is characterised by being situated into various changing circumstances and conditions. This situatedness (1991) also implies that 'the voice of the person' might be impossible to catch by listening only to individuals. To address this complexity, our ambition with this book is to present material and research that meets the need to further knowledge on what 'engagement in everyday life' can be, and how service delivery can meet the challenges from situated involvement in everyday life.

While we need to distinguish between conceptual and policy-related terminology and processes, ICF has contributed strongly to the increased interest for participation, not only as a broad value, but also as a more tangible objective for health services, and to the perceived relevance of participation for health professionals, health services and health policies. This book is particularly inspired by the distinction between the medical and the social model of human functioning, and the merging of these two models into ICF. While still facing some criticism for upholding the link between health and disability, and with inherent weaknesses that will be discussed in later chapters, the ICF model might be an important step towards a conceptual understanding that can be useful beyond the sphere of disability and health. Importantly, participation entails a key role in the model as the outcome of the interaction between the individual and his/her environment, with health and welfare services comprising one element of the environment. A human rights perspective underlies ICF, understanding participation in daily and social life as the desired outcome of service interventions.

This book is about participation and the role healthcare and social welfare can play in stimulating participation as a key outcome of service delivery. The changes in the patient/user–provider interface provides an opportunity for individuals to become less dependent on healthcare providers, to increase their control over treatment, their own health and daily life. Implicit in such a development is also an understanding of patients, users, service recipients, etc. as participating actors and resources on different levels. This includes daily life, family and social life, but also reaches deeper into service delivery, either as taking control of one's own treatment and/or as playing active roles in others' daily and social lives with implications for service delivery in general (Berwick 2009). Our perspective is thus not primarily various forms of user involvement and related concepts, but rather how healthcare and social welfare can live up to the general ambition of impacting on the ability and opportunities of patients/users to participate more broadly in their daily life and in society. This is in line with how we understand participation in the ICF framework: participation as engagement in life situations. While the conceptual development of participation outside service delivery is the main interest for the majority of the contributions (chapters), participation inside and outside of service delivery both belong to the concept of participation in this book.

The shift towards participation as a core goal for health and welfare services can be grounded in different ways. From the perspective of healthcare providers and the need to meet the challenges and increased costs resulting from demographic changes, user participation may be seen as a tool for producing more effective services. Collins et al. (2007) point to improved patient satisfaction, co-operation, enhanced patient–provider relationship, management of disease, improved appropriateness, safety and outcome of care and a reduction in complaints, as possible outcomes of enhanced user participation. Some attention has also been given to participation as an antidote to services themselves forming barriers against participation as engagement in life situations (Barnes and Cotterell 2012; Vik and Eide 2012). Another contributing factor in the shift to participation is more ideological: linked to the rights of citizens to be active agents in local matters, cultures and circumstances. This use of the concept stems from disability movements and user organisations, and highlights other dimensions in everyday life and functioning for people facing the consequences of disease and marginalisation. Uggerhøy (2014) further highlights participation as key for preventing and handling marginalisation. A human rights perspective on health, with health equity as a key concept and goal, is also reflected in, for instance, the EC White Paper 'Together for Health' (EC 2007b). A third use of the concept is prominent among healthcare practitioners focusing on the actual opportunities for people facing the consequences of disease to engage and participate in everyday practices, such as work, leisure and self-care (Witzø, Eide and Vik 2010; Vik and Eide 2011).

Barnes and Cotterell (2012) trace the history of user involvement in health and social care in the UK at least as far back as the early 1970s. While the concept of user involvement is rather diffuse, with many different meanings at different levels ranging from policy to service delivery, the development of user involvement over the years, broadly speaking, belongs to two distinct traditions. One is driven by the services themselves, inviting service users and citizens to take part in service delivery and policy processes. The other is driven by service users and citizens as autonomous movements, and more often has a broader sociopolitical purpose than specific services. While a 'consumerist' version of user involvement is occupied with improving services, a 'democratic' version is embedded with ideals of participatory democracy and peoples' control over their own lives (Barnes and Cotterell 2012). The shape of user involvement in health and social services must be seen in relation to the prevailing theoretical and ideological backdrop, with consumerism, citizenship and rights/empowerment as major trends influencing welfare state development. The notion of the 'active citizen' is embraced by current policies in a wide range of sectors, including health and social care. Newman and Tonkens (2011, p. 9) describe three dimensions of citizen activation that influence the current welfare state transformation: choice in the marketplace of welfare services, extended responsibility for individuals and families, and participation in service delivery, policymaking and the polity.

The democratisation and activation of citizens as political ambitions form part of the backdrop of intensified efforts to engage and include service users in developing service delivery. The importance of user involvement in order to effectively meet diversified needs is widely recognised, and impacts on the development of health and social care services (Collins et al. 2007; Warren 2007; Berwick 2009). While both the 'democratic' and the 'effectiveness' arguments are drivers of user participation, Uggerhøy (2014) underlines the importance of the rationale for participation, and that any kind of welfare service rationality is able to produce both increased participation and marginalisation. Defining individuals as patients, clients or users may easily contribute to sidelining and pacifying, and turn participation into tokenism or simply a tool for improved effectiveness, without strengthening engagement in life situations. This is an important reason for pursuing in-depth knowledge about conditions for daily life participation.

While 'welfare services' is increasingly being used as a term covering both health and welfare services (Matthies 2014), the current text largely distinguishes between health services and welfare services. A majority of the chapters draw on experiences and research in health and care-related practice, but the intention of the book is to contribute to a discussion that is relevant across the two. This poses certain challenges due to differences in terminology between disciplines (such as the term 'user' vs. 'patient'). Even more challenging, however, is the somewhat blurred distinction between user involvement and related concepts on the one hand, and participation in daily and social life or engagement in life situations on the other. We have attempted to draw this distinction as clearly as possible, but it still poses challenges due to the fact that one (user participation) can be seen as an element of the other (daily life participation). Also, it is not entirely clear what is meant by 'involvement in a life situation'. Here we need a critical discussion on what a life situation can be from the 'everyday perspective' that is highlighted in this book. An everyday perspective is suggested as an addition to existing participation theory and practice, and we address possible dilemmas and opportunities with such an addition (Hemmingsson and Jonsson 2005).

Research challenges

As there is no consensus on how to understand participation conceptually or how to work with participation as a central value or principle in professional practice and service delivery (Cornwall 2008), the concept is used imprecisely, at a generalised level and not defined, leaving it up to the reader to create meaning. When translated into the context of service delivery, this leads either to a variety of professional practices, or to non-implementation. While we do not claim that there is one definition or framework that is superior to others, and whether participation is understood as everyday life, daily life activity, social participation, user involvement in service delivery, or influence on service delivery more generally, it is necessary to clarify the applied understanding. This is important not least in order to establish a platform for research or a research agenda that positions various contributions in relation to each other. Bearing this in mind, it is possible that ICF has specific benefits, primarily because of the ambition to establish a cross-disciplinary mutual language, building a bridge between medical and social sciences.

Different disciplines and scientific paradigms contribute with unique knowledge and understandings. While the two tracks of research on daily life participation differ on a range of issues, including epistemology, values, research methods, etc., it is argued that a combination of an 'insider' perspective and the 'ICF track' has the potential to progress participation research theoretically, and to lay the groundwork for research-based development of participation as a key objective for health and welfare services. While the potential to establish a common language is acknowledged, the above text has also indicated the complexity of participation. By incorporating an everyday perspective as well as the ICF terminology of 'engagement in daily life' and the subjective experience and understanding of participation into the theoretical fundament, we are dealing with different conditions for understanding and use between the everyday life and the professional level. While participation research currently takes place within different disciplines, mostly separated by established scientific disciplines, professions and (health and welfare) systems, a main challenge will be to build a joint framework that can enhance the generation of knowledge that is needed to guide health and welfare services in the endeavour to stimulate participation in mainstream society.

Participation – a review of literature

The following review of how participation has been understood and applied within different scientific traditions and disciplines is intended as a backdrop to the analysis of the complexity and multidimensionality of the concept, and as a further contribution to the framework for the discussion on participation. We carried out a broad search among contemporary literature, including articles published during the past ten years with a main focus on participation, or including reflections or discussions on participation. The concept is discussed within the framework of three main perspectives. The review of the literature is not complete in that it does not give a full overview of all literature and all empirical research focusing on participation. Neither does it contain an assessment of the scientific quality of the literature. Rather, the purpose has been to include literature that can contribute to the discourse on participation and, we hope, stimulate a more conscious and consistent use of participation in clinical practice and service delivery. The review is further intended as a framework for responding more easily and understandably to the various challenges linked to defining and analysing participation, and to relate the different contributions in this book to these challenges.

To illustrate variation in the use of participation in clinical practice, the following describes how different perspectives and understandings might play out at a meeting at a health and social centre discussing the vision and overall aim of the service, which is formulated as 'participation for all':

NURSE *With participation I mean patient-participation, or as we say, user-participation, meaning that I try to include the patients in the rehab process through their own decisions and to get them to control their own individual plan.*

MANAGER *Including participation in my work means that our service users are represented on our board and our consumer committee, which give advice to our service. Empowerment is an important part of this work.*

SOCIAL WORKER *I think autonomy is the concept that is closest to my understanding of participation; I try to stimulate the clients to make their own decisions even though the person is not able to execute the tasks. But my role is also to stimulate the social network or environment to be more inviting, and to include the main person.*

PHYSIOTHERAPIST *To reach the goal of participation, you have to have a repertoire of body functions. Therefore, my contribution is to assist the person in improving motor actions, e.g. balance, mobilisation, strength, etc., which are important for daily living.*

OCCUPATIONAL THERAPIST *Meaning is my key word – the person has to experience meaning while doing, e.g. moving or reaching has to be part of daily activities and experienced as important. My challenge is to discover, along with the client, what he or she is experiencing as meaningful. That is participation.*

CLIENT *User organisations claim that participation is a human right supported by the UN, and in some countries regulated by anti-discrimination law. Universal design is one way to reach full participation for all.*

PHYSICIAN *I want patients who are well-informed and who are able to understand what I say, so that they can make their decisions together with me and thus increase adherence to treatment.*

The statements above are drawn from Ness (2011) and slightly edited by the authors to demonstrate how background and position of different professionals or non-professionals in the health services might affect the understanding of the concept of participation, perhaps in spite of a mutual understanding at a more generalised level, and with likely consequences also for practice. The statements differ in terms of the level of explanation as well as a concrete description of participation. Nevertheless, they illustrate how the varying use of the concept can be explained by professional identity and the nature of the work, as well as the professional level on which the individual actor is operating. The statements are also largely in line with how participation is conceptualised in the literature. This is important, as it is at the interface between clients/users/patients that the policies are implemented and shaped.

Participation as a human right

The advent and development of discourses on human rights are mainly linked to either a disability movement perspective focusing on equal participation and citizens' rights for people with disabilities, or the Social Model of Disability (Oliver 1996), focusing on the environment (contextual, social and physical) as more or less disabling and thus the main explanatory factor for disability in any society. A role for individuals with disabilities as active, participating and contributing members of society follows from this understanding. This is in accordance with the right of people with disability to participate in society as formulated in international declarations, resolutions and conventions. The UN Convention on the Rights for Persons with Disabilities (CRPD) (UN 2008) describes one of the basic principles as 'Full and effective participation and inclusion in society' (art. 3c), which is described as a political right connected to all areas of human life.

The initiatives from disability rights organisations and the UN have brought forward participation together with equality, citizenship and inclusion as fundamental human rights (e.g. UN 2008), and thus influenced legal regulations and social change related to areas like education, work, health and social care, anti-discrimination, etc. The view of participation as a right has influenced both rehabilitation policy and policy for the disabled in many countries.

Participation as an invitation from the environment

Within this perspective, an accessible and adaptable physical environment and attitudes are seen as important factors that could invite participation. One example of this is when Bricout and Gray (2006) use the term 'community receptivity', including both social and physical environments defined as 'willingness, values and knowledge of people in the community that facilitate the participation of people with disabilities in valued activities and events including: social events, religious worship, employment, entertainment, travel outside home'. Another example is when Yeatman (2000) identified two related conditions: first, the person's sense of self that permits self-action and thus participation skills. Second, relevant others have to act in ways that invite the person to participate by providing ongoing recognition of individual selfhood in how an individual acts. Yeatman argues that 'no one can participate in the conduct of their life except as they are invited by relevant others to participate' (p. 189). Yeatman also reasons that participation has to be thought of as appropriate for all individuals in all contexts of social actions and this 'draws attention to the bilateral character of individual participation, that it depends on willingness and capacity of others' (p. 200).

Related to viewing participation as an invitation from the environment are studies on environmental barriers and facilitators for participation. Researchers from different scientific traditions such as, for instance, Hammel et al. (2015) and Levasseur et al. (2015), have highlighted a range of relevant factors that could be integrated in public health interventions to stimulate participation.

Participation as an outcome of rehabilitation services

Participation is described as the ultimate goal (UN 1994) or as a long-term goal (Magasi 2012) of rehabilitation services (United Nations Standard Rules). However, some authors make a distinction between the medical and the rehabilitative perspective that influences how the concept of participation is used. In a medical perspective, Stucki (2005) argues that functioning and health are seen as the unidirectional outcome or consequence of a disease or condition and that the medical models do not address the relationship between participation and environment. According to Stucki, Ewert and Cieza (2002), medical interventions tend to target the disease process, while rehabilitation interventions are targeting a person's functioning and health. This is an important difference in focus; a rehabilitation focus gives attention to other dimensions of participation, such as activities of daily living (ADL), vocational assessment and re-education, functional rehabilitation (training of body function), as well as individual adaptations and assistive devices with the aim of independent living.

On the one hand, while it may be useful to distinguish between medical and social rehabilitation in order to reach conceptual clarity, this distinction is not clear-cut, as indicated by the use of the term 'medical social rehabilitation'. It is argued that ICF will continue to influence this distinction and contribute further to a broad understanding of rehabilitation as relevant for all dimensions in ICF, including participation. Not least is this relevant for the bulk of the rehabilitation process that takes place outside of the specialised health services, i.e. in the local community.

On the other hand, a causal and linear approach from the medical model as well as the predecessors of ICF are also echoed in the way the concept of participation is used within this functional rehabilitation approach, where body functions and structures (muscle control, joint movement, grip, cognitive functions, etc.) or specific activities are trained with the aim of achieving independence and participation. It could be argued that the close link between a medical and a rehabilitation approach might make the role of participation unclear, both as a goal and as a process of active participation. Participation, in this view, is more a linear outcome of functional competencies or activities than process, where the client is perceived as the actor in a context.

Participation as an individual experience (agency and belonging)

Our analysis revealed that attention has started to be directed to the concept of participation from the perspective of the individual. Also, theoretical discussions have recently paid more attention to the perspective of the individual. These studies fall into two categories: one that relates participation to autonomy, agency or control, and another that describes participation, for example, as an individual's experience of belonging, being something for others and/or engagement.

One example of this is when Cardol argues that autonomy (literally, self-rule) is the fundamental prerequisite for participation (Cardol, de Jong and Ward 2002). She distinguishes between decisional and executional autonomy. Decisional autonomy is defined as 'the ability to make decisions without external restraint or coercion, e.g. deciding when and how to get dressed' (p. 970). Executional autonomy also implies the actions to be carried out, and is defined as 'the ability and freedom to act on a basis of decisional autonomy, e.g. actually dressing oneself as one wishes' (p. 972). In line with Cardol, other empirical research has described how regaining agency and being in control of occupations and daily life is important in individuals' experiences of participation. Cardol, de Jong and Ward (2002) claimed that the ultimate goal of rehabilitation is to regain and retain the highest possible level of autonomy, in order to maximise participation. Consequently, participation may (should) 'be understood primarily in terms of individual preferences, rather than in terms of general competencies' (p. 973). Thus, the focus is on an individual's opportunity, motivation and capacity to make decisions and execute agency, rather than the functional ability to perform activities.

An understanding of participation, which includes autonomy, has for example been shown in the development of recent outcome measures in relation to participation. However, empirical research has documented that, among older adults who receive home-based services, agency has come forward as a strong feature of participation (Vik et al. 2008; Vasunilashorn et al. 2012; Witsø, Vik and Ytterhus 2012).

Further attention has been given to how people with a disability experience participation. The experience of being a part of one's social environment has for example been seen as important. Asbjørnslett and Hemmingson (2008) found that among teenagers at school, it was more important to be where things actually happen than doing the same activities with others. Or, as in Borell et al. (2006), participation among adults living with chronic pain was experienced as doing something social and doing something for others. Furthermore, participation as engaging in evolving daily life could be seen as an important aspect among older adults (Vik et al. 2008; Witsø, Vik and Ytterhus 2012). Hammel et al. (2008) found that participation was conceptualised as a cluster of values that included active and meaningful engagement/being part of, choice and control, access and opportunity, personal and societal responsibilities, having an impact and supporting others.

Understanding participation solely as a subjective experience might give in-depth insights into a person's own experiences. However, it has also been argued that this approach might reinforce 'tragic' stereotypes of disabled people, and blur the political importance of participation as a human right. Barron (2001) discusses autonomy and points to the contradiction that those who have the greatest need for support, in order to ensure autonomy and self-determination in everyday life, risk being the least likely to benefit if individuals' voices are foregrounded. In line with such argumentation, subjective experience is not included in ICF, and it is explicitly stated that 'participation should be distinguished from the subjective experience of involvement' (WHO 2001, p. 13). It may be argued that seeing autonomy as a prerequisite to participation and a key concept in client-centred rehabilitation is failing to take cultures outside Western societies into consideration. Autonomy and independence correspond to an individualistic liberal view, perhaps relevant in some European countries and the US, but not universally endorsed. Cats and Itzkovich (2002) present the same argument and instead suggest more appreciation of the functional capacity and of achieving maximal functioning. Saadah (2002) argues that the principal purpose of healthcare should centre on the needs of patients and on designing an environment to humanise patient care. Bearing in mind such critical viewpoints, it is argued that the individual perspective on participation is key to understanding the mechanisms enhancing or hindering participation.

Participation as a facilitator of the relationship between person and society

The third dimension on participation that we have foregrounded in our analysis is the interactional perspective, which includes an integration of the individual and the social perspective (Fougeyrollas 1997; WHO 2001). Such a perspective might more clearly incorporate the dialectics between the person and the environment. Not only is the environment contributing to participation for the individual, but the individual is also contributing to participation for his/her environment by being somebody for someone.

Fougeyrollas et al. (1999) developed the systemic Disability Creation Process (DCP), which was influential in the development of ICF (Desrosiers 2005). In DCP, participation is explained by life habits which are daily activities and social roles valued by the person and his/her sociocultural context and which ensure the survival, development and well-being of the person in society throughout his/her life. According to Desrosiers (2005), social roles are not defined in the typical way (e.g. as mother, student, worker, etc.), but as observable activities carried out in society, usually required for development and well-being. Participation is conceptualised as the result of an interaction between individual and contextual factors (Noreau and Fougeyrollas 2000). Consequently, this interpretation of participation might be regarded as a process created by the person and his/her environment; participation will thus always be variable and modifiable (Cott 2005).

According to ICF, participation can be interpreted as a dynamic process between the person and his/her environment; participation is the person's actual performance of a task or action in his or her current environment (WHO 2001). Participation is described as the individual involvement in a life situation. The definition of 'involvement' incorporates taking part, being included or engaged in an area of life, being accepted, or having access to required resources. The concept of involvement is, in this regard (ICF), distinguished from the subjective experience of involvement (the sense of belonging). Participation is linked to the dimension activity, which is defined as 'the execution of a task or action by an individual' (WHO, 2001, p. 10). Participation and activity share common domains divided into: learning and applying knowledge, general tasks and demands, communication, mobility, self-care, domestic life, interpersonal interactions and relationship, major life areas and community, social and civic life. Molin (2004) analysed and explored the definition of participation according to ICF, identifying different forms of participation and arguing that participation be regarded as a relationship between the individual and his/her social and physical environment. Participation includes internal conditions (will and capacity to participate) and external conditions (accessibility and opportunity). Nordenfelt (2003) argues that there is confusion between the capacity for action and the actual performance of an action, and that the distinction between activity and participation is not coherent. This particular distinction (between activity and participation as defined by the ICF model) is also discussed by Jette et al. (2003) and Eide et al. (2007), both bringing some support to the distinction between the two dimensions. Nordenfelt (2003) suggests that ICF is in need of an action-theoretical reconstruction. This might include inner: resources or capacity; and outer: external possibilities or opportunities. The amalgam of the person's capacity and opportunities in the environment is the person's practical possibilities for action.

Medical, social and interactional models

The medical, social and interactional models of disability and human functioning represent different dimensions with a distinct scientific and philosophical basis. While this may contribute to complicating communication and practice involving participation as a key target, the three dimensions also represent unique contributions to our understanding of the complexities of participation.

The main message from this review is that the three dimensions all have an impact on how participation is understood, and thus also on how participation as an important target for health and welfare services is interpreted and how it influences practice. A first important step is therefore to initiate a discussion about participation that includes the different perspectives. A second step will be to concretise the meaning of the concept within service delivery. And a third step will be to develop a common language or frame of reference about participation that takes the different dimensions into consideration. ICF may well make an important contribution in this regard as it is already a serious attempt to merge a medical, a social and an interactional dimension.

Participation, as described above and by different client groups, is multifaceted but also operates on different levels: individual, group or societal. Understanding participation as a creation or interaction between person and environment might have consequences for practice by service providers, but it requires a conscious discussion within each service. First of all, this might give a better understanding of the aspects of participation that are influencing service provision, depending on the needs of the service receiver and the objectives of the service system.

Several studies among those mentioned above show the importance of control related to participation. This has to do with a person's own decisions, autonomy, and the invitation from the environment, including health services, to take control. Furthermore, in all the publications reviewed, participation is directly or indirectly linked to activity, or a 'doing' aspect. While participation is generally treated as positive and involving all humans, the issue of control and activity will eventually challenge the established power relationship between service providers and those who depend upon services, as well as the content of the services.

Participation is neither an individual aspect nor an environmental phenomenon. Rather, it takes place between the person and the environment, and in fact also in encounters with the occupation or activity participated in by individuals. It might be easier to see participation as part of a three-element system. Different services and different service providers might prioritise different aspects of participation.

The content of the book

The purpose of this book is to describe, explain and discuss the relevance of participation as a research area to the challenges facing health and welfare services, in particular in industrialised countries with an ageing population, and a substantial number of people being marginalised or at risk of exclusion. The aim is further to contribute to the discussion of possible challenges and opportunities that the inclusion of engagement in daily life as a component of participation might involve. This introduction has drawn on diverse literature in order to demonstrate the complexity of the term. We have argued that ICF is a potentially useful frame of reference for the discourse on participation and participation research. We have also argued that it has evident weaknesses, not least by discarding the subjective experience of participation. While the main topic is daily life activity and social participation, we acknowledge the relevance and useful contributions from the broad literature on participation seen as user involvement. This book is primarily interested in participation as it evolves outside of the user–provider context, and the role of health and welfare services in promoting, or perhaps hindering, daily life participation. There are, however, overlaps between daily life participation and participation in services, and the content and form of health and welfare services will have an influence on capabilities and opportunities for daily life participation. This is particularly true for large groups of people who, for different reasons, are long-term or permanently dependent on services.

The book brings together contributions from different research traditions in order to promote a cross-disciplinary approach which is necessary to fully address such a complex social phenomenon as participation. Rapidly changing solutions for communication between patients and providers, easy access to information as well as technological progress, are challenging the traditional roles of patients and providers, and the book's ambition is to critically discuss and analyse participation as a key component in the discourse on health and health services. It is argued that there is a need to further develop a scientific basis for participation as a concept, tool and aim for health services broadly. We further need to translate research so that this knowledge base may be interpreted into professional paradigms as well as the public understanding of participation which are at work in health services.

Following this introduction, which defines the purpose and objectives of the book and discusses participation as a professional concept and everyday lived experience in view of a review of relevant literature, Chapter 2 explores the possibilities and limitations inherent in the participation dimension of the ICF. The author, in particular, discusses weaknesses in its relational perspective, and the need for combining an insider perspective and a more theoretical approach in order to strengthen the relational approach to participation. Chapter 3 aims at expanding the understanding of an insider perspective, i.e. how individuals and groups use and understand the concept of participation. A subjective understanding is then compared with contemporary definitions of participation. Chapter 4 concentrates particularly on the environmental component in ICF, and studies environmental determinants of the quality of participation in healthcare settings among persons with mobility impairments. The authors analyse the relative importance of the different variables reported in the literature that are barriers to participation in healthcare at healthcare facilities. In Chapter 5, the topic is the relationship between culture and participation, proposing that health services have to take into account users' cultural context as well as their cultural identity in order to promote their participation in daily and social life. Culture has an impact on individual identity, which substantially influences participation. Understanding the cultural aspects of individuals' choices and preferences is therefore necessary in order to understand how services can promote participation. Chapter 6 aims to explicate and explore a user-led approach, including its origins and some of its different expressions, and to look at the barriers in its way, how these barriers may be overcome, and why this is especially important for the development of effective and sustainable services. The chapter highlights how welfare service user movements have placed a new emphasis on how services can have a role in enabling people's participation in mainstream society. In Chapter 7, the authors explore how participation is perceived and how it takes place in the context of home-based care services. A comparative analysis of the perspectives on participation among older service users and providers is presented. Chapter 8 studies the participation of clients in the interface with welfare service, expanding on the relational perspective in ICF. A transactional perspective is used to explain how individual and contextual aspects change and adapt to each other over time. In Chapter 9, the authors highlight differences between hospital and municipal rehabilitation services. The ICF model is used to illuminate challenges in collaboration between hospital and municipal rehabilitation services and how this impacts on participation among service users. Chapter 10 outlines how the increasing interest in the position of parents as collaborators and partners in child welfare takes place within a service attempting to resolve the tension between coercion and voluntarism. The author raises the question of whether dominant participation models in the field of health and welfare services, including ICF, need to develop more theoretical concepts in order to grasp the complexity of a process-oriented perspective. The aim of Chapter 11 is to discuss how political, social, personal and economic factors may impact on working-life participation among persons with mental health disability. The complexity and nuances of facilitators of work participation are highlighted by contrasting the situation of persons with and without work. Chapter 12 explores how engagement in creative activities can enhance active agency and participation in everyday activities among persons in vulnerable life situations. Chapter 13 describes and discusses what meaning participation may have for social identity and mental health. The authors describe and discuss theories and two empirical examples of how social identity, empowerment and opportunities to receive recognition should be considered central principles for developing mental health services that are based on participation. Chapter 14 investigates participation in the everyday life of young disabled people in relation to ICTs through an interactional perspective. The purpose is to analyse how young disabled persons' use or non-use of assistive information and communication technology influence their social participation. The purpose of Chapter 15 is to unpack the practice of participation, specifically aiming to describe how participation works in the everyday lives of individuals. The authors aim to uncover how participation happens in everyday life. This is applied to expand on the understanding of ongoing processual qualities of the way in which participation is conceptualised and understood. Chapter 16 explores how time use in everyday life activities, in combination with environmental factors, influence participation for young adults with disabilities, using a time-geographic perspective and method. Chapter 17 reports on a multi-country study exploring mental health service users' experience of social inclusion and participation, and links the themes emerging from the qualitative analysis to ICF categories. In the Epilogue, we return to the aim of this book and reflect on breaches and possibilities that emerge from the different contributions of this book on the concept of participation and its use.

References

Alford V M, Ewen S, Webb G R, McGinley J, Brookes A, Remedios L J (2016) The use of the international classification of functioning, disability and healht to understand the health and functioning experiences of people with chronic conditions from the person perspective: A systematic review. *Disability and Rehabilitation*, 37(8): 655–666. DOI: 10.3109/09638288.2014.935875.

Asbjørnslett M, Hemmingson H (2008) Participation at school: Experienced by teenagers with physical disabilities. *Scandinavian Journal of Occupational Therapy*, 15(3): 153–161.

Barnes M B, Cotterell P (Eds.) (2012) *Critical perspectives on user involvement*. Bristol: Policy Press.

Barron, K (2001) Autonomy in everyday life, for whom? *Disability & Society*, 16(3): 431–447.

Berwick D M (2009) What 'patient-centered' should mean: Confessions of an extremist. *Health Affairs*, 28(4): 555–565.

Borell L, Asaba E, Rosenberg L, Schult M-L, Townsend E (2006) Exploring experiences of 'participation' among individuals living with chronic pain. *Scandinavian Journal of Occupational Therapy*, 13: 76–85.

Bricout J C, Gray D B (2006) Community receptivity: The ecology of disabled persons' participation in the physical, political and social environments. *Scandinavian Journal of Disability Research*, 8(1): 1–21.

Cardol M, de Haan R J, van den Boos G A M, de Jong B A, de Groot I J M (1999) The development of a handicap assessment questionnaire: the impact on participation and autonomy (IPA). *Clin Rehabil*, 13(5): 411–19. DOI:10.1191/026921599668601325.

Cardol M, de Jong B, Ward C D (2002) On autonomy and participation in rehabilitation. *Disability and Rehabilitation*, 24(18): 970–974.

Cats A, Itzkovich M (2002) On autonomy and participation in rehabilitation. *Disability and Rehabilitation*, 24(18): 996–998.

Cerniauskaite M, Quintas R, Boldtd C, Raggi A, Cieza A, Bichenbach J E, Leonardi M (2011) Systematic literature review on ICF from 2001 to 2009: Its use, implementation and operationalization. *Disability and Rehabilitation*, 33(4): 281–309.

Collins S, Britten N, Ruusuvuori J, Thompson A (2007) Understanding the process of patient participation. In: S Collins, N Britten, J Ruusuvuori and A Thompson (Eds.), *Patient participation in health care consultations*: *Qualitative perspectives* (pp. 3–21). Berkshire: McGraw-Hill, Open University Press.

Conklin A, Morris Z, Nolte E (2012) What is the evidence base for public involvement in health-care policy? Results of a systematic scoping review. *Health Expectations*, 18: 153–165.

Cornwall A (2008) Unpacking 'participation': Models, meanings and practices. *Oxford University Press and Community Development Journal*, 43(3): 269–283. DOI:10.1093/cdi/bsn010.

Cott C A (2005) *Conceptualizing and measuring participation* (p. 51) Toronto: Particiaption Team Working Report.

Desrosiers J (2005) Participation and occupation. *Canadian Journal of Occupational Therapy*, 72(4): 195–203.

Eide A H, Jelsma J, Loeb M E, Maart S, Ka' Toni M (2007) Exploring ICF components in a survey among Xhosa speakers in Eastern and Western Cape, South Africa. *Disability and Rehabilitation*, 30(11): 819–829.

EU (2007a) Treaty of Lisbon. Amending the treaty on European Union and the treaty establishing the European Community (2007/C 306/01). Bruxelles: European Union.

EU (2007b) White Paper. Together for health: A strategic approach for the EU 2008–2013. COM (2007) 630 final. Bruxelles: European Commission of the European Communities.

European Commission (2005). A common agenda for integration: Framework for the integration of third-country nationals in the European Union.

Flaskerud J H, Winslow B J (1998) Conceptualizing vulnerable populations health-related research. *Nursing Research*, 47: 69–78.

Fougeyrollas P (1997). The influence of the social participation of people with disabilities. In: C Christiansen and C M Baum (Eds.), *Occupational therapy: Enabling, function and well-being* (pp. 379–388). Thorofare: Slack Incorporated.

Fougeyrollas P, Cloutier R, Bergeron H, Cote J, St Michel G (1999) *Quebec classification, disability creation process*. Lac St Charles, Quebec: CSICIDH.

Gray D B, Hollingsworth H H, Stark S L, Morgan K A (2006) Participation survey/mobility: psychometric properties of a measure of participation for people with mobility impairments and limitations. *Arch Phys Med Rehabil*, 87(2): 189–97.

Hammel J, Magasi S, Heinemann A, Gray D B, Stark S, Kisala P, Carlozzi N E, Tulsky D, Garcia S F, Hahn E A (2015) Environmental barriers and supports to everyday participation: A qualitative insider perspective from people with disabilities. *Archives of Physical Medicine and Rehabilitation*, 96: 578–588.

Hammel J, Magasi S, Heinemann A, Whiteneck G, Bogner J, Rodriguez E (2008) What does participation mean? An insider perspective from people with disabilities. *Disability and Rehabilitation*, 30(19): 1445–1460.

Haraway, D (1991) *Simians, cyborgs and women*. New York: Routledge.

Hemmingsson H, Jonsson H (2005) An occupational perspective on the concepts of participation in the international classification of functioning, disability and health – some critical remarks. *The American Journal of Occupational Therapy*, 59(5): 569–576.

Hurley M, Dudziec M, Kennedy B, Anderson L, Jackson I, Koskela S, Gallagher W, Jones F (2014) Increasing the health, activity and participation levels of people attending day centres. *International Journal of Therapy and Rehabilitation*, 21(7): 310–317.

Jette A M, Haley S M, Kooyookijan J T (2003) Are the ICF activity and participation dimensions distinct? *Rehabilitation Medicine*, 35: 145–149.

Lee E O, Emanuel E J (2013) Shared decision making to improve care and reduce costs. *The New England Journal of Medicine*, 368: 6–8. DOI:10.1056/NEJMp1209500.

Levasseur M, Cohen A A, Dubois M-F, Genereux M, Richard L, Therien F-L, Payette H (2015) Environmental factors associated with social participation of older adults living in metropolitan, urban and rural areas: The NuAge study. *American Journal of Public Health*, 105: 1718–1725. DOI:10.2105/AJPH.2014.302415.

Magasi S (2012) Negotiating the social service system: A vital yet frequently invisible occupation. *Occupation, Participation and Health*, 32(1): 25–33.

Matthies A-L (2014) How participation, marginalization and welfare services are connected. In: A-L Matthies and L Uggerhøj (Eds.), *Participation, marginalisation and welfare services* (pp. 3–19). Surrey: Ashgate.

Matthies A-L, Uggerhøj L (2014) The powerful meeting between social workers and service users: Needs, barriers and possibilities in participation processes in agency settings.

In: A-L Matthies and L Uggerhøj (Eds.), *Participation, marginalization and welfare services: Concepts, politics and practices across European countries* (pp. 201–217). Farnham: Ashgate.

Molin M (2004) Delaktighet inom handlikappområdet – en begreppsanalys. In: A. Gustavsson (Ed.), *Delaktighetens språk* (pp. 61–81). Lund, Studentlitteratur (Swedish language).

Ness N E (2011) *Hjelpemidler og tilrettelegging for deltagelse. Et kunnskapsbasert grunnlag.* (Norwegian language). Trondheim: Tapir Akademisk Forlag.

Newman J, Tonkens E (Eds.) (2011) *Participation, responsibility and choice. Introduction.* Amsterdam: Amsterdam University Press.

Nordenfelt L (2003) Action theory, disability and ICF. *Disability and Rehabilitation,* 25: 1075–1079.

Noreau L, Fougeyrollas P (2000) Long-term consequences of spinal cord injury on social participation: The occurrence of handicap situations. *Disability and Rehabilitation,* 22: 170–180.

Oliver M (1996) *Understanding disability. From theory to practice.* New York: Palgrave.

Petersen K, Hounsgaard L, Nielsen C V (2008) User participation and involvement in mental health rehabilitation: A literature review. *International Journal of Therapy and Rehabilitation,* 15(7): 306–313.

Rickard N, Clarke C (2015) The involvement of older people in their rehabilitation: Generating a substantive grounded theory. *International Journal of Therapy and Rehabilitation,* 22(8): 361–369.

Saadah M A (2002) On autonomy and participation in rehabilitation. *Disability and Rehabilitation,* 24(18): 977–982. DOI:10.1080/09638280210152021.

Shakespeare T (2006) *Disability rights and wrongs.* London: Routledge.

Stucki G (2005). International classification of functioning, disability, and health (ICF). *American Journal of Physical Medicine & Rehabilitation,* 84: 733–740.

Stucki G, Ewert T, Cieza A (2002). Value and application of the ICF in rehabilitation medicine. *Disability and Rehabilitation,* 24(17): 932–938.

Uggerhøy L (2014) Participation or marginalisation: How different perspectives lead towards a democratic direction. In: A-L Matthies and L Uggerhøj (Eds.), *Participation, marginalisation and welfare services* (pp. 277–295). Surrey: Ashgate.

UN (1994) *The standard rules on the equalization of opportunities for persons with disabilities.* New York: United Nations.

UN (2006) *Development Goals Report 2006.* New York: United Nations.

UN (2008) *Convention on the rights of persons with disabilities.* New York: United Nations. www.un.org/disabilities/convention/facts.shtml.

Vasunilashorn S, Steinman B A, Liebig P S, Pynoos J (2012) Aging in place: Evolution of a research topic whose time has come. *Journal of Aging Research,* 2012 (2012): 6 pp. DOI: 10.1155/2012/120952.

Vik K, Eide A E (2011) Older adults that receive home-based services, on the verge of passivity: The perspective of service providers. *International Journal of Older People Nursing.* DOI: 10.1111/ j.1748–3743.2011.00305.x.

Vik K, Eide A H (2012) The exhausting dilemmas faced by home-care service providers when enhancing participation among older adults receiving home care. *Scandinavian Journal of Caring Science,* 26: 528–536.

Vik J, Josephsson S, Borell L, Nygård L (2008) Agency and engagement: Older adults experiences of participation in occupation during home-based rehabilitation. *Canadian Journal of Occupational Therapy,* 75: 262–271.

Warren J (2007) *Service user and carer participation in social work*. London: Sage.

WHO (2001) *International classification of functioning, disability and health*. Geneva: World Health Organization.

WHO (2002) Active ageing. A policy framework. WHO/NMH/NPH/02.8. Geneva: World Health Organization. http://www.who.int/ageing/publications/active_ageing/en/

WHO (2004) *International plan of action on ageing: Report on implementation* (p. 5). Geneva: World Health Organization.

Witsø A E, Vik K, Ytterhus B (2012). Participation in older home care recipients: A value based process. *Activities, Adaptation & Aging*, 36: 297–316. DOI:10.1080/01924788.2 012.729187.

Witzø A U, Eide A H, Vik K (2010) Professional carers' perspectives on participation for older adults living in place. *Disability and Rehabilitation*, 33: 557–568.

Yeatman A (2000). What can disability tell us about participation? In: M Jones and L A B Marks (Eds.), *Explorations on law and disability in Australia* (pp. 181–202). Annandale, NSW: Federation Press.

2 International classification of functioning, disability and health in the context of participation

Annelie Schedin Leiulfsrud

Introduction

Over the years, the WHO has developed a number of health classifications. The International Classification of Functioning, Disability and Health (ICF) is one of three current WHO classifications (http://www.who.int/classifications/en/).

The 1990s saw increased interest among member states and experts in the WHO system and the United Nations in the contextualization of health and disability within a disability, human rights and social policy framework (Bickenbach et al 1999; Cerniauskaite et al 2011). Civil society organizations, including disability organizations and disability rights advocates, contributed to the development of the ICF in an effort to change previous medical definitions.

The main aim of this chapter is to explore the possibilities and limitations inherent in the participation dimension of the ICF. The claim made is that the ICF is a model with several paradoxes with respect to how participation is presented theoretically and as a contextualizing concept. As we turn our attention to paradoxes and ambiguities in the way participation are presented in the ICF, we avoid the problem of seeing the ICF as a fixed model. It is also suggested that this may enable us to open up the discussion with respect to limitations and potential usages of the ICF framework.

The ICF is presented in seemingly neutral language (referred to as "etiological neutrality") without an explanatory theory. This presentation reflects an attempt both to unify the languages of disability and health and to translate this language into a scientific vocabulary that unifies practitioners, researchers, policymakers and clients. The ICF fits well with Mary Douglas's description of how socially inspired classifications are often translated into scientific classifications: "The striving for objectivity is precisely an attempt not to allow socially inspired classifications to overwhelm the inquiry" (Douglas 1987: 59).

In contrast to previous WHO classifications, such as the International Classification of Impairments, Disabilities and Handicaps (ICIDH), which are rooted in a negative understanding of deficiency and loss, the new classification emphasizes participation, empowerment and ability. This emphasis is congruent with different versions of what is commonly referred to as "the social model of disability" in terms of the goals of breaking social barriers and giving prominence to empowerment and ability (Barrow 2008). However, the ICF is primarily framed in a context of the social integration of people with disabilities, whereas the social model is framed in a narrative of their social exclusion and social oppression. Consequently, leading advocates of the social model may have a more critical view of the societal transformation that is necessary to achieve these goals (Oliver 1990; Barnes and Mercer 2010) compared with the technocratic view found in the ICF. The idea of a seemingly neutral model of health and disability may illustrate an ideological position in its own right with respect to how we explain systematic differences in participation levels within a society. For others, it may represent the "ICF's major strength in terms of its applicability as a universally acceptable framework" (Stücki, Reinhardt and Bickenbach 2011: 1739). Whereas some view the ICF as a paradigm shift in rehabilitation research (Reinhardt 2012), others promote its use in tandem with the International Classification of Diseases (ICD-10) (Kohler et al 2012).

The WHO is explicit in its policy recommendation that the ICF should be a tool to establish health policies that include all people and groups, not primarily people with a medically defined impairment. With this approach, disability is viewed not on the basis of how society shapes us as individuals, but on how we as actors (individuals or groups) with various impairments and obstacles are able to participate in society (WHO 2001).

Body structures and body functions are well described in the ICF model. Activity and participation are seen as outcomes of the interaction between a person's health condition and relevant environmental factors (WHO 2001; Schneidert et al 2003).

One of the main arguments in this chapter is that we need to develop a more theoretical discussion of the interrelationship between the participation dimension and environmental factors in the ICF model. Unless we primarily see participation as an outcome of the environment in which it is situated, we must develop an understanding of the agency that produces participation. This argument may be viewed as an attempt to incorporate the people/groups involved in different types of participation roles. A person is not merely determined by social factors but is able to act as a reflexive entity with agency of his or her own in activity and participation. This concept is consistent with attempts to incorporate theories and models of participation from rehabilitation, social work and community-based services, which emphasize the actor's point of view and interests (Mallinson and Hammel 2010; Magasi et al 2015).

The ICF – a model based on actors participating in environmental systems

Every classification has implications for how we understand the main concepts and the relationships among the concepts. Each classification is also based on a language and an underlying order, which enable the determination of meaningful classifications (Franzosi 2004; Sohlberg and Sohlberg 2014). Although the ICF manual published in 2001 is important, it is only an initial version of a new model of disability that will be further developed in the years to come.

The main purpose of the ICF "is to provide a unified and standard language and framework for the description of health and health-related states" (WHO 2001: 3). The main difference between the ICF and previous health classifications (including WHO's ICIDH) is the aim to classify health and impairment in terms of "functions" and how these functions relate to activities and participation in different areas of life, including work, family, friendships and community, social activities and leisure activities (see the ICF model in Figure 2.1).

In the ICF model, *body functions* refers to physiological and psychological functions (WHO 2001). The body refers to all aspects of the human organism, including its structures and anatomical parts, which are classified according to relevant organ systems.

Activity is understood in the ICF model as the execution of tasks or actions performed by an individual. It is based on an idea of the person's capacity to perform various tasks (which is based on a view of activity that can be measured with clinical instruments in for example a hospital ward). *Participation* is understood as the performance of tasks and actions in the environment in which people actually live and requires some type of personal involvement beyond the activity itself. In the ICF framework, participation is primarily understood as the person's involvement in their life situation. Because the technical/clinical aspect of activity is easier to measure and already exists in previous classifications, it is not surprising that this aspect is more developed in the ICF literature (Noonan et al 2009; Dijkers 2010).

In the ICF model, *function* is viewed either as a factual description of body function, activity and participation, or in terms of deviances that restrict such functions and are referred to as "disability". In this model, function and disability

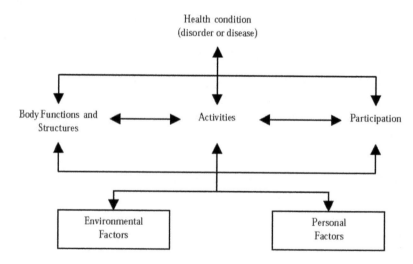

Figure 2.1 Interactions between the components of ICF

(*Source*: WHO 2001: 18)

are seen in a dynamic interplay between health conditions and contextual factors. Health condition, depicted at the top of Figure 2.1, is technically classified as it is in ICD-10, but it is interpreted as the outcome of interrelated ICF factors, namely, body functions and the ability to perform activities and participate in the local community and in society.

Environmental factors in the ICF refer to five different areas (which are described as chapters in the ICF): (1) the products and technology in a person's immediate environment; (2) the natural environment and human-made changes to the environment; (3) support and relationships in the person's environment or in daily activities; (4) attitudes, including norms, beliefs and value systems in the environment; and (5) the services, systems and policies found in various sectors of society (Schneidert et al 2003).

Facilitators or barriers (described as hindrances in the model) refer to factors that enable or disable persons in their daily lives. In certain cases and countries, the hindrances are expected to be substantial (for example, a lack of technical aids to promote mobility or the absence of public and community support for disabled people). In other instances, general welfare systems and disability-friendly policies may reduce the number of obstacles in people's daily lives (WHO 2001).

Personal factors are included in the general ICF model but are more or less excluded from the operationalization presented by the WHO in 2001. Several codes,[1] measurement instruments and attempts to capture psychological-personal factor domains have been developed to fit the ICF model (Geyh et al 2011). However, surprisingly little has been written about how personal factors explain differences in functioning, disability and health outcomes for people with identical types and levels of injuries. In a similar vein, we also detect a pattern of prioritizing instruments that measure objective aspects of activity/participation.

Actors in participation and action situations

One of the main obstacles encountered when operating with highly standardized models of behaviour is what Ellinor Ostrom (2005: 32) refers to as an "action situation": "Whenever two or more individuals are faced with a set of potential actions that jointly produce outcomes". In Ostrom's model of action situations, we are asked to specify the set of participants; their status and positions; possible actions and outcomes; each individual's degree of control, information, and control over actions and outcomes; and costs and incentives. The message of the model is that various situations may trigger a range of actions by an individual. None of these specifications are made explicit in the original version of the ICF model.

Given the design of the ICF categories, it is tempting to refer to an underlying "belief" among modern, empowered clients who are in charge of their own lives (Foucault 2002; Vabø 2003). Other roles in the context of the ICF model are the person as a social citizen with a number of basic rights, and the person as a client and consumer of services. In the philosophy upon which the ICF model is based, we find an underlying idea that the obstacles preventing the integration of people with impairments must be regulated to optimize the inbuilt potential of those people (WHO 2001: chapter 1; WHO 2011).

It is almost unnecessary to refer to norms and discrimination as important in a discussion of social participation (for Stinchcombe 1997; Elster 2007; this position also reflects the ICF perspective), but the definition of successful participation in society remains unclear. Is this definition restricted to the domains operationalized in the ICF manual, or are there certain societal domains that are more important than others? If certain domains are given priority, which of them should be included? Is prioritization merely a matter of the questions posed by the observer (researcher, expert or service provider)?

An alternative to the realist approach to actors typically found in the ICF literature is a more phenomenological approach that views the actors as "constructed entities", similar to actors in a theatre with scripted identities engaging in scripted actions (Meyer 2010: 3–4).

ICF is interesting in terms of its liberal idea that societies ultimately must eliminate hindrances/barriers and identify facilitators that promote full integration regardless of disability, race, gender, religion, etc. (see UN 2006; WHO 2011; Bickenbach 2014). The underlying idea is that discrimination is unfair and violates basic human rights. Those more concerned about social policy would also say that it is unproductive and a waste of human capital to exclude anyone with a productive potential.

Whether we see the social environment as limited, with binding rules that restrict our actions (e.g. Ostrom 2005; Henrich and Henrich 2007), or pay attention to complex meaning systems (Berger and Luckmann 1966; Meyer 2010: 3–4) depends on the research topic. For example, investigations of participation conducted in a clinical ward are not automatically relevant to how we meaningfully approach participation in people's local environments, as consumers, or in interactions with the public welfare system.

Recent developments in clinical research and practice

If the aim is to find commonalities in individual behaviour, it may be fruitful to take a realist approach. However, if the aim is to explore meaning systems, agency and identity instead of, for example, the participation of individuals and groups, it may be more reasonable to find inspiration in a phenomenological approach (see also Chapter 1 in this volume).[2]

The actor's point of view is mainly explored in qualitative interviews with patients or people with disabilities to hear their voices and their descriptions of difficulties in becoming fully integrated in society. This information may be used either as a voice counter to that of the informed experts (Hammel et al 2008; Schedin Leiulfsrud et al 2014) or (more commonly) as valuable data for further development of the ICF categories and domains or appropriate measurement tools (Heinemann et al 2010; Reinhardt and Post 2010). Although the two approaches are not necessarily mutually exclusive, there is an important distinction between viewing qualitative data as valuable information in its own right, and viewing these data primarily as a tool to move from the generation of analytical categories and mechanisms to the development of measurement instruments and numbers (Franzosi 2004).

Numerous ICF articles and reviews illustrate the shift towards measuring activity limitations and participation restrictions. One of the main problems in measuring how activity limitations and participation restrictions potentially affect each other may be stated as follows: "There is so little differentiation within and between impairments, functional limitations, activity limitations, and participation restrictions that it is . . . impossible to create a simple taxonomy" (Dijkers 2010: 7). One common method of measuring participation is to assess actual role performance or the time spent in actual role performance. This parameter may be operationalized through concrete activities and daily life measures or based on psychometric models for measuring participation in major life activities. One of the obvious difficulties with most available participation instruments is that participation is essentially understood as an outcome of individual factors. Consequently, for example, the centre of interest has not been what employment contributes in terms of overall participation in the community and in society, but on the impact of individual attributes on participation.[3]

The introduction of the ICF has broadened the view of participation from body and mind to the interaction between the person and the environment. This expanded view is expressed through the inclusion of a broader range of life activities and ICF domains. In some cases, this view is also supplemented with questions about barriers and facilitators and the importance of the activity, choice, satisfaction, etc. (Gray et al 2006). Finally, the broader view of participation is also seen in a more nuanced discussion of the transactions taking place among the person, task and environment (Mallinson and Hammel 2010).

In a more traditional rehabilitation context, appropriate measurements of participation are often expressed as involvement and engagement in a life similar to that before the injury or assessed through comparisons with non-disabled peers.

Various attempts have been made to incorporate the individual's priorities and norms into activity and participation measurements; examples include the COPM (Carswell et al 2004; Parker and Sykes 2006) and inventories of environmental factors, such as the Craig Handicap Assessment and Reporting Technique (CHART), which measures participation on a scale ranging from 1 to 100 with the non-disabled population as a reference (Whiteneck 2010). Almost regardless of the merits of these instruments, participation is largely interpreted without considering how to study society where participation takes place.

From classification towards a theory of participation?

One of the advantages of treating the ICF primarily as a classification without an explanatory theory is that it may be incorporated and applied to a number of theoretical frameworks, ranging from various types of actor/person-based perspectives on participation that emphasize the ability to involve or distance oneself from roles and actions, to ecologic and systems-based theories that focus on understanding the transactions that take place in concrete participation processes (Mallinson and Hammel 2010).

Most health professionals and ICF advocates probably agree on the importance of developing relevant "opportunity qualifiers" to understand external facilitators and barriers to activity and participation.

A major challenge in the concrete operationalization of the ICF is determining what to include in the activity dimension. If activity is limited to the optimal capacity to perform actions regardless of environment, norms and institutions, we could easily end up with a very instrumental understanding of activity. If participation is understood as performance that is guided by norms, values and the culture in which we live, it may be difficult to make a proper distinction between participation and activity. This criticism has been expressed by Lennart Nordenfeldt (2003, 2006), who suggests that we abolish the distinction between participation and activity and replace it with the concept of action. In addition, Nordenfeldt criticizes the ICF model for not paying enough attention to the actors engaged in the actions and the actors' potential to perform actions despite bodily limitations. This argument is based on a utilitarian view of actors being able to do things rather than a view of disability as a negative outcome of activity/participation. Despite their differences, both Nordenfeldt and his critics in the field of rehabilitation medicine (de Klein-de Vrankrijker 2006; McPherson 2006; Scherer, McAnaney and Sax 2006) agree that the concepts of activity and participation in the ICF must be further developed in terms of the actors' goals, preferences, will and opportunities. This argument is mainly based on a discussion regarding individuals and their abilities and capacities to control or live the life they want.

An alternative means of developing the ICF into a more theoretically elaborated framework is to go back to its theoretical foundation in biology and adopt a view of participation that goes beyond individual actions taking place in a social environment. This view is consistent with traditional systems theory and reflects the WHO's (2001) original presentation of the ICF model as a holistic bio-psychosocial framework for human functioning. The main question is not whether we accept the claim of a holistic model, but whether we should treat each factor in the ICF model as mutually dependent or as having different functions depending on the question asked.

Theory without reference to individuals or people as actors is rare in disability studies.[4] Few scholars have chosen to omit individual action altogether in their treatment of the ICF. One way to handle the bio-psychosocial systems is to refer to actors in terms of "whole people" taking part in multiple roles. To distinguish people from animals, it is more or less taken for granted in the ICF framework that a person has a will of his or her own and intends to perform different roles and to shape his or her life story (Solli and da Silva 2012: 283).

One major problem with the ICF view is that activity and participation may be used interchangeably. The notion that the two concepts should be replaced by a single concept of action (Nordenfeldt 2003, 2006) is that we can easily lose track of the meaning of participation or how it may be understood. One alternative proposed by Solli and Da Silva (2012) is to regard participation primarily as a normative and political concept. In this view, the main norm is the ideal of full participation in all areas of life by people with disabilities. This view also resonates well with human rights and the political struggle to break down social barriers based on discrimination and the social exclusion of certain citizens to the benefit of the majority population (Alves, Fazzi and Griffo 2012; Bickenbach 2014). The problem with the notion of participation proposed by Solli and Da Silva is that it focuses mainly on a narrow understanding of the roles and rights of social citizenship; it is less concerned with community participation or participation in the labour market as consumers, e.g. the bulk of everyday participation in society.

The norms and culture that guide us in our everyday lives and actions are not restricted to human rights; rather, they include part of what we define as people's environment in any society. If we want to incorporate the actors into actions, we must do so in a way that is related to how we as humans see ourselves, how we relate to others, and how we respond to how other people and groups perceive and treat us. These elements constitute the practice of being a participating person. Taking part in activities with others, how we perceive ourselves and how we like to be perceived and socially recognized by others are essential components of participation in any type of social environment. In other words, participation is not only of interest with respect to norms but with respect to all types of social actions and interactions with other people, groups or organizations. One productive way to view this concept of participation is to consider multiple intersections between person, tasks and the environment, and focus on participation as "a pattern of life that is personally relevant, acceptable, meaningful, and supported by society" (Mallinson and Hammel 2010: 30).

Discussion and conclusion

In contrast to the many years of revision work on the ICIDH, the ICF was not initially an evidence-based model. Rather, the ICF was a model of disability and health based on a compromise among numerous interest groups, including human rights and disability advocates and experts. The WHO introduced the ICF as a brand new model of disability and health with a strong emphasis on people's abilities as opposed to their disabilities. The ICF was framed within a view of activity and participation as highly contingent and situational, not fixed. The ICF was also introduced with a view of disability as relational, depending on the interaction between the person and the environment, which resembles the view found in Nordic disability research (Gustavsson, Tøssebro and Traustadottir 2005; Shakespeare 2006; Tøssebro 2010).

Surprisingly few entities have discussed or criticized the theoretical foundation of the ICF model. Contrary to what might be expected, the leading representatives of what has come to be known as the social model of disability have been very quiet or have simply treated the ICF as a continuation of the ICIDH. The researchers and ambassadors of the ICIDH, who lost the battle to have ICIDH established as the WHO's new gold standard, have gained ground mainly in Canada, with a revised model of disability and health resembling the ICF. Although the final Canadian model was also developed in established

WHO milieus, it is seldom referenced in international journals or discussions. This lack of attention is even more remarkable because the Canadian competitor, the Disability Creation Process (DCP) model, is more developed with respect to the purposeful engagement of individuals in activity and participation (Levasseur, Desroisiers and St-Cyr Tribble 2007). The lack of attention paid to alternative models of relevance for the research questions asked, supports Meyer's idea that an international standard such as the ICF is not merely a classification but also a program that provides experts with scientifically based legitimacy (Meyer 2010). If we want to develop the ICF as a scientific tool, we cannot take it for granted; instead, we must reflect upon its strengths and deficiencies.

As Meyer (2010) suggests, the spread of standards such as the ICF model may serve many functions beyond the obvious ones related to practical applications in clinical work, the bureaucratic manipulation of health costs and priorities, and research. Such models also encourage actors to apply for research funds and bestow prestige and scientific legitimacy upon the people and organizations actively involved in their preparation.

The ICF represents a very ambitious effort by transnational organizations (such as the WHO and the UN) to force nation states and health organizations to unite the concepts of disability and human rights. If the ICF is referenced primarily in the public rhetoric but not followed by nation states, hospitals and health professionals may continue to maintain the status quo.

For the WHO, it is important to build a model based on human rights. The WHO's policy is thus to promote the societal integration of active, participating individuals and to counter discrimination based on sex, religion, ethnicity and socioeconomic status. However, most socioeconomic dimensions remain absent from the ICF framework.

The link between disability and human rights in the ICF project is a good example of how the WHO incorporates a new domain into its definition of disability. On the surface, the ICF resembles a social model of disability, given its emphasis on human rights and social inclusion. However, in reality, the ICF is not a social model but a more liberal framework, wherein the role of the individual is emphasized (Bickenbach et al 1999; Üstün et al 2003). In this less-politicized version of disability, it is easier for medical experts, economists, philosophers and social scientists to find common ground than it was in previous models characterized by a sharp distinction between the biomedical and social models of disability.

Despite potentially conflicting approaches to using and understanding standards such as the ICF, the WHO may actually gain legitimacy, maintain its identity and prove its adaptability to new ideas by allowing a discrepancy between the ICF in theory and the ICF in practice (see also Eriksson-Zetterquist 2009: 5). According to the WHO's view that the ICF may be used according to questions of relevance, practitioners are allowed to conduct business as usual as long as they refer to the official script and gold standards (ibid.).

For those engaged in the therapeutic process, the "client's choice, action, and experience" are of crucial importance (Kielhofner 2008: 4). To develop the

ICF as a disability and health model, we must engage in an ongoing exploration of commonalities and differences across individuals' worlds of action and meaning.

Notes

1 Each code is accompanied by a *qualifier* that indicates the severity of the health problem (WHO 2001: 21).
2 It is also interesting to see how established rehabilitation models that resemble ICF have gradually shifted from activity and participation framed in a realist language towards an interest in the phenomenology of everyday life and in the actors' understanding, motivation and interest in participating in various action situations. This shift clearly occurred in the development of the "Model of Human Occupation" introduced by Gary Kielhofner and colleagues (1985, 2008). It is also evident in models such as the Canadian Occupational Performance Model (COPM), which has an interest in patient- and client-defined primary goals for being active and participating in their everyday lives after an injury (Carswell et al 2004; Parker and Sykes 2006).
3 One reason indicators such as employment, education, family status and participation in religious activities are used is that such factors may be explained by common latent traits and empirically correlated (Dijkers 2010: 9).
4 Inspired by Niklas Luhmann's system theory, Dimitris Michailakis's (2003) discussion of the concept of disability is an exception to individual- or person-centred models of disability. Michailakis's argument is that the distinction between individual and society, "which constitutes the basis of the well-known scheme of observed differences between impairment, disability and 'handicap', is a distinction based on a naive realism and obscures the problems within disability research" (p. 209). In line with this argument, Michailakis asserts that all categories and concepts are based on distinctions that are relative to the system or model used and to the observer's perspective. The original version of Gary Kielhofner's Model of Human Occupation (MOHO) was also heavily influenced by systems theory from the field of psychology (Kielhofner 1985).

References

Alves I, Fazzi L, Griffo G (2012). Human rights, UN convention, and the international classification of functioning, disability and health – Collecting data on persons with disabilities. *American Journal of Physical Medicine and Rehabilitation*, 91(2, suppl).

Barnes C, Mercer G (2010). *Exploring Disability*. Cambridge: Polity Press.

Barrow FH (2008). The international classification of functioning, disability and health (ICF), a new tool for social workers. *Journal of Social Work in Disability & Rehabilitation*, 5(1): 65–73.

Berger P, Luckmann T (1966). *The Social Construction of Reality. A Treatise in the Sociology of Knowledge*. London: Penguin Books.

Bickenbach J (2014). Reconciling the capability approach and the ICF. *ALTER, European Journal of Disability Research*, 8: 10–23.

Bickenbach J, Chatterji S, Badley EM, Üstun TB (1999). Models of disablement, universalism and the international classification of impairments, disabilities and handicaps. *Social Science and Medicine*, 48: 1173–1187.

Carswell A, McColl MA, Baptiste S, Law M, Polatajko H, Pollock N (2004). The Canadian occupational performance measure: A research and clinical literature review. *Canadian Journal of Occupational Therapy*, 71(4): 210–222.

Cerniauskaite M, Quintas R, Boldt C, Raggi A, Cieza A, Bickenbach JE, Leonardi M (2011). Systematic literature review on ICF from 2001 to 2009: Its use, implementation and operationalization. *Disability & Rehabilitation*, 33(4): 281–309.

De Klein-de Vrankrijker MW (2006). On health, ability and activity: Comments on some basic notions in the ICF. Response on some issues raised by Nordenfeldt. *Disability & Rehabilitation*, 28(23): 1475–1476.

Dijkers MP (2010). Issues in the conceptualization and measurement of participation – An overview. *Archives of Physical Medicine Rehabilitation*, 91(1): S5–S16.

Douglas M (1987). *How Institutions Think.* London: Routledge and Kegan Paul.

Elster J (2007). *Explaining Social Behavior.* New York: Cambridge University Press.

Eriksson-Zetterquist U (2009). *Institutionell teori – ideer, moden, forandring.* Stockholm: Liber.

Foucault M (2002). *Forelesninger om regjering og styringskunst.* Oslo: J.W. Cappelens forlag AS.

Franzosi R (2004). *From Words to Numbers- Narrative Data, and Social Science.* Cambridge, UK: Cambridge University Press.

Geyh S, Muller R, Peter C, Bickenbach JE, Post MWM, Stucki G, Cieza A (2011). Capturing the psychologic-personal perspective in spinal cord injury. *American Journal of Physical Medicine and Rehabilitation*, 90(suppl): S79–S96.

Gray DB, Hollingsworth HH, Stark SL, Morgan KA (2006). Participation survey/mobility: Psychometric properties of a measure of participation for people with mobility impairments and limitations. *Archives of Physical Medicine Rehabilitation*, 87: 189–197.

Gustavsson A, Tøssebro J, Traustadottir R (2005). Introduction: Approaches and perspectives in Nordic disability research. In Gustavsson A, Sandvin J, Traustadottir R, Tøssebro J (Eds.) *Resistance, Reflection and Change: Nordic Disability Research* (pp. 23–39). Lund, Sweden: Studentlitteratur.

Hammel J, Magasi S, Heinemann A, Whiteneck G, Bogner J, Rodriguez E (2008). What does participation mean? An insider perspective from people with disabilities. *Disability & Rehabilitation*, 30(19): 1445–1460.

Heinemann AW, Tulsky D, Dijkers M, Brown M, Magasi S, Gordon W, DeMark H (2010). Issues in participation measurement in research and clinical applications. *Archives of Physical Medicine and Rehabilitation*, 91(9): S72–S76.

Henrich J, Henrich N (2007). *Why Humans Cooperate. A Cultural and Evolutionary Explanation.* Oxford: Oxford University Press.

Kielhofner G (1985). *A Model of Human Occupation.* Baltimore: Williams and Wilkins.

Kielhofner G (2008). *Model of Human Occupation. Theory and Application.* Fourth ed. Philadelphia: Lippincott Williams and Wilkins.

Kohler F, Selb M, Escorpizo R, Kostanjsek N, Stucki G, Riberto M (2012). Towards the joint use of ICF and ICF: A call for contribution. *Journal of Rehabilitation Medicine*, 44: 805–810.

Levasseur M, Desroisiers J, St-Cyr Tribble D (2007). Comparing the disability creation process and international classification, disability and health models. *Canadian Journal of Occcupational Therapy*, 74(special issue): 233–236.

Magasi S, Wong A, Gray DB, Hammel J, Baum C, Wang CC, Heinemann AW (2015). Theoretical foundations for the measurement of environmental factors and their impact on participation among people with disabilities. *Archives of Physical Medicine and Rehabilitation*, 96: 569–577.

Mallinson T, Hammel J (2010). Measurement of participation: Intersecting person, task and environment. *Archives of Physical Medicine and Rehabilitation*, 91(1): S29–S33.

McPherson K (2006). What are the boundaries of health and functioning – And who should say what they are? *Disability & Rehabilitation*, 28(23): 1473–1474.

Meyer JW (2010). World society, institutional theories, and the actor. *The Annual Review of Sociology*, 36: 1–20.

Michailakis D (2003). The systems theory concept of disability: One is not born as a disabled person, one is observed to be one. *Disability & Society*, 18(2): 209–229.

Noonan VK, Kopec JA, Noreau L, Singer J, Dvorak MF (2009). A review of participation instruments based on the international classification of functioning, disability and health. *Disability & Rehabilitation*, 31(23): 1883–1901.

Nordenfeldt L (2003). Action theory, disability and ICF. *Disability and Rehabilitation*, 25(18): 1075–1079.

Nordenfeldt L (2006). On health, ability and activity: Comments on some basic notions in the ICF. *Disability & Rehabilitation*, 28(23): 1461–1465.

Oliver, M. (1990). *The Politics of Disablement.* Basinstoke: Macmillan.

Ostrom E (2005). *Understanding Institutional Diversity*. Princeton, New York: Princeton University Press.

Parker DM, Sykes CH (2006). A systematic review of the Canadian occupational performance measure: A clinical practice perspective. *British Journal of Occupational Therapy*, 69(4): 150–160.

Reinhardt JD (2011). ICF, theories, paradigms and scientific revolution. RE: Towards a unifying theory of rehabilitation. *Journal of Rehabilitation Medicine*, 43: 271–273.

Reinhardt JD, Post MWM (2010). Measurement and evidence of environmental determinants of participation in spinal cord injury: A systematic review of the literature. *Top Spinal Cord Injury Rehabilitation*, 15(4): 26–48.

Schedin Leiulfsrud A, Reinhardt JD, Ostermann A, Ruoranen K, Post MWM (2014). The value of employment for people living with spinal cord injury in Norway. *Disability & Society*, 29(8): 1177–1191.

Scherer M, Mc Ananey D, Sax C (2006). Opportunity is possibility; performance is action: Measuring participation. (Commentary) *Disability & Rehabilitation*, 28(23): 1467–1471.

Schneidert M, Hurst R, Miller J, Ustun B (2003). The role of environment in the international classification of functioning, disability and health (ICF). *Disability & Rehabilitation*, 25(11–12): 588–595.

Shakespeare T (2006). *Disability Rights and Wrongs*. London and New York: Routledge.

Sohlberg P, Sohlberg B-M (2014). *Kunnskapens former*. Stockholm: Liber.

Solli HM, da Silva AB (2012). The holistic claims of the biopsychosocial conception of WHO's international classification of functioning, disability and health (ICF): A conceptual analysis on the basis of a pluralistic-holistic ontology and multidimensional view of the human being. *Journal of Medicine and Philosophy*, 37: 277–294.

Stinchcombe AL (1997). On the virtues of the old institutionalism. *Annual Review of Sociology*, 23: 1–18.

Stücki G, Reinhardt JD, Bickenbach JE (2015). Re: Theoretical foundations for the measurement of environmental factors and their impact on participation among people with disabilities. *Archives of Physical Medicine and Rehabilitation*, 96: 1739–1740.

Tøssebro J (2010). *Hva er funksjonshemming?* Oslo: Universitetsforlaget.

United Nations General Assembly (2006). *Conventions on the Rights of Persons with Disabilities.* 61/106.

Üstün TB, Chatterji S, Bichenbach J, Kostanjsek N, Schneider M (2003). The international classification of functioning, disability and health: A new tool for understanding disability and health. *Disability and Rehabilitation*, 25(11–12): 565–571.

Vabø M (2003). Forbrukermakt i omsorgstjenesten – til hjelp for de svakeste? In Widding Isaksen, L. (Ed.) *Omsorgens pris. Kjønn, makt og marked i velferdsstaten* (pp. 102–121). Oslo: Gyldendal Forlag AS.

Whiteneck GG (2010). Issues affecting the selection of participation measurement in outcomes research and clinical trials. *Archives of Physical Medicine Rehabilitation,* 91(1): S54–S59.

World Health Organization (2001). *International Classification of Functioning, Disability and Health (ICF).* Geneva: WHO Publishing.

World Health Organization (2011). World report on disability. http://www.who.int/disabilities/world_report/2011/en/ http://www.who.int/classifications/en/. http://www.en.wiki pedia.org/wiki/Occupational_therapy.

3 Participation from the perspective of the user

From subjective experiences to lived experiences

Margareta Lilja and Staffan Josephsson

Introduction

The word 'participation' is used in everyday language for various purposes and with different meanings. We might ask if a friend is going to participate in the spring cleaning of the local neighbourhood, or if a colleague is participating in a new seminar series at the workplace. Like with most everyday words, we do not define it every time we use it; instead, its different nuances are part of lived situations and the everyday communication resources which language offers. The considerable meaning and resonance the word participation has for people in everyday life are also reasons why participation has become a professional concept. Policymakers and professional members of user organisations have been eager to widen the definition of health to not only signifying the absence of disease, but also involvement in everyday situations where people live and act. In this process, the word participation has been put forward as a concept relating to health and including everyday situations, and in this way encompassing more than the absence of disease. However, when classifications and official definitions are concerned, the concept turns its back on the everyday connotations of fluidity in meaning and use, and addresses the need for clarity and boundaries in meaning. If we take the official definition of participation as expressed in the International Classification of Functioning, Disability and Health (ICF) as 'involvement in a life situation' (WHO, 2001: 10) and put this definition alongside meanings the word has acquired in everyday life, there will be differences, tensions, but also opportunities in applying the range of meanings of participation in different contexts. For example, for a health professional, the term might be used for the performance of activities which are required in order to live independently; while for the service user, the term might mean, for example, being included in decisions, or being part of social networks. There are opportunities for use of participation within healthcare, as well as for individuals and groups striving for space, engagement and influence in various life contexts.

In this chapter, we want to expand the understanding of how individuals and groups use and understand the concept of participation. We also aim to address the relationship and tensions between everyday use and alternative understandings of the concept.

From a subjective to a social understanding of the life world

In the title of this chapter, we use the term 'subjective'. In many ways, that framing can be misleading. When connecting the discussion to a dichotomy of subjective-objective, we relate to a theoretical understanding of language, separating the world in terms of 'not real' and 'real', a conceptualisation that is not very useful (Piškur et al., 2013). We will therefore, from here on, use the term 'lived experience' for the dimension of participation we are addressing. We use the term lived experience for the direct experience of the world which orientates a person's self-conception and around which individuals organise their lives. We argue that it is through the lived experience that the complex layers of meaning of particular life stories unfold. As the attentive reader might notice, we differ somewhat from traditional notions of the life world as an individual entity. This position is central, since it differs from an understanding of meaning as singular and instead opens up meaning to be seen as an ongoing dialogue between alternatives. We argue that stressing the individual perspective alone is too limited a framing of the life world in order to portray the various meanings of participation.

In this chapter, the story of Linda is used as a resource to exemplify our reasoning. The story emerges from narratives collected in a research study about aging and life projects conducted in Sweden. Even if the main focus of the project was not on participation per se, the stories told by the participants included lived experiences of everyday situations. By exploring Linda's story in relation to participation, salient issues about the concept will be situated and interpreted with theory. This way, different meanings of participation in the lived experience of everyday life will be outlined.

Linda's story – lived experience of participation

At 17, Linda moved from the countryside to live in a local town, studying to be a teacher. After graduating, she got a job as a teacher in the same town. She got married, and after the birth of their first child, she and her husband moved to an apartment in the suburbs. This was not an easy decision since both of them had lived in the town for many years and their closest friends lived in the same area. One reason for the move was the possible closure of the school where Linda was working, and her fear of losing her job. She had already got a job in a school where they were going to live. Another reason was that her husband had just lost his job, and since they now had a child to care for, it was essential for at least one of them to have a secure income.

After the move, much of Linda's participation in activities was through her children and her work as a teacher. Her husband, who shortly after they moved got a job as an engineer on an oil platform, worked three weeks abroad and was then at home for two weeks. This meant that Linda was often alone at home, and was the one creating and keeping up their social life. As a teacher, she got involved in the life of the school and often met with other teachers and supported school-related charitable activities, for instance, children's bike rides, skiing or other activities. During the years when her child was growing up, the school and the parents organised a lot of events and activities open to the whole community: as Linda said, 'the school always tried to get everyone together and join in with things, which is lovely'. Linda was asked to join the school committee. She really wanted to, but she declined because she had a negative impression of it, which had put her off the idea of committees in general: 'I didn't want to be a part of it because it all just seemed like they were having committee meetings and spending time talking about other mums'.

A major event in Linda's life was when her daughter went to Australia to work as an au pair. Many of the activities Linda had been engaged in had been related to her daughter, and she now found herself being forced to work out what she wanted to do besides working as a teacher. This led to her reducing the number of hours she worked, and getting slightly 'itchy feet', saying she needed 'to influence things' and make changes in her life. She would never have made this decision if her husband had not supported her. Actually, he encouraged her since it meant that when he was at home from his work, they could spend more time together.

Since her work was in the public sector and she had been involved with a project about the environment and sustainability as a teacher, she knew that this was something that interested her. She made a conscious decision to make more of an active life locally for herself as she now had a bit more space and time. Linda joined a fair trade group and worked in their local shop, which was something of a hub in the area, where people were friendly and welcoming, and where neighbours could find someone to help them out. This resulted in Linda doing a lot of informal helping, participating in different social events and getting new friends. She really enjoyed this way of participating and influencing the community, and at the same time socialising with all her new friends. Her only regret was that she hadn't made these changes earlier in her life, but as she said, 'this was not something I thought of until my daughter moved to Australia, which got me thinking that I should get engaged in something different to what I was doing before'.

Another turning point was when Linda's husband retired. Because of his work on an oil platform, he could retire when he was 55 years old. For many years, they had organised their activities more or less around his three weeks at the oil platform and two weeks at home. The year before he retired, they bought a summerhouse where they now spent a lot of time together. During the summer, they almost moved out to the summerhouse, and it kept them busy with gardening and socialising with their neighbours. They loved travelling, and undertook a trip every year to a new place, experiencing new adventures. They had two grandchildren, but since their daughter was living in Australia with her family, they only spent time together with them twice a year. This was something that Linda missed, and she used Skype to keep in regular touch and thereby feel that she was participating in their everyday life. Sometimes they even had dinner 'together' on Skype.

Linda's story might seem one of a rather ordinary life for the reader of this chapter, and that is precisely the point. It is in everyday situations that we participate. However, it suffices as material for a discussion on how participation as lived experience emerges over time. Before entering into a discussion on that, however, we will present possible theoretical resources to ground the understanding of participation.

Theoretical resources

In the literature on the meaning of everyday life, different theoretical resources have been used. Phenomenology based on Husserl's reasoning on the life world has had a great influence in how meaning has been understood in healthcare practices (Husserl, 1970). The notion of the life world, the world as immediately or directly experienced in the subjectivity of everyday life, has been influential in how meaning has been conceived in health and social care, both in education and practice. Central in phenomenology is that the understanding that comes through the individual's life world needs interpretation to make sense and have meaning (Merleau-Ponty, 2012 [1945]). The use of interpretation in phenomenology stems from the hermeneutical tradition, with its origin in the interpretation of texts (Bleicher, 1980). The idea of the life world has often been used to conceptualise meaning as individual in nature, and for example to identify meaning of disease as different from generic diagnosis. Drawing on phenomenology or hermeneutics implies an understanding of meaning as active, evolving and dynamic.

The interest in the everyday is also a focus in the philosophical tradition of pragmatism that emerged at the end of the 19th century, and which, with the everyday in focus, moved interest from representation and description, or existential questions, to everyday problem-solving and action. Even if meaning is not a central focus of pragmatism, this philosophy and its resonance in contemporary health and social care practice, such as occupational therapy and social work, links meaning to the everyday practical world rather than to existential issues on a philosophical level. In these practices, issues related to meaning are connected to the everyday practical world rather than to existential issues on a philosophical level (Dickie, Humprey and Cutchin, 2006).

A somewhat different thread in the conceptualisation of meaning stems from social science and the notion of the social construction of meaning. In the framework of social science, and grounded in influential sources such as Berger and Luckman's book *The social construction of reality* (1966), this tradition of conceptualising meaning highlights the shared and interconnected way that people create meaning.

Finally, in this short review of theoretical resources central to contemporary use of the term 'meaning', the narrative turn in social and health sciences (that is, the interest in using narrative theory and practice to explain various aspects of human life) needs attention (Mattingly, 1998). Drawing from different sources, such as phenomenology and social constructivism, the notion of meaning as narratively constructed has furthered the understanding of the term. Narrative theory can explain how meaning in everyday situations simultaneously draws on one's own narrative emplotment of material and situations, and on existing meaning structures within culture. That is, the individual makes individual meaning of situations and material by emplotting this material in storied structures rooted in culture.

To make a generic statement on what the meaning of the everyday is and how it can be conceptualised is, of course, impossible, but it could be stated that the notion that humans construct meaning in life by drawing on both generic cultural resources and individual negotiation and emplotment of situations in everyday life represents a contemporary understanding reasonably well. When theoretical resources are applied to how humans construct meaning in the lived experience of participation, we might say that the lived experience of participation can be characterised by being situated in individuals' ongoing lived emplotment of resources and situations.

Participation as lived experience – personal and context tied

In this section, we will explore the lived experience of participation by drawing on some of the resources outlined above.

Meaning of participation as social construction

Linda's story follows known storylines in everyday culture on how life emerges in a Western cultural context, such as her struggle to combine her professional life and family, as well as how emerging migration issues impact on her participation. Her story is placed within contemporary societal and cultural structures, framing her participation in the everyday. Thus, when she gives meaning to her participation by telling her life story, it comes out as something people recognise and sympathise with. However, this function of making meaning of participation, drawing from existing structures in culture, is within Linda's story melded with her own unique perspectives. This function of participation in the everyday, being simultaneously unique and generic, characterise the lived experience of Linda's participation in life as shown in her story. In line with how meaning-making is understood in narrative theory, Linda's participation is not a tale of her static conditions, but rather portrays the negotiations she has to make in order to make sense in her everyday and to find ways to participate. Her story illustrates how the meaning of participation in everyday life plays out as socially constructed, taking colour from local situations and circumstances as well as larger cultural resources. One example is how Linda and her daughter participated in each other's daily lives. Because of the geographic distance between them, they used Skype as a tool for taking part in everyday situations, being a grandmother and even 'having dinner together'. Today, the Internet as a place for participation has almost become a norm. This is an illustrative example of how changes in the environment shape the material for meaning in the everyday and the forms these meanings take. How it takes shape is formed by the actual situation and how the persons involved react and act in response to the situation.

Meaning of participation as fluid and multifaceted

When reading Linda's story, it is clear how the meaning that she attaches to her participation is multifaceted and has a capacity to change over time as well as in everyday situations, depending on how these play out. In other words, her participation should not be regarded as a capacity or a trait that she possesses which can be measured in similar ways as, for example, cognition or motor functions. Rather, it takes a fluid form with the capacity to adjust to circumstances, but also to be a resource in Linda's hope and ambition to influence her life. When she was asked to join the school committee, which was in line with her ambition to influence the committee's work at the school, she knew she had the capacity and she wanted to accept, but she declined because she had a negative impression of the other members on the committee. The meaning of her participation and her choice not to participate cannot be conceptualised and understood as based only on individual choice and preferences. Such understanding falls short when it comes to situations involving more people and various contexts, as shown in Linda's story.

Linda's meaning of participation as fluid and multifaceted was also shown in those critical moments and turning points or transitions revealed in her life story – for instance, when her daughter moved to Australia, when she herself quit her job and when her husband retired. These kinds of life changes might influence what people participate in or not (Womack, Isaksson, & Lilja, 2016). It is important to highlight that this is seldom a straightforward decision. It is about how meaning in everyday situations simultaneously draws on one's own narrative emplotment of situations and existing meaning structures within one's culture, for example seeing new opportunities when children move away from home or when getting a summerhouse after retirement (Nyman, Josephsson & Isaksson, 2012). It is about back and forward discussions and negotiations with oneself and others. It is about moving beyond an individualistic view that situates a single person and his/her capacity to act in relationship to the environment towards a consideration of lived experiences as situations in which temporal/historical aspects, multifaceted contextual factors, and varied meanings both influence and emerge from what is occurring.

Some consequences for service delivery

A number of trends and policy shifts that are promoting greater participation by the user in service delivery can be identified. However, the reasoning above on the lived experiences of participation and the theoretical resources to ground this reasoning has consequences for practice and service delivery. For instance, a person's Activities of Daily Living (ADL) performance is a frequently performed measure in health and social services, and is assessed in various outcomes such as 'can or does perform an activity'. After the introduction of the ICF, participation has gained prominence as an outcome or therapeutic goal. But is it even possible to measure participation? There is no **one** pattern or cluster of activities that represents participation. Nor would a record of activities with which each instance of participation was performed tell us what participation meant to individuals (Dijkers, 2010; Hammel et al., 2008). If the lived experience of participation is more to be seen as a verb, something you do, then the core of assessment shifts from measurement to active collaboration and dialogue. Participation becomes a quality and a right for the individual person, and service delivery needs to find ways to ensure that these rights are catered for. Listening to the individual and providing space and opportunities for the individual to talk about how he/she wants to participate and the meanings he/she gives to the concept must be central. This implies that the current plethora of assessments of participation might be supplemented with ongoing communication with users over time.

One aspect of participation and service delivery is the connection with contemporary ambitions on client-centred or person-centred work (Law, Baptiste & Mills, 1995). These ambitions have been put forward as ways of making clients participate in decisions about their own service. It is important to realise, however, that the meaning which clients give to their participation in everyday life might not be easily understood. When in need of services, the client is often in a new, demanding situation, and thereby in new lived everyday experiences which haven't even been explored yet. Nevertheless, they are often expected to make choices about treatment, services and highly valued occupations without being grounded in the individual meaning of their situation. We need to be aware that when clients express the meanings they attach to their participation, these expressions are situated within the context they are experiencing and take meaning from the approaches used. Therefore, grounding a service within the client's understanding of participation needs ongoing negotiation, including the meaning the client gives to everyday participation and opportunities to try out how they want to participate.

Another aspect is that service delivery is often directed towards one individual, aiming to solve a problem experienced by that person. Moreover, as an outcome, individual performance is often seen as a primary and defining characteristic of participation. Nevertheless, the service is often delivered in the person's home environment, in everyday situations, where other family members live and act. This means that spouses, partners, children and families are a part of that person's experienced everyday life (Van de Valde et al, 2010; Womack, Isaksson & Lilja, 2016). Participation must therefore also be understood from a social or family-oriented perspective, situated as a social-relational concept influencing their decision-making process, and signifying the ways in which these couples/families participate in everyday life.

This chapter's point of departure was subjective experiences of participation. To validate that, some theoretical resources on meaning and people's creation of meaning were presented as key components in the understanding of the concept. The discussion presented on how the reception of the concept takes on various meanings among different groups and across cultures, is multifaceted and incorporates ambiguity. A consequence of our argumentation is that participation within service delivery for people with varying needs cannot be confined to portraying the meaning individuals and their social networks attach to their current participation and their desires to participate. The focus moves towards active dialogue and negotiations with service users. Other chapters in this book will provide examples of how this can be accomplished.

References

Berger, P., and Luckman, T. (1966) *The social construction of reality.* London: Penguin Group.

Bleicher, J. (1980) *Contemporary hermeneutics: Hermeneutics as method, philosophy and critique.* London and Boston: Routledge & Kegan Paul.

Dickie, V., Humprey, R., and Cutchin, M. (2006) Occupation as transactional experience: A critique of individualism in occupational science. *Journal of Occupational Science*, 13(1): 83–93.

Dijkers, M.P. (2010) Issues in the conceptualization and measurement of participation: An overview. *Archives of Physical Medicine and Participation*, 91(9 Suppl 1): S5–16.

Hammel, J., Magasi, S., Heinemann, A., Whiteneck, G., Bogner, J., and Rodriguez, E. (2008) What does participation mean? An insider perspective from people with disabilities. *Disability and Rehabilitation*, 30(19): 1445–1460.

Husserl, E., editor. (1970) *The crisis of European sciences and transcendental phenomenology. An introduction to phenomenology.* Evanstone, IL: Northwestern University Press.

Law, M., Baptiste, S., and Mills, J. (1995) Client-centred practice: What does it mean and does it make a difference? *Canadian Journal of Occupational Therapy*, 62: 250–257.

Mattingly, C. (1998) *Healing dramas and clinical plots: The narrative structure of experience.* Cambridge and New York: Cambridge University Press.

Merleau-Ponty, M. (2012) *Phenomenology of perception* (original: *Phénoménologie de la perception*, 1945). London: Routledge.

Nyman, A., Josephsson, S., and Isaksson G. (2012) Being part of an enacted togetherness: Narratives of elderly people with depression. *Journal of Aging Studies*, 26(4): 410–418.

Piškur, B., Daniëls, R., Jongmans, M.J., Ketelaar, M., Smeets, R., Norton, M., and Beurskens, A. (2013) Participation and social participation: Are they distinct concepts? *Clinical Rehabilitation*, 28(3), 211–220. DOI: 10.1177/0269215513499029.

Van de Valde, D., Brackec, P., Van Hoveb, G., Josephsson, S., and Vanderstraetena, G. (2010) Perceived participation, experiences from persons with spinal cord injury in their transition period from hospital to home. *International Journal of Rehabilitation Research*, 33(4), 345–355. DOI: 10.1097/MRR.0b013e32833cdf2a.

WHO (2001) *International classification of functioning, disability and health (ICF).* Geneva: World Health Organization.

Womack, J.L., Isaksson, G., and Lilja, M. (2016) Care partner dyad strategies to support participation in community mobility. *Scandinavian Journal of Occupational Therapy*, 23(3): 220–229.

4 Environmental determinants of quality of participation in healthcare settings among people with impairments and limitations

Jessica Dashner, Holly Hollingsworth, Jade Gross and David B. Gray

Introduction

Currently, 54 million – or more than one in five – Americans live with a disability (U.S. Department of Health and Human Services [USDHHS] 2005; Census Bureau 2010), which is above the 15% stipulated by the World Health Organisation (WHO 2011). In addition, 87% of people with disabilities report living with at least one preventable, secondary condition (Kinne, Patrick, & Lochner Doyle 2004). Commonly reported secondary conditions include, but are not limited to, fatigue, pain, and weight problems or obesity. Furthermore, people with disabilities are also more likely to report poorer overall health, less access to adequate healthcare, more smoking, and less physical activity than those without a disability. Information gathered directly from individuals with disabilities is necessary to further understand the user involvement and the factors that influence participation in healthcare activities. This type of information is essential to determine the influence of barriers to accessing health services and to begin to understand how to improve access for individuals with disabilities. The purpose of this chapter is to further investigate participation of people with disabilities inside service delivery with a specific focus on access to healthcare.

Disability, or decreased ability to participate, occurs when there is a mismatch between the individual and the environment in which the activity occurs. As described in earlier chapters, the environment is multidimensional and includes aspects such as physical/architectural elements, policies, culture, and social interactions with others. Environmental factors can either facilitate or create barriers to participation. The social model emphasises the need to remediate the environment to decrease the expression of disability and promote participation in activities. Community receptivity refers to the willingness, values and knowledge of people in the community who facilitate the participation of people with disabilities in valued activities and events (Bricout & Gray 2006). To date, environmental-based policies and interventions have focused more on aspects of the physical environment and less on improving social interactions or receptivity. The World Health Organization's (WHO's) International Classification of Functioning, Disability and Health (ICF) (WHO 2001) provides a framework for further understanding the factors that contribute to the expression of disability (see Chapter 2). While the ICF creates a framework for looking at various factors that influence participation, the specific relationships between different variables described as barriers to participation in specific activities, such as healthcare, have not been examined.

Access to healthcare is imperative to the well-being for all individuals and particularly for people with disabilities, but healthcare access barriers have been cited as a leading cause of poor health outcomes among people with disabilities (Neri & Kroll 2003). Compared to the general population, people with disabilities report more unmet health needs, are less likely to receive routine healthcare, and are less likely to receive preventive services (NOD 2004; Chevarley et al. 2006). High occurrences of negative experiences can contribute to a reduction in the frequency of participating in healthcare-related activities. Another study has shown that people with disabilities report up to three times as many unmet healthcare needs compared with people without a disability (McColl, Jarzynowska, & Shortt 2010).

The World Disability Report (WHO 2011) explicitly addresses access to healthcare as a key service priority for individuals with disability. The publicly identified need to increase healthcare access and to improve the understanding of healthcare needs of people with disabilities in the United States was also emphasised in a Surgeon General's Call to Action to 'improve the health and wellness of persons with disabilities' (USDHHS 2005). The specific objectives called for were: increasing public health provider knowledge and understanding regarding disability, treating the whole person versus the disability, promoting health and wellness for people with disabilities, and increasing access to needed healthcare services for people with disabilities (USDHHS 2005). Despite this Call to Action and an increase in public awareness, few efforts have been made to implement changes and increase health and wellness.

Most of the published studies on barriers to healthcare access are based on qualitative data. People with disabilities report a large number of environmental and social barriers to the maintenance and improvement of their health (Scheer et al. 2003; Iezzoni et al. 2004; Drainoni et al. 2006; Kroll et al. 2006; Kirschner, Breslin, & Iezzoni 2007; Manns & May 2007; Carmona et al. 2010). Common barriers to healthcare access for people with disabilities are categorised as environmental, structural, or delivery process barriers. Environmental barriers include access to transportation, inaccessible facilities, inaccessible medical equipment, difficulty accessing preventive services such as mammograms, and lack of provider recommendations for preventive services (Nosek & Simmons 2007; Yankaskas et al. 2010). Structural barriers consist of limitations in health plan benefits, therapy services, durable medical equipment, and mental health services. Delivery process barriers involve lack of provider knowledge, provider insensitivity and lack of respect, untimely appointments, and difficulty with appointment scheduling (Scheer et al. 2003; Drainoni et al. 2006; Kroll et al. 2006). An analysis of the accessibility of 62 primary physicians' surgeries revealed that 18% of the physicians could not serve people with disabilities due to noncompliance with Americans with Disabilities Act (ADA) regulations (Grabois, Nosek, & Rossi 1999). The lack of provider knowledge and training, and the inaccessibility of healthcare offices and equipment, are risk factors for patient safety and quality of care (Kirschner, Breslin, & Iezzoni 2007). Using the Scale of Attitudes Toward Disabled Persons, a sample of 338 health professional students was found to have negative attitudes toward disability (Tervo, Palmer, & Redinius 2004). Individuals with hearing impairments cite communication difficulties with their provider during physical examinations and procedures, medication safety, and difficulties interacting with office staff in person and over the phone as barriers (Iezzoni et al. 2004). In 2012, Cupples et al. described case studies reporting that individuals with visual impairment and blindness experience difficulty reading information about appointments and treatment, navigating unfamiliar environments, and difficulty with communication and consultation skills.

This chapter uses a structural equation modelling approach to estimate the relationships of social and environmental barriers with participation at the doctor's surgery. A prior study by Hollingsworth and Gray (2010) used a similar methodology to quantify the relationship between aspects of the environment and participation. This study used a measure of participation (PARTS/M) to examine environmental and personal contributors to leisure participation by people with mobility limitations. This analysis was based on participation in leisure activities undertaken in a variety of settings over a 30-day time period. For the analysis described in this chapter, a different measure, the Survey of Participation and Receptivity in the Community (SPARC), was used to collect data based on the specific site of participation rather than the general activity of participating in healthcare (Gray et al. 2006). This approach allows for further examination of the influence of the environment and facilitators and barriers to participation in context. To examine the differential weights of healthcare access barriers for people with disabilities, a structural equation model was used. The goal of this project was to increase awareness of the relative importance of the various variables reported in the literature that are barriers to participation at healthcare facilities. By understanding the factors that impact participation at doctors' surgeries by people with mobility, vision, and hearing impairments, healthcare facilities and practices in the healthcare services can be prioritised for remedial attention.

Methods

Participants

The participants included in this study were between the ages of 18 and 75, lived in the community, could access a computer or telephone, and read at or above the sixth-grade level. They were able to enter responses into a web-based survey or to direct another individual to enter their responses into a web-based survey, and they had a self-identified mobility, visual, or hearing impairment. Individuals who had a developmental disability or emotional impairment, or who reported that they were blind or deaf, were excluded from this study.

A convenience sample of 692 individuals was recruited nationally from a variety of organisations that advocate for or serve people with disabilities. Invitations to participate in the study were sent to individuals on LISTSERVs of the organisations and were posted on disability-related websites. All study procedures were reviewed and approved by the Washington University School of Medicine Human Research Protection Office. The data discussed in this study include 311 individuals with mobility, vision, and hearing impairments who responded to a survey indicating that they go to doctors' surgeries.

Table 4.1 Sample demographics

	Total Population	Percentages per Group				
	N=311	*PW (N=85)*	*MW (N=61)*	*CCW (N=54)*	*LV (N=59)*	*HofH (N=52)*
Group Breakdown by %	*100.0*	*27.3*	*19.6*	*17.4*	*19.0*	*16.7*
Test age						
Mean	47.0	46.2	44.5	50.6	44.9	50.1
Range	19–74	21–73	19–68	23–69	21–74	21–71
Gender						
Male	34.1	40.0	47.5	16.7	30.5	30.8
Female	65.9	60.0	52.5	83.3	69.5	69.2
Race						
American Indian/Alaskan Native	3.9	3.5	4.9	5.6	3.4	1.9
Asian	1.0	1.2	1.6	0.0	0.0	1.9
African American/Black	5.1	0.0	4.9	9.3	11.9	1.9
Native Hawaiian/ Other Pacific Islander	1.3	1.2	3.3	0.0	0.0	1.9
White	86.5	91.8	85.2	85.2	78.0	90.4
Other	4.5	3.5	4.9	5.6	6.8	1.9
Prefer not to answer	1.3	2.4	0.0	1.9	1.7	0.0
Hispanic/Latino Origin						
Yes	4.5	4.7	3.3	5.6	6.8	1.9
Marital Status (>1 option)						
Married	38.3	23.5	39.3	46.3	40.7	50.0
Divorced/ Widowed/ Separated	23.2	18.8	21.3	29.7	17.0	32.7
Never Married	34.1	50.6	32.8	24.1	35.6	17.3
Member of Unmarried Couple	8.4	12.9	9.8	3.7	6.8	5.8
Prefer not to answer	1.0	1.2	3.3	0.0	0.0	0.0
Annual Income						
< $15,000	29.9	38.8	24.6	38.9	23.7	19.2
$15,000 to < $35,000	30.2	32.9	27.9	35.2	33.9	19.2

	Total Population	Percentages per Group				
	N=311	*PW (N=85)*	*MW (N=61)*	*CCW (N=54)*	*LV (N=59)*	*HofH (N=52)*
Group Breakdown by %	*100.0*	*27.3*	*19.6*	*17.4*	*19.0*	*16.7*
$35,000 to < $55,000	15.1	11.8	18.0	3.7	16.9	26.9
$55,000 to < $75,000	9.3	8.2	16.4	1.9	5.1	15.4
≥ $75,000	5.8	3.5	6.6	7.4	5.1	7.7
Don't know/ Prefer not to answer	9.6	4.7	6.6	13.0	15.3	11.5
Highest Level Education						
Grade 1–11	1.3	1.2	3.3	1.9	0.0	0.0
Grade 12 or GED	11.6	15.3	14.8	11.1	5.8	5.8
College 1–3 y	27.7	25.9	23.0	37.0	25.0	25.0
College ≥ 4 y	59.2	56.5	59.0	50.0	69.2	69.2
Prefer not to answer	0.3	1.2	0.0	0.0	0.0	0.0

Abbreviations: PW: Power Wheelchair; MW: Manual Wheelchair; CCW: Cane/Crutches/Walker LV: Low Vision; HofH: Hard of Hearing; GED: General Educational Development diploma.

Measures

The Characteristics of the Respondent (CORE) was administered to obtain demographic information (Gray et al. 2008). Data collected includes benefits received, any disabling primary diagnosis, any current or past secondary conditions, type of assistive device used, and personal assistance used.

The Survey of Participation and Receptivity in Communities (SPARC) is a location-based measure of community participation from the perspective of people who have mobility impairments, low vision, or are blind, hard of hearing, or deaf. The SPARC was developed by combining items from three other valid and reliable measures: Participation for People with Mobility Impairments and Limitations – PARTS/M (Gray et al. 2006); Facilitators and Barriers to Participation – FABS/M (Gray et al. 2008), and Community Health Environment Checklist – CHEC (Stark et al. 2007). Seventeen sites were included in this study of community participation, doctors' surgeries being one site. All response options use a four-point or five-point Likert scale with scale direction from low to high. One site in the SPARC is referred to as the SPARC-DO (doctor's surgery). The questions included in the SPARC-DO provide a self-report of the quality of participation in healthcare at the participant's own doctor's surgery, and barriers and facilitators to healthcare that impact participation. The SPARC-DO takes approximately 15 minutes to complete.

The SPARC-DO includes items about community participation with respect to the evaluative factors influencing the quality of participation (importance, control, choice, and satisfaction) (Table 4.2). Evaluative Quality of Participation (EQOP) was assessed by examining the mean scores for the importance (scale of 1–4), choice (scale of 1–4), control (scale of 1–4), and satisfaction (scale of 1–4) items for each site. Importance represents how much value the participant places on performing activities in each site. Choice denotes the number of options available for where one participates. For example, does a person have the option of visiting any of the five clinics in his/her community? Control refers to the level of flexibility over when one is able to participate in the community. Finally, satisfaction items allow the respondent to report the level of enjoyment he/she derives from doing activities in the community. The SPARC measures the influence of environmental factors, including the physical accessibility of the site, the receptivity of employees toward the person, and the support he/she used to participate (i.e. use of personal assistance and use of assistive devices). The physical accessibility features of doctors' surgeries include equipment in the examination room and features of the building (Table 4.2).

Community receptivity, or how individuals in the sample perceived they were treated, was assessed using eight questions. The community receptivity items were developed through key informant interviews and focus groups and were vetted by a sample of people with disabilities. Examples of communication receptivity

Table 4.2 Items included in the SPARC to examine participation at doctors' offices

---

Evaluative Quality of Participation – Participation intrinsic variables
How *important* is participating in healthcare activities at your doctor's offices?
   (1) Very unimportant (2) Unimportant (3) Important (4) Very important
How much *choice* did you have when you selected this doctor's office?
   (1) No choice (2) Little choice (3) Some choice (4) A lot of choice
How much *control* do you have over when you go to this doctor's office?
   (1) No control (2) Little control (3) Some control (4) A lot of control
How *satisfied* are you with your participation in healthcare activities at this doctor's office?
   (1) Very dissatisfied (2) Dissatisfied (3) Satisfied (4) Very satisfied

Environment – Participation extrinsic variables
Equipment and Building Features – Accessible Exam Table, Accessible Scale & Counter

Direct Receptivity – Do people working in your doctor's office . . .
Help you in a timely manner? Look directly at you? Speak directly at you? Avoid you?
   (1) Never (2) Rarely (3) Often (4) Always

Indirect Receptivity – Do people working in your doctor's office . . .
Solve problems for you without asking? Control the conversation? Make decisions or choices for you? Treat you as a child?
   (1) Never (2) Rarely (3) Often (4) Always

---

items are whether the employee looks directly at the visitor, speaks directly to him/her, and attends to the visitor without delay; if the employee engages in these actions, the communication style is characterised as direct and positively receptive. If the employee treats the visitor like a child, avoids the person, or controls the conversation, then the communication style is considered to be indirect and to have negative receptivity (see Table 4.2).

Procedure

Individuals recruited for the study completed a web-based screener survey. If eligible, the individual received a link to the CORE and SPARC-DO web-based surveys via email. Individuals who did not have access to a computer were offered the opportunity to complete the survey with the assistance of a research team member, who called and read the survey questions to the participant. Individuals were reimbursed by cheque or gift card for their time spent completing the surveys.

Statistical analysis

Reported descriptive statistics were computed using SPSS version 22 (IBM 2013), and structural equation models were computed using EQS 6.3 for Windows, Multivariate Software Inc. (2016). Data analysis proceeded in two steps. The first step used confirmatory factor analysis to determine the dimensions of receptivity as a latent variable. This step indicated that the manifest variables of receptivity reduced to two factors: a direct factor and an indirect factor. The second step involved testing the hypothesised structural relationships among the variables shown in Figure 4.1. Model integrity was determined by examining the solution estimates of the observed and latent variables, the model fit indices, and the pattern of standardised residuals (Browne & Cudeck 1993).

Results

The structural model provided a reasonable fit to the data based on fit statistics [$\chi^2 = 341.24$, $p = 0.00$, confirmatory factor analysis (CFI) = 0.83, root mean square error of approximation (RMSEA) = 0.10]. Overall, the receptivity variables accounted for nearly 70% of the variance in quality of participation of people with disabilities at their doctors' surgeries.

The standardised coefficients for quality of participation were all statistically different from zero ($p < 0.05$). The standardised coefficients for the manifest variables are importance, 0.14; choice, 0.62; control, 0.62; and satisfaction, 0.76. The standardised coefficients for receptivity were all statistically different from zero ($p < 0.05$). The latent trait, direct receptivity (standardised

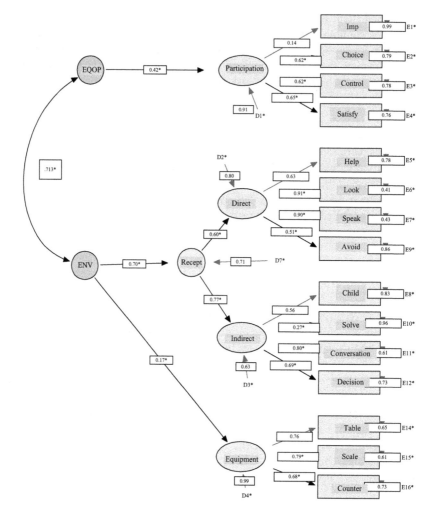

Figure 4.1 EQS 6 md_office diagram 040416.eds: Chi Sq. = 341.24, P = 0.00, CFI = 0.83, RMSEA = 0.10

coefficient of 0.60), is represented by four manifest variables: (1) employees help you in a timely manner, 0.63; (2) employees look directly at you, 0.91; (3) employees speak directly to you, 0.90; and (4) employees avoid you, 0.51. The latent trait, indirect receptivity (standardised coefficient of 0.77), is also represented by four manifest variables: (1) employees solve problems for you without asking, 0.27; (2) employees control the conversation, 0.80; (3) employees make decisions or choices for you, 0.69; and (4) employees treat you like a child, 0.59.

Accessible equipment inside the doctor's surgery was included in the model with receptivity to judge its relative contribution to the environment. Accessible examination tables, scales, and counters all had a significant relationship with the latent equipment variable: 0.76, 0.79, and 0.68, respectively. However, the latent variable had a significant but low relationship – 0.17 – with environment. According to this model, the attribute of receptivity is a more important feature of the environment than accessible equipment when evaluating the relationship between the environment and the quality of participation in the doctor's surgery.

Discussion

The results of this study indicate that perceived attitudes are more important to the quality of participation than accessible equipment at doctors' surgeries. The lower relationship between EQOP and equipment features may be due to building standards and the ADA accessibility guidelines. For example, few individuals with disabilities would choose or be able to go to a physically inaccessible healthcare facility. There is a strong relationship between the EQOP for people with mobility, vision, and hearing limitations and the perceived receptivity in a doctor's office. Receptivity accounts for nearly 70% of the variance of the environment.

The latent trait of importance has a non-zero contribution to the quality of participation but is relatively small due to the evaluative latent trait. The contribution is statistically small because there is little variation to the response of how important it is for the individual to go to his/her doctor's surgery. Going to a doctor's surgery is an important activity for all individuals, so there was minimal variability in the response options. The evaluative latent trait is composed of three manifest variables – choice, control, and satisfaction – that all contribute about equally to the trait. Participation is a complex construct and can be measured multiple ways. Assessing the quality of participation is an effective strategy to thoroughly understanding the experience of individuals with disabilities. This is a first step in being able to identify the environmental factors with the greatest influence on the quality of participation at doctors' surgeries.

There are two latent traits associated with receptivity: direct and indirect receptivity. The results indicate that both latent traits contribute about equally to the trait of receptivity at the doctor's surgery, but that the indirect component is perceived to be more of a concern for people with mobility, vision, and hearing impairments. The latent trait of indirect receptivity is composed of four manifest variables that contribute differentially to the trait. The standardised coefficients for 'control the conversation', 'make decisions or choices', and 'treat you like a child' are about equal in magnitude. The coefficient for 'solves problems for you without asking' is smaller than the other coefficients. This may be due to patients' expecting employees at the doctor's surgery to solve problems without asking, whereas at other sites in the community, respondents may be offended by the same level of interaction.

The latent trait of direct receptivity is composed of four manifest variables that contribute differentially to the trait. The manifest variables for employees looking directly at the patient and speaking directly to the patient have nearly equal and positive standardised coefficients. Educating healthcare providers, possibly during their career training, could be a step that is needed to improve receptivity. Particularly in the doctor's surgery, this can be an issue due to people commonly having someone accompany them for support. Communication is often directed towards the other person instead of directly to the person with a disability. The manifest variables of employees helping in a timely manner and avoiding the patient have standardised coefficients of the same magnitude.

The results from this study indicate the importance of improving receptivity and communication between healthcare providers and individuals with disabilities. Interventions designed to improve the social environment and improve the interactions between individuals with disabilities and healthcare providers are needed. Improving these interactions can increase the quality of participation at doctors' surgeries for people with disabilities and make the environments more receptive. The purpose of this investigation was to determine the relationship between environmental factors and the quality of participation at doctors' surgeries. While the results have determined the strongest relationship was between perceived receptivity and not the accessible equipment, having access to accessible equipment is additionally important for maintaining health. Further research is needed to determine the influence of environmental features on health and wellness in addition to the quality of participation for individuals with disabilities.

While this chapter was being written, Professor David B. Gray passed away. He was a pioneer in the research on participation of people with disabilities. His leadership will be missed, but his influence will continue through the many people he engaged. This chapter has been dedicated in his memory.

References

Bricout, J, & Gray, D. 2006. Community receptivity: The ecology of disabled persons' participation in the physical, political, and social environments, *Scandinavian Journal of Disability Research*, vol. 8, no. 1, pp. 1–21.

Browne, M, & Cudeck, R. 1993. Alternative ways of assessing model fit, in KAL Bollen, JS Long (eds.), *Testing Structrual Equation Models*, Newbury Park: Sage, pp. 136–162.

Carmona, RH, Giannini, M, Bergmark, B, & Cabe, J. 2010. The surgeon general's call to action to improve the health and wellness of persons with disabilities: Historical review, rationale, and implications 5 years after publication, *Disability and Health Journal*, vol. 3, no. 4, pp. 229–232.

Census Bureau: Facts for Features 20th Anniversary of the Americans with Disabilities Act: July 26. Published online May 26, 2010. https://www.census.gov/newsroom/releases/archives/facts_for_features_special_editions/cb10-ff13.html.

Chevarley, FM, Thierry, JM, Gill, CJ, Ryerson, AB, & Nosek, MA. 2006. Health, preventive health care, and health care access among women with disabilities in the 1994–1995 national health interview survey, supplement on disability, *Women's Health Issues*, vol. 16, pp. 297–312.

Cupples, ME, Hart, PM, Johnston, A, & Jackson, AJ. 2012. Improving healthcare access for people with visual impairment and blindness, *BMJ*, vol. 344, p. e542.

Drainoni, ML, Lee-Hood, E, Tobias, C, Bachman, SS, Andrew, J, & Maisels, L. 2006. Cross-disability experiences of barriers to health care access, *Journal of Disability Policy Studies*, vol. 17, no. 2, pp. 101–115.

EQS 6.3 for Windows. 2016. Multivariate Software Inc.

Grabois, EW, Nosek, MA, & Rossi, CD. 1999. Accessibility of primary care physicians' offices for people with disabilities, *Archives of Family Medicine*, vol. 8, pp. 44–51.

Gray, DB, Hollingsworth, HH, Stark, S, & Morgan, KA. 2006. Participation survey/mobility: Psychometric properties of a measure of participation for people with mobility impairments and limitations, *Archives of Physical Medicine and Rehabilitation*, vol. 87, no. 2, pp. 189–197.

Gray, DB, Hollingsworth, HH, Stark, S, & Morgan, KA. 2008. A subjective measure of environmental facilitators and barriers to participation for people with mobility limitations, *Disability and Rehabilitation*, vol. 30, no. 6, pp. 434–457.

Hollingsworth, H, & Gray, DB. 2010. Structural equation modeling of the relationships between participation in leisure activities and community environments by people with mobility impairments, *Archives of Physical Medicine and Rehabilitation*, vol. 91, pp. 1174–1181.

IBM. 2013. SPSS Statistics Version 22. USA: IBM.

Iezzoni, LI, O'Day, BL, Killeen, M, & Harker, H. 2004. Communicating about health care: Observations from persons who are deaf or hard of hearing, *Annals of Internal Medicine*, vol. 140, no. 5, pp. 356–363.

Kinne, S, Patrick, DL, & Lochner Doyle, D. 2004. Prevalence of secondary conditions among people with disabilities, *American Journal of Public Health*, vol. 94, no. 3, pp. 443–445.

Kirschner, KL, Breslin, ML, & Iezzoni, LI. 2007. Structural impairments that limit access to health care for patients with disabilities, *The Journal of the American Medical Association*, vol. 297, no. 10, pp. 1121–1125.

Kroll, T, Jones, GC, Kehn, M, & Neri, MT. 2006. Barriers and strategies affecting the utilization of primary preventive services for people with physical disabilities: A qualitative inquiry, *Health and Social Care in the Community*, vol. 14, no. 4, pp. 284–293.

Manns, PJ, & May, LA. 2007. Perceptions of issues associated with the maintenance and improvement of long-term health in people with SCI, *Spinal Cord*, vol. 45, pp. 411–419.

McColl, MA, Jarzynowska, A, & Shortt, SED. 2010. Unmet health care needs of people with disabilities: Population level evidence, *Disability and Society*, vol. 25, no. 2, pp. 205–218.

National Organization on Disability. 2004. *Landmark disability survey finds pervasive disadvantages*. http://www.2010disabilitysurveys.org/pdfs/surveyresults.pdf.

Neri, MT, & Kroll, T. 2003. Understanding the consequences of access barriers to health care: Experiences of adults with disabilities, *Disability and Rehabilitation*, vol. 25, no. 2, pp. 85–96.

Nosek, MA, & Simmons, DK. 2007. People with disabilities as a health disparities population: The case of sexual and reproductive health disparities, *California Journal of Health Promotion*, vol. 5, special issue, pp. 68–81.

Scheer, J, Kroll, T, Neri, MT, & Beatty, P. 2003. Access barriers for persons with Disabilities, *Journal of Disability Policy Studies*, vol. 13, no. 4, pp. 221–230.

Stark, S, Hollingsworth, HH, Morgan, KA, & Gray, DB. 2007. Development of a measure of receptivity of the physical environment, *Disability and Rehabilitation*, vol. 29, no. 2, pp. 123–137.

Tervo, RC, Palmer, G, & Redinius, P. 2004. Health professional student attitudes towards people with disability, *Clinical Rehabilitation*, vol. 18, pp. 908–915.

United States Department of Health and Human Services [USDHHS]. 2005. *The Surgeon General's Call to Action to Improve the Health and Wellness of Persons with Disabilities*. Retrieved from http://www.surgeongeneral.gov/library/disabilities/calltoaction/healthwellness.html.

World Health Organisation. 2001. *The International Classification of Functioning, Disability and Health*. Geneva: World Health Organisation.

World Health Organisation. 2011. *World Disability Report*. Geneva: World Health Organisation.

Yankaskas, BC, Dickens, P, Bowling, M, Jarman, MP, Luken, K, Salisbury, JH, & Lorenz, CE. 2010. Barriers to adherence to screening mammography among women with disabilities, *American Journal of Public Health*, vol. 100, no. 5, pp. 947–953.

5 Culture and participation

Skender Redzovic and Arne H. Eide

Introduction

The individual is unique, rational, has personal volition and goals, as well as the ability to make independent choices (Bellah et al. 1985; Markus & Kitayama 1991; Triandis 1995). On the other hand, it is today widely recognised that our way of thinking is also bounded (Simon 1991). Social influence theory, with its roots in the early studies of group attitude and perceptual convergence, suggests that homo sapiens is also homo sociologicus (Sheriff 1936) – we need others in order to define ourselves and our existence, to gain approval, avoid rejection and maintain a positive self-concept (Turner 1991).

Although there are many hypotheses about the nature of the symbiosis between the individual and the group, one thing is clear: individuals' doing is influenced by others through social norms, and to a large extent we all conform to social norms (Turner 1991). Studies underline that processes of influence inherent in social relationships create and maintain implicit pressure for agreement, even without instructions to agree or explicit group membership (Festinger 1950; Turner 1991). This informal pressure for agreement is also about members' behaviour in a group – 'this is how things are done around here'. Therefore, culture has a bearing on our participation.

The International Classification of Functioning, Disability and Health (ICF) recognises participation as a major contributor to health, and defines it as 'involvement in a life situation' (WHO 2001, 2007). Enabling users' participation in health services is crucial in order to promote both their health and control over their own treatment and everyday life (Berwick 2009). Studies have shown that social participation is associated with lower rates of heart disease and cancer (Kawachi et al. 1997), better physical and mental health, happiness and self-reported health (Nummela et al. 2008; Myroniuk & Anglewicz 2015). Participation in physical activities is also associated with various health benefits, including the prevention of cardiovascular diseases, diabetes, cancer, hypertension, obesity, depression, osteoporosis and premature death (Warburton, Nicol & Bredin 2006). Scholars describe participation as multidimensional (Granlund 2013; Imms et al. 2015).

According to Eide et al. (Chapter 1), individual, social and interactional perspectives on participation yield different terminology and understandings. As Vik et al. (2007) argued, participation is both an individual and an environmental phenomenon – it emerges in the interaction between environment and the individual through our doing. Culture is embedded both in the environment, and in the self of individuals – ergo it influences our participation from both the outside and the inside. However, current models on participation do not consider how culture influences individuals' preferences, understandings and behaviour.

The aim of this chapter is to provide a theoretical elaboration of the relationship between culture and participation in order to shed light on how culturally sensitive health services can enable user participation in services and in daily life. Culture emerges and develops through continuous interaction and communication between individuals as they meet up through various activities in everyday life, or through the use of information and communications technology. Consequently, a web of cultural preferences emerges within various large and small groups, even within societies we used to call homogeneous. Therefore, an elaboration of the relationship between culture and the participation of individuals is needed, in order to increase consciousness about the culturally sensitive choices that service providers have to make in order to design health services that enable users to participate. Second, the process of globalisation, access to new information and communications technology, as well as emigration, have created a context where people with different cultural backgrounds live together, or share their ideas from a distance. It is a world of opportunities, but also of challenges. It is vital to promote participation in multicultural societies as it promotes integration and contributes to the build-up of social capital. Studies have demonstrated that social integration boosts one's overall mental health and sense of autonomy (Rose 2000; Cattell 2001). That, in turn, presumes knowledge of how culture draws boundaries for the participation of individuals.

In his widely cited book *Culture's Consequences*, Hofstede (1980) differentiated country-level individualism from power distance, masculinity and uncertainty avoidance. The typology of individualistic versus collectivistic cultures is extensively studied. For that reason, we are using the typology in order to illustrate our reasoning.

Defining culture

The concept of culture has its origin in anthropology (Reichers & Schneider 1990). Both symbolic interactionism and social constructivism have had influence on the conceptual development. The roots of the concept can be found in ethnographies by Jacques (1951), Dalton (1959) and Rohlen (1974), including Mead's work (1910). Many definitions of culture exist despite substantial research within a wide array of social sciences. Indeed, the definition has gradually become more complex with the development of science. However, there is no consensus about what culture is, whether it can be generalised and how it should be understood and studied. Such issues are the target of a fuelled discussion between multiple research traditions (Martin 2002). As early as the 1950s, Kroeber and Kluckhohn (1952) identified 164 definitions of culture. Edward Tylor, in his work *Primitive*

Culture (Tylor 1920/1871: p. 1), gave one of the earliest definitions. According to him, culture 'is that complex whole which includes knowledge, belief, art, morals, law, custom, and any other capabilities and habits acquired by man as a member of society'. Mead (1937) made a distinction between 'culture' and 'a culture'. She stated that

> Culture means the whole complex of traditional behavior which has been developed by the human race and is successively learned by each generation. A culture is less precise. It can mean the forms of traditional behavior which are characteristic of a given society, or of a group of societies, or of a certain race, or of a certain area, or of a certain period of time.
>
> (Mead 1937: p. 17)

Kroeber and Parsons (1958) defined culture as 'transmitted and created content and patterns of values, ideas, and other symbolic meaningful systems as factors in the shaping of human behavior and the artefacts produced through behavior' (p. 583). Hofstede (2001) described culture as the collective programming of the mind that distinguishes the members of one group or category of people from another (p. 9). Culture determines the uniqueness of a human group, just as personality determines the uniqueness of an individual. The uniqueness of the group is provided by both practical, specific solutions embedded in its culture – giving the group the ability to cope with the environment – and by individual psychological adaptations needed in order to maintain those solutions (Hofstede 2001).

Culture and participation

Scholars have different approaches to the construct of participation, and in many studies, a conceptual or operational definition of participation is not provided (see Chapter 1) (Imms et al. 2015). The word 'participation' refers to taking part in some action – often where other people are involved. User participation in health services, for instance, implies collaborative effort between the user and service providers in a process designed to help the user to attain better health, to get well from, or live with, a condition, or more broadly to cope with his/her life. Thus, participation can only make sense in a context – an environment. According to Maxwell et al. (2012), participation is situated within environmental contexts, including dimensions such as availability, accessibility, affordability, accommodability and acceptability. Culture is part of the environment and has a bearing on all those dimensions, especially accommodability and acceptability.

A study showed that participation was experienced by users as 'being confident', 'comprehending' and 'seeking and maintaining a sense of control'; non-participation was experienced as 'not understanding', 'not being in control', 'lacking a relationship' and 'not being accountable' (Eldh, Ehnfors & Ekman 2004). A recent review study (Imms et al. 2015) showed that attendance and involvement are the most common words used to define and measure participation. Being confident, being able to comprehend the context, seeking and maintaining a sense of control and ensuring involvement and even attendance, requires an understanding of the role that culture plays in our participation. While there are a large number of definitions of culture, several assumptions that are shared in those definitions emphasise the bearing culture has on participation.

'This is how we think and do things around here'

Culture is a group phenomenon (Mead 1937; Kroeber & Kluckhohn 1952; Hofstede 2001). The compound construct of culture refers to created, shared and transmitted patterns of ideas, assumptions and values, as well as more tangible culture manifestations such as behavioural prescriptions, rituals, symbols and definition of heroes, and other symbolic meaningful systems (Kroeber and Kluckhohn 1952; Hofstede 2001). It creates informal expectations about how we should think and behave in our everyday life. As Hofstede (2001) emphasised, it is the identity of a group. For instance, individualistic and collectivistic cultures are defined as two distinctive dimensions (Hofstede 1980; Hui 1988), or as world views that differ in the issues they make salient (Kagitcibasi 1997). Individualistic cultures emphasise individual independence, rights, uniqueness, goals, self-fulfilment and control (Hsu 1983; Bellah et al. 1985; Markus & Kitayama 1991; Triandis 1995; Kagitcibasi 1997). Individuals in collectivistic societies from birth onwards are integrated into strong, cohesive in-groups, often extended families and/or clans, ethnic, religious or other groups (Hui 1988; Triandis 1995) which offer protection in exchange for unquestioning loyalty. In-groups as social units with a common fate, diffuse and mutual obligations and expectations based on ascribed statuses (Schwartz 1990), common goals and common values, are centralised. Individual independence, uniqueness, goals and control have secondary priority. Loyalty within a group is always important; harmony is to be maintained while confrontation is to be avoided.

Consequently, culture influences users' participation through deep assumptions about what is right and wrong, as well as through concrete prescriptions about our behaviour, symbols we should use, rituals we should attend, and who we have to become in order to be looked up to. For instance, in individualistic cultures, participation will be oriented toward the person. 'How do I see myself and my participation?' would be the default question of people with an individualistic culture mindset (Yoon 1994). On the other hand, in collectivistic cultures, participation would be oriented toward social context, the situation and social roles. 'How am I and my participation seen by others?' would be the default question of people living in collectivistic cultures (Yoon 1994). Within an individualistic culture, users would be expected to be active in their choices and participate in activities that are meaningful to them in order to fulfill their personal achievement. It is thus acceptable and even expected for a patient or a user of health services to contribute to the service delivery by presenting his or her own premises and choices. Within collectivistic cultures, users would be expected to follow recommendations from service providers as authorities. Furthermore, participation in health and social services and in everyday life would, to a greater extent, be influeced by the attitudes of their family and/or in-group beyond the family. Therefore, it is crucial that service providers are consciuous about possible cultural patterns in the environment which guide users' motivation and choices with regard to participation, both in their life and in health and social services.

Informal sanctions and participation

Culture is viewed by many scholars as informal social control. It is widely recognised that cultural patterns have the ability to sustain their 'ought' or 'must' quality in a group, mostly through informal sanctions (O'Reilly 1996; Falk, Fehr & Fischbacher 2005; Jensen 2010). Informal psychological sanctions are actions by peers or groups and can include ridicule, frowning, smiling, rejection, condemnation, sarcasm, gossip, criticism, avoidance, insults, etc. Informal sanctions remind others that their behaviour is displeasing and that they have to comply with cultural prescriptions in order to be accepted by the group. Studies have shown that both co-operators who share cultural prescriptions and defectors who reject them use informal sanctions against each other (Jensen 2010; Redzovic 2014).

Through the possibility of formal and informal sanctions, culture encourages participation which is in accordance with cultural prescriptions. Participation which is contrary to cultural prescriptions can both hinder participation, and, even worse, trigger exclusion and discrimination. Studies have shown that discrimination and exclusion can bring additional risks to the health of individuals (Corrigan & Penn 1997; Craig et al. 2007). This can create 'damned if you do and damned if you don't' situations if a user participates in a context with different cultural expectations. For instance, for a user with collective cultural preferences, being active and independently contributing to his/her situation in the user's interaction with service providers can trigger informal sanctions by the user's family and other members of that group. If he/she complies with their expectations and finishes the practice, service providers with individualistic values would understand his/her practice as irresponsible. That can trigger informal sanctions by service providers and the community around. It is crucial that service providers understand the ability of culture to create and maintain implicit pressure for agreement through sanctions, even without instructions to agree or explicit group membership (Festinger 1950; Turner 1991). Thus, adherence to health service ideals – or lack of it – can trigger sanctions that could further complicate an already challenging situation.

Individual culture and participation

Another core assumption about culture is that it is learned through everyday interaction and relationships (Hofstede 2001). Whether consciously or not, individuals are socialised in a cultural environment. Cultures have the ability to shape individual psychological processes within their ecological context, which in turn shapes the self of individuals – their identity, their own sense of who they are (Nisbett 2003). Let us return to studies which elaborate on the differences between individualistic and collectivistic cultures.

The self-concept of individuals in individualistic cultures implies creating and maintaining a positive sense of self (Baumeister 1998), an appreciation of feeling free and good about oneself, personal success, and having many unique or distinctive personal opinions (Oyserman & Markus 1993; Triandis 1995) as well as abstract characteristics (Fiske et al. 1998). The pursuit of individual interests and rewarding personal success is legitimate (Hsu 1971). The view of the self in collectivistic cultures is of a connected, flexible, fluid self, commited to others (Markus & Kitayama 1991). The pursuit of socially desirable and culturally mandated achievements characterises the socially oriented self (Luo & Gilmour 2004). In a study (Tafarodi et al. 2004), the following question was presented to Canadian and East Asian women: 'Do you believe that you know yourself more accurately than any other living person in your life knows you?' Eighty-six percent of the Canadian women answered yes, while only 40% and 52% of the women in Japan and China, respectively, did the same. Suh (2002) reported that Korean self-views, for example, vary more than those of Americans, and identity consistency was less predictive of social well-being in Korea than in the US. Other empirical studies have shown that the content of self-descriptions changed more across contexts and roles among Japanese than among Americans (Cousins 1989). Kashima et al. (2004) stated that the true self in Japan is believed to be self-in-context.

Participation in accordance with our cultural identity provides us with a feeling of coherence, belonging, safety, meaningfulness and well-being. A user with individualistic culture would probably find little meaning in participating in accordance with collectivistic norms, despite the fact that he/she moved to a place with collectivistic cultural norms. The user would find himself/herself alienated if his/her participation was more about being a part of a group. The same could happen with a user with collectivistic cultural identity if the user's participation was more about his/her own success and defining his/her own distinctiveness from others.

Health services have to take into account users' individual cultural identity in order to assess and promote their participation, referring both to their own health and to the relationship with health and social service providers. Such services will always represent majority culture and may easily disregard or fail to understand how cultural identity could lead to different preferences and even the ability to participate. This can produce misunderstanding and wrong interpretations among both providers and clients, which in turn can be counterproductive to health and well-being. The role and understanding of participation may differ substantially depending on cultural preferences and identity, for instance, between majority and minority cultures and between carers and individuals who depend on health services.

Cultural variation and participation

Although the construct of culture is widely recognised and studied, many scholars have addressed a wide array of critical issues. It is crucial to pay attention to those critical views in order to avoid misunderstandings regarding the role culture has on users' participation.

Culture is associated with consensus – something that is shared. The understanding is that culture is shared by individuals within a group and it is an unambiguous phenomenon. However, studies have shown that culture often contains assumptions that are blurred, unconscious, ambiguous or even paradoxical, further complicated by the existence of subcultures (Martin 2002; Redzovic 2014). An approach with emphasis on consensus tends to have a static view of culture, focusing on the differences of the end product – not on how culture evolves like it does. Hofstede's (1980) cultural model has successfully brought people's attention to cultural differences in the past decades. However, the model can be criticised for emphasising alienation without considering the social processes that construct cultural differences. It addresses the construct of culture as a snapshot. Culture always evolves within a historical and structural setting where different groups with different cultures in their dominant and subordinate positions struggle to define 'what is the right thing to think and do' (Clark et al. 1975). The evolution of a certain culture can be the result of groups struggling over, rather than sharing, understandings. Service providers should adopt an approach that emphasises a process perspective for the understanding of culture, including its influence on users' participation. Such an approach would imply studying culture and participation as an ongoing dynamic process where different layers of culture are being created and reshaped in social interactions.

Defining the cultural identity of a group is an arduous task, as it is difficult to find meaningful parameters that precisely define the boundaries of the group. Should that be religion, nation state, a civilisation, a local football club, generational belonging, gender, disability, or simply what is shared (Martin 2002; Redzovic 2014). As a consequence of this challenge, many – often ambiguous – terms are used to describe a culture, such as Norwegian, Nordic, Western, Eastern, African, Christian, Muslim, etc. Drawing conclusions about individuals' participation from such constructs can often be a habitual simplification, if not directly stigmatisation. Moreover, it is obvious that economic, social and cultural globalisation, propelled by access to new information and communications technology, has created a context where people from all over the world can interact and exchange their ideas in no time. Such interaction leads to the blurring of boundaries between cultures. Culture is less bound to a geographical area, country, race or religion – as was traditionally studied in anthropology. Today, it is appropriate to speak of the culture of online communities. Consequently, understanding how culture enables participation requires a balanced approach. Failing to do so would lead to misunderstandings, wrong decisions, prejudices, and in the worst cases, stigmatisation and exclusion. Such a scenario would be contrary to all good intentions and lead to further complication with users' participation.

Further, our cultural identity is being influenced by a web of different cultures as individuals are members of multiple large and small online and real-world groups, with different cultures in their dominant and subordinate positions. They all struggle to define the assumptions of our existence, what is right and wrong, morally accepted and meaningful. Some cultural assumptions and behaviour prescriptions may be shared at a national level, but individuals within that nation would still hold different cultural preferences. Norwegian culture appreciates walking in the countryside, but the truth is that many Norwegians do not like that. Women's right to have an abortion is widely recognised in Norway, but there are groups opposing it.

Studies have shown that service providers act as gatekeepers of users' participation as they have the power to encourage or hinder their participation (Schoot et al. 2005; Tutton 2005; Frank et al. 2009). One of the fundamental preconditions for users' participation is their relationship to service providers (Helgesen, Larsson & Athlin 2010; Latimer, Chaboyer & Gillespie 2013). Moreover, the ability of service providers to provide users with information (Mitcheson & Cowley 2003; Almborg et al. 2009), as well as their knowledge about participation, have a bearing on users' participation (Sahlsten 2005; Angel & Frederiksen 2015). Service providers need to gain cultural competence in order to have the ability to effectively deliver healthcare services that meet the personal, social, cultural and linguistic needs of patients (Betancourt, Green & Carillo 2002). Even more important, because of the constantly changing nature of cultural patterns, cultural competence is something that has to be continuously maintained. Cultural competence means that service providers have knowledge, awareness and understanding of how culture influences users' participation in their everyday life as well as in health services (Burchum 2002; Purnell & Paulanka 2003). However, that might encourage rigid thinking about cultures and individuals, legitimising cultural stereotypes and increasing prejudice (Eiser & Ellis 2007; Jenks 2011). Therefore, service providers need to develop cultural sensitivity on how culture may influence users' participation, and in particular the relationship with providers of health and social services (Schim & Doorenbos 2010; Perng & Watson 2012), as well as cultural skills (Willis 1999; Gozu et al. 2007). Cultural sensitivity and skills are key elements of their cultural competence in service provision, particularly in multicultural contexts. Studies have demonstrated significant links between user-perceived service provider cultural sensitivity and adherence to provider treatment recommendations (Tucker et al. 2011). This implies that they need to use their cultural skills in order to be responsive to users' cultural attitudes and circumstances, including how they influence their participation. That, in turn, will enhance their ability to show support and respect in interactions with users, use empathy and project warmth. Studies have shown that users' satisfaction with their healthcare providers is positively associated with such abilities (Beach, Saha & Cooper 2006).

Conclusion

The compound construct of culture refers to created, shared and transmitted patterns of ideas, assumptions and values, as well as more tangible cultural manifestations such as behavioural prescriptions, rituals, symbols and definition of heroes, and other symbolic meaning systems. It creates informal expectations in users' environments about how they should think and behave. Therefore, it has a bearing on users' participation in everyday life. Formal and informal sanctions can be applied by other group members if users' participation fails to follow cultural prescriptions. The cultural environment, in turn, impacts our cultural identity – our sense of who we are, what we believe in and what we want to be, which has a substantial influence on our participation, even when the environment no longer has such expectations.

Understanding culture is therefore necessary in order to understand participation, including how health services can promote users' participation. Increased awareness and knowledge of the influence of culture on individual understanding and choices are thus crucial. However, knowledge about the potential biases which a culture perspective can bring into health services is crucial. Studies have demonstrated that it is difficult to define boundaries of a group and its culture. Traditional stereotypes might emerge and get sustained, leading to wrong perceptions of who and what a user is, and about their participation. Moreover, the construct of culture focuses on consensus, which makes the construct too static. The reality is rather one of ongoing struggles between different ideas where culture is continuously being shaped, especially in a world where communication and interaction between people is propelled by access to new information and communications technology.

Service providers are advised to gain cultural competence in order to cope with cultural complexity and avoid static group perceptions, cultural stereotypes and prejudice. Cultural competence requires both cultural awareness, knowledge and understanding, and cultural sensitivity and skills. Cultural sensitivity is needed at all levels in order to promote users' participation in everyday life and healthcare services. Future theory-building and research on participation should unwrap both positive and negative roles which different layers of culture can have for users' participation, including the consequences for service providers and health services.

References

Almborg, AH, Ulander, K, Thulin, A & Berg, S 2009, 'Patients perceptions of their participation in discharge planning after acute stroke', *Journal of Clinical Nursing*, vol. 18, no. 2, pp. 199–209.

Angel, S & Frederiksen, KN 2015, 'Challenges in achieving patient participation: A review of how patient participation is addressed in empirical studies', *International Journal of Nursing Studies*, vol. 52, pp. 1525–1538.

Baumeister, R 1998, 'The self', in *Handbook of social psychology*, vol. 1, eds D Gilbert, S Fiske & G Lindzey, Oxford University Press, New York, pp. 680–740.

Beach, MC, Saha, S, & Cooper, LA 2006, *The role and relationship of cultural competence and patient-centeredness in health care quality*, Commonwealth Fund, New York.

Bellah, R, Madsen, R, Sullivan, W, Swidler, A & Tipton, S 1985, *Habits of the heart: Individualism and commitment in American life*, University of California Press, Berkeley.

Berwick, DM 2009, 'What "patient-centered" should mean: Confessions of an extremist', *Health Affairs*, vol. 28, no. 4, pp. 555–565.

Betancourt, J, Green, A & Carillo JE 2002, *Cultural competence in health care: Emerging frameworks and practical approaches*, The Commonwealth Fund, New York, pp. 1–30.

Burchum, JLR 2002, 'Cultural competence: An evolutionary perspective', *Nursing Forum*, vol. 37, pp. 5–15.

Cattell, V 2001, 'Poor people, poor places, and poor health: The mediating role of social networks and social capital', *Social Science and Medicine*, vol. 52, no. 10, pp. 1501–1516.

Clark, J, Hall, S, Jefferson, T & Roberts, T 1975, 'Subculteres, cultures and class', in *Resistance through rituals*, eds S. Hall & T. Jefferson, Routledge, London, pp. 100–111.

Corrigan, PW & Penn, D 1997, 'Disease and discrimination: Two paradigms that describe severe mental illness', *Journal of Mental Health*, vol. 6, pp. 355–366.

Cousins, SD 1989, 'Culture and self-perception in Japan and the United States', *Journal of Personality and Social Psychology*, vol. 56, pp. 124–131.

Craig, M, Burns, T, Fitzpatricl, R, Pinfold, V & Priebe, S 2007, 'Social exclusion and mental health, conceptual and methodological review', *British Journal of Psychiatry*, vol. 191, pp. 477–483.

Dalton, M 1959, *Men who manage*, Wiley, New York.

Eiser, AR & Ellis, G 2007, 'Cultural competence and the African American experience with health care: The case for specific content in cross-cultural education', *Academic Medicine*, vol. 82, no. 2, pp. 176–183.

Eldh, AC, Ehnfors, M & Ekman, I 2004, 'The phenomena of participation and non-participation in health care-experiences of patients attending a nurse-led clinic for chronic heart failure', *European Journal of Cardiovascular Nursing*, vol. 3, no. 3, pp. 239–246.

Falk, A, Fehr, E & Fischbacher, U 2005, 'Driving forces of informal sanctions', *Econometrica*, vol. 73, no. 6, pp. 2017–2030.

Festinger, L 1950, 'Informal social communication', *Psychological Review*, vol. 57, pp. 271–282.

Fiske, AP, Kitayama, S, Markus, HR & Nisbett, RE 1998, 'The cultural matrix of social psychology', in *Handbook of social psychology*, 4th ed., vol. 2, eds D Gilbert, S Fiske & G Lindzey, McGraw-Hill, Boston, pp. 915–981.

Frank, C, Asp, M, & Dahlberg, K 2009, 'Patient participation in emergency care – A phenomenographic analysis of caregivers'conceptions', *Journal of Clinical Nursing*, vol. 18, no. 18, pp. 2555–2562.

Gozu, A, Beach, MC, Price, EG, Gary, TL, Robinson, K, Cooper, LA 2007, 'Self-administered instruments to measure cultural competence of health professionals: A systematic review', *Teaching and Learning in Medicine*, vol. 19, pp. 180–190.

Granlund, M 2013, 'Participation – Challenges in conceptualization, measurement and intervention', *Child Care Health Development*, vol. 39, pp. 470–473.

Helgesen, AK, Larsson, M & Athlin, E 2010, 'Patient participation in everyday activities in special care units for persons with dementia in Norwegian nursing homes', *International Journal Older People Nursing*, vol. 5, no. 2, pp. 169–178.

Hofstede, GH 1980, *Culture's consequences: International differences in work-related values*, Sage Publications, Beverly Hills.

Hofstede, GH 2001, *Culture's consequences: Comparing values, behaviors, institutions, and organizations across nations*, Sage, Thousand Oaks.

Hsu, FLK 1971, 'Psycho-social homeostasis and Jen: Conceptual tools for advancing psychological anthropology', *American Anthropologist*, vol. 73, pp. 23–44.

Hsu, FLK 1983, *Rugged individualism reconsidered*, University of Tennessee Press, Knoxville.

Hui, CH 1988, 'Measurement of individualism–collectivism', *Journal of Research in Personality*, vol. 22, pp. 17–36.

Imms, C, Adair, B, Keen, D, Ullenhag, A, Rosenbaum, P & Granlund, M 2015, "Participation": A systematic review of language, definitions, and constructs used in intervention research with children with dissabilities', *Developmental Medicine & Child Neurology*, vol. 58, pp. 29–38.

Jacques, E 1951, *The changing culture of a factory*, Tavistock Institute, London.

Jenks, AC, 2011, 'From "list of traits" to open-mindedness: Emerging issues in cultural competence education', *Culture, Medicine and Psychiatry*, vol. 35, no. 2, pp. 209–235.

Jensen, K 2010, 'Punishment and spite, the dark side of cooperation', *Philosophical Transactions of the Royal Society*, vol. 365, pp. 2635–2650.

Kagitcibasi, C 1997, 'Individualism and collectivism', in *Handbook of cross-cultural psychology: Vol. 3. Social behavior and applications*, eds JW Berry, MH Segall & C Kagitcibasi, Allyn & Bacon, Boston, pp. 1–49.

Kashima, Y, Kashima, M, Farsides, T, Kim, U, Strack, F & Werth, L 2004, 'Culture and context-sensitive self: The amount and meaning of context-sensitivity of phenomenal self differ across cultures', *Self and Identity*, vol. 3, pp. 125–141.

Kawachi, I, Kennedy, BP, Lochner, K & Prothrow-Stith, D 1997, 'Social capital, income inequality, and mortality', *American Journal of Public Health*, vol. 87, no. 9, pp. 1491–1498.

Kroeber, AL & Kluckhohn, C 1952, *Culture: A critical review of concepts and definitions*. Papers of the Peabody Museum of American Archeology and Ethnology (vol. XLVII, no. 1), Harvard University, Cambridge.

Kroeber, AL & Parsons, T 1958, 'The concept of culture and of social system', *American Sociological Review*, vol. 23, no. 5, pp. 582–583.

Latimer, S, Chaboyer, W & Gillespie, B 2013, 'Patient participation in pressure injury prevention: Giving patient's voice', *Scandinavian Journal of Caring Science*, vol. 28, no. 4, pp. 648–656.

Luo, L & Gilmour, R 2004, 'Culture and conceptions of happiness: Individual oriented and social oriented swb', *Journal of Happiness Studies*, vol. 5, no. 3, pp. 269–291.

Markus, HR & Kitayama, S 1991, 'Culture and the self: Implications for cognition, emotion, and motivation', *Psychological Review*, vol. 98, no. 2, p. 224.

Martin, J 2002, *Organizational culture: Mapping the terrain*, Sage Publications, London.

Maxwell, G, Alves, I, & Granlund, M 2012, 'Participation and environmental aspects in education and the ICF and the ICF-CY: Findings from a systematic literature review', *Developmental Neurorehabilitation*, vol. 15, no. 1, pp. 63–78.

Mead, GH 1910, 'Social consciousness and the consciousness of meaning', *Psychological Bulletin*, vol. 7, pp. 397–405.

Mead, M 1937, *Cooperation and competition among primitive peoples*, 1st ed., New York, London: McGraw-Hill Book Company.

Mitcheson, J & Cowley, S 2003, 'Empowerment or control? An analysis of the extent to which client participation is enabled during health visito/client interactions using a structured health needs assessment tool', *International Journal of Nursing Studies*, vol. 40, no. 4, pp. 413–426.

Myroniuk, T & Anglewicz, P 2015, 'Does social participation predict better health? A longitudinal study in rural malawi', *Journal of Health and Social Behavior*, vol. 56, no. 4, pp. 552–573.

Nisbett, RE 2003, *The geography of thought: How Asians and westerners think differently . . . and why*, The Free Press, New York.

Nummela O, Sulander, T, Rahkonen, O, Karisto, A & Uutela, A 2008, 'Social participation, trust and self-rated health: A study among ageing people in Urban, semi-urban and rural settings', *Health & Place*, vol. 14, no. 2, pp. 243–253.

O'Reilly, CA & Chatman, JA 1996, 'Culture as social control: Corporations, cults, and commitment', *Research in Organizational Behavior*, vol. 18, pp. 157–200.

Oyserman, D & Markus, HR 1993, 'The sociocultural self', in *The self in social perspective*, eds J Suls, Erlbaum, Hillsdale, pp. 187–220.

Perng, SJ & Watson, R 2012, 'Construct validation of the nurse cultural scale: A hierarchy of abilities', *Journal of Clinical Nursing*, vol. 21, pp. 1678–1684.

Purnell, LD & Paulanka, BJ 2003, 'The purnell model for cultural competence', in *Transcultural health care: A culturally competent approach*, 2nd ed., eds LD Purnell & BJ Paulanka, PA Davis, Philadelphia, pp. 8–39.

Redzovic, S 2014, *"This is how we do it around here". Exloring the influence of organizational norms on subjective well-being at work in individualistic and collectivistic cultures*, Ph.D. thesis, Norwegian University of Science and Technology.

Reichers, AE & Schneider, B 1990, 'Climate and culture: An evolution of constructs', in *Organizational climate and culture*, eds B. Schneider, Jossey-Bass, San Francisco, pp. 5–39.

Rohlen, TP 1974, *For harmony and strength: Japanese white-collar organization in anthropological perspective*, University of California Press, Berkeley.

Rose, R 2000, 'How much does social capital add to individual health?', *Social Science and Medicine*, vol. 5, no. 9, pp. 1421–1435.

Sahlsten, M 2005, 'Patient participation in nursing care: An interpretation by Swedish registered nurses', *Journal of Clinical Nursing*, vol. 14, no. 1, pp. 35–42.

Schim, SM & Doorenbos, AZ 2010, 'A three-dimensional model of cultural congruence: A framework for intervention', *Journal of Social Work in End-of-Life & Palliative Care*, vol. 6, pp. 256–270.

Schoot, T, Proot, I, Meulen, RT & De Witte, L 2005, 'Actual interaction and client centeredness in home care', *Clinical Nursing Research*, vol. 14, no. 4, pp. 370–393.

Schwartz, SH 1990, 'Individualism-collectivism: Critique and proposed refinements', *Journal of Cross-Cultural Psychology*, vol. 21, no. 2, pp. 139–157.

Sheriff, M 1936, *The psychology of social norms*, Harper, New York.

Simon, HA 1991, 'Bounded rationality and organizational learning', *Organization Science*, vol. 2, no. 1, pp. 125–134.

Suh, EM 2002, 'Personality processes and individual differences – Culture, identity consistency, and subjective well-being', *Journal of Personality and Social Psychology*, vol. 83, no. 6, pp. 1378.

Tafarodi, RW, Lo, C, Yamaguchi, S, Lee, WWS & Katsura, H 2004, 'The inner self in three countries', *Journal of Cross-Cultural Psychology*, vol. 1, no. 35, pp. 97–117.

Triandis, HC 1995, *Individualism and collectivism*, Westview Press, Boulder.

Tucker, CM, Marsiske, M, Rice, KG, Jones, JD & Herman, KC 2011, 'Patient-centered culturally sensitive health care: Model testing and refinement', *Health Psychology*, vol. 30, no. 3, pp. 342–350.

Turner, JC 1991, *Social influence*, Open University Press, Buckingham.

Tutton, EMM 2005, 'Patient participation on a ward for frail older people', Journal Advanced Nursing, vol. 50, no. 2, pp. 143–152.

Tylor, E 1920/1871, *Primitive culture*, JP Putnam's Sons, New York.

Vik, K, Lilja, M & Nygård, L 2007, 'The influence of the environment on participation subsequent to rehabilitation as experienced by elderly people in Norway', *Scandinavian Journal of Occupational Therapy*, vol. 14, pp. 86–95.

Warburton, DER, Nicol, CW & Bredin, SSD 2006, 'Health benefits of physical activity: The evidence', *Canadian Medical Association Journal*, vol. 174, no. 6, pp. 801–809.

Willis, WO 1999, 'Cultural competent nursing care during the perinatal period', *Journal of Perinatal and Neonatal Nursing*, vol. 13, pp. 45–59.

World Health Organisation 2001, *International classification of functioning, disability and health*, World Health Organisation, Geneva.

World Health Organisation 2007, *International classification of functioning, disability and health: Children and youth version (ICF-CY)*, World Health Organisation, Geneva.

Yoon, TR 1994, 'The Koreans, their culture and personality', in *Psychology of the Korean people: Collectivism and individualism*, eds G Yoon & C Sang-Chin, Dong-Ah Seoul, Korea, pp. 15–26.

6 A participatory approach to services and support

Peter Beresford

A key domain for participation is the involvement of service users in service delivery. Writing in the second decade of the twenty-first century, when concepts like user involvement, empowerment and co-production have become commonplace, it is easy to forget how recent a development this actually is. But it is important not to do this. Such involvement only became a requirement in UK health and social care with legislation at the beginning of the 1990s. Social work, a pioneer in this field, had only started to seek the views of service users, let alone involve them, in 1970 (Meyer and Timms, 1970). There is, at the most, no more than thirty years, or a generation, of public service and professional engagement with the perspectives of service users. Yet those same services and professions have much longer histories and cultures, stretching back in some cases to at least the nineteenth century, if not before. Thus, a discussion of inter-professional and inter-agency practice, which seeks to build seriously on service user perspectives, has two developments in complex relation to deal with. It must not only advance our understanding of inter-professional and inter-agency practice. It must also provide an adequate basis for understanding and engaging with service users, their organisations and their aims and objectives, in order to do so. This chapter has a particular concern to help with this second task.

Service users and their movements

Human services historically have tended to see the people who use them as individuals, family members or possibly members of broader groups and communities. But from the 1970s, a growing range of such service users began to organise collectively and get together in their own organisations and movements. A number of reasons for this development can be identified. These include dissatisfaction with the services and support they were receiving, a new assertiveness linked with more liberatory political times and the emergence of broader movements, as well as new political challenges to the welfare state coming from both the new political right and the radical left. Many different groups organised in this way, starting with the disabled people's movement but also embracing people with learning difficulties, older people, mental health service users/survivors, people living with HIV/AIDS, young people who had been brought up in state care and so on (Beresford and Croft, 1993).

While it would be wrong to overstate the impact of these movements, it has been significant. It has led to major changes in ideas, culture, practice, policy, processes and legislation on a global scale. Groups that had previously often been hidden have gained a greater individual, as well as political and cultural, presence in societies. In countries like the UK, their viewpoints have begun to permeate the mainstream, just as they have made major steps on the long road to inclusion and equal rights (ODI, 2008). It is also an international development, finding various expression in North America, Europe and the majority world (Coleridge, 1993; Campbell and Oliver, 1996; Morris, 1996; Oliver, 1993, 1996; Aspis, 1997; Charlton, 1998; Priestley, 1999).

All these service-user movements have placed an emphasis on people's right to live on equal terms in mainstream society and to speak for themselves. They seek to challenge discrimination and to ensure appropriate and adequate support over which they are able to exert greater choice and control (Campbell, 1996; Campbell and Oliver, 1996; Carter and Beresford, 2000). Each of these movements has a particular history, character, culture and traditions. However, they also seem to have some important things in common. All highlight the importance they attach to:

- Service users speaking and acting for themselves;
- Working together to achieve change;
- Having more say over their lives and the support that they receive;
- Challenging stigma and discrimination;
- Having access to alternatives to prevailing medicalised interventions and understandings;
- The value of user-controlled organisations, support and services;
- A focus on people's human and civil rights and their citizenship, which emerged later, but is increasingly evident in the survivors' movement;
- Being part of mainstream life and communities, able to take on responsibilities as well as securing entitlements (Beresford and Harding, 1993; Campbell, 1996; Campbell and Oliver, 1996; Beresford, 1999).

Services versus lives

One of the themes running through service user groups and movements is that people define themselves not in terms of services or practitioners, but rather in terms of their lives and their overall identity. Indeed, there is no agreed terminology for people in this field. There are no existing words that adequately embrace all the groups and individuals who are included in these groups and movements. While 'service user' is the term most often used, many individuals dislike this term, because they feel it defines them passively and solely in relation to services they use, rather than taking account of their overall identity. This may include being a parent, a worker, a student, a volunteer, a partner and much more (Beresford, 2005). This desire to be framed in terms of your life, rather than the services that can impact on it, is epitomised by the name chosen by one British service user organisation and network, *Shaping Our Lives*.[1] This explicitly places an emphasis on people's lives rather than their services, framing them accordingly and highlighting the desire they have to shape their lives for themselves.

Thus, service users understandably tend to take a holistic view of themselves and their situation. They do not frame themselves in terms of the particular services and professions that may interact with them and impact on their lives. This can make divisions that exist between such policies, services and professions particularly difficult and unhelpful for service users. It means that they need to learn what their boundaries and different roles and cultures are, how to negotiate them and what to expect of them. It means life can become like 'pass the parcel', where one agency or practitioner passes the individual on to another, and it is difficult to pin down where responsibility lies and how to secure the help and support that is needed.

Problems with traditional professional and service approaches

Working to move to more inter-professional and inter-agency approaches to practice also raises many complex issues from service users' perspectives. It is worth looking at some of these issues, if effective ways of overcoming them are to be developed by and for practitioners. The knowledge and experience of service users and their organisations are likely to have a helpful role to play in supporting better integrated and coordinated practice in human services.

Administrative barriers to integrated practice

Long-term human-service users can frequently be on the receiving end of at least four different major services: health, social care, housing and benefits. Like the rest of us, they are also likely to turn to and have contact with many more. Not only do workers in these four specific services have separate, different training, but many may not have training at all. There are differences in professional power and status. Each of these services has different histories, cultures and traditions, goals, organisational structures, chains of command and philosophical approaches. Some may be locally provided, others under central control. They fall under different government departments, as well as different local organisations and systems. All these issues have implications for the practice of their particular practitioners, as well as for integrated and inter-professional and inter-agency practice. Thus, the National Health Service is still essentially a universalist service, free at the point of delivery. Local authority social care in England, on the other hand, continues to be a means and needs-tested residual service. There have long been serious shortages of housing provision, and its provision and management have increasingly been outsourced. Meanwhile, benefits policy and practice has increasingly been framed in terms of containing 'abuse' and reducing the numbers in receipt of incapacity benefits. These different approaches, principles and organisational arrangements have major implications for the various practitioners, for the potential for cooperation and coordination between them, and of course for the support that service users are able to access.

But from service users' experience, there are other significant consequences for practice and coordination created by the different locations and professional backgrounds of practitioners. One of these is the tendency of services to divide service users into administrative categories and to be structured and organised accordingly. But this does not take account, for example, of the fact that disabled people may also be parents, and children include disabled children. Thus, while people in practice frequently cross over such bureaucratic divides – they may have physical impairments, as well as use mental health services, or be deaf and have learning difficulties – their allocation to different departments, services and practitioners creates barriers and divisions between practitioners and between practice and service users. Another problem occurs during times of transition, for example when an individual moves from the status of child and young person to adult, or from adult to 'older person'. At such points, the professionals working with people, and often the entitlements they have, may change. Services are notoriously inept at ensuring continuity and good support through these periods.

The complex and overlapping nature of people's actual identities is one of the reasons why *Shaping Our Lives* and a number of other service user-controlled organisations have come to work with a wide range of service users, instead of working with just one group, like mental health service users, or being 'impairment specific', as many traditional disability charities have been. This has made it possible for them to see the many things these different groups have in common, as well as differences which distinguish them.

There are undoubtedly tensions between the commonalities and differences that may exist between different individuals and groups. The trend in services like health and social care, however, seems to have been towards specialism and away from genericism, justified by the argument that this is most likely to recognise and serve the particular needs of different groups. Service users have mixed views about this (Beresford, 2007). However, lines of demarcation tend to be drawn according to professional and organisational issues rather than service-user preferences. Obtaining the views of service users on service reorganisation – both within and between agencies – is therefore important in meeting service users' preferences and needs in relation to how services are reworked. Key issues to be asked in such reviews might be how sharing information, and with what consent, is to take place and by what means; and how the different groups propose to put the interests of service users at the centre of their inter-professional activities, and how this will be reviewed, by whom, when, and in what ways.

Service users also highlight the tendency of services and professionals to see people as sets of isolated symptoms or 'needs' rather than recognising and relating to the whole person. This is sometimes encouraged by both the structuring and value base of occupational roles in human services. Trends towards the division of labour and narrowing of caring roles can discourage people from being seen in the round. Thus, recent tendencies, for example in policing, nursing and social care, have all contributed to the narrowing of professional roles to more managerialist organising functions and the creation of ancillary roles having a more 'hands-on' role. Yet from service users' experience, it is often the routine and mundane ongoing contact that they can have with workers which encourages the relationships that they tend to see as fundamental to positive practice.

What these organisational, professional and structural issues highlight from service users' perspectives is that, if agencies and practitioners are to work better together, high-level change, different kinds of roles, and changed face-to-face relationships are *all* likely to be needed if service users are to be ensured appropriate, seamless and uninterrupted support.

The dominance of medicalised individual models

It is not only the ways in which agencies and professions are organised which can affect and limit their ability to work well together. The values and philosophies underpinning them also have an important bearing. Health and social care have tended to be based predominantly on individualised understandings of people and their problems. Over the twentieth century, these were increasingly overlaid with medicalised understandings. Such medicalised individual interpretations and explanations of people, with their origins in physical and psychiatric medicine, have spread to dominate public services much more generally, although this is often implicit rather than explicit in their working. Historically, understandings of groups like disabled people, mental health service users, older people, people with chronic and life-limiting conditions and people with learning difficulties have tended to be framed in terms of them having a personal problem, in terms of their incapacity, deficiencies and pathology. They tend to be understood in terms of what they can't do rather than what they can do. This has had massive ramifications for human-service practice. We can see it institutionalised in the increasing trend to respond to problems experienced and identified in children and young people through their inclusion in a growing range of psychiatric diagnostic categories like ADHD ('attention-deficit hyperactivity disorder') and the evidenced over-prescription of major tranquilisers to older people in institutional provision.

Such service users' historical experience of public provision has tended to be characterised by two features. First is the tendency to segregate and lump people in such groups together in separate, often institutional, provision. Thus, they have often been cut off from more mainstream services, reinforcing prevailing assumptions and stereotypes about them among their workers. Second, dedicated services and professions, and occupations which have been developed to work with them, have tended to frame their understanding of them in individualistic terms as needing help and care because of their 'incapacity' and 'vulnerability'. Such individualistic interpretations have also encouraged the making of moral judgements, often implicitly in occupational and professional practice. This has particularly applied to groups, where an element of culpability has been felt to explain their failure to conform, notably among young and unemployed people and people living on welfare benefits.

Such individualised interpretations of people may not only offer only a partial picture, placing a disproportionate emphasis on the individual, rather than taking account of them in their broader context and circumstances; but it can also create underlying tensions between different professional perspectives. This is particularly highlighted in the case of social work, although it is also evident in the competing approaches of psychiatry and psychology. Service users value the social approach of social workers, but they quickly become aware that this is not the prevailing model in use and that human-service workers coming from other perspectives tend not to attach the same emphasis or have the same understanding of broader social and situational issues. This leads to a related and no less important issue that service users repeatedly highlight, particularly in the context of multidisciplinary and multi-agency work. This is the operation of a hierarchy of power and credibility between different professionals. This is frequently talked about in relation to community mental health teams (CMHTs), but applies in many other contexts too. Here, service users are conscious of the professional dominance of psychiatry, the tendency for nursing staff to be subordinate, and for social workers often to challenge such inequalities of status and power and to come into conflict with other professionals for this reason. Some teams work in much more egalitarian ways, but traditional medical dominance reflected in differentials in reward and recognition continue to operate to create more fundamental barriers to truly collaborative and equal working. Such inequalities still seem to be perpetuated in professional education and training, reinforcing inequalities for the future.

Many service users particularly value the social workers' role as advocate, with both their own and other agencies and with other professionals. They frequently align themselves with social workers' perspectives, especially since, in a field like mental health, for instance, they are not as directly involved in actual medical treatment aspects of their experience of services – which may, for example, include the administration of major tranquillisers and depot injections, both willingly and against their will.

Ways forward for collaborative practice

As we have seen, a number of overarching obstacles to positive inter-agency and inter-professional practice can be identified from the perspectives of service users. These include:

- Administrative and organisational barriers;
- The reduction of service users to abstracted needs and characteristics;
- The dominance of the medical model and the subordination of social approaches;
- Inequalities of power and status between professions and occupations.

All of these can lead to tensions and conflicts between different agencies, services and workers, which in turn can have damaging and disruptive effects for service users.

Including service users

Service users, however, not only offer a critique of the barriers facing collaborative practice. They also offer ways forward from their own ideas and discussions for overcoming these difficulties and developing a unified and unifying approach to practice.

A different way of approaching collaborative working between agencies and professions is for both to be shaped much more by service users and their organisations. This approach offers a key route to harmonising them all with the rights and wants of service users, and in turn, with each other. The perspectives of service users:

- Offer common core values and principles;
- Reflect shared goals and objectives;
- Make it possible to build on shared user experience and knowledge.

Several key components for change emerge. All are key elements in the theory and practice of service-user organisations and movements. They include:

- Developing social/barriers-based models to underpin practice;
- The philosophy of independent living;
- Rights, responsibilities and entitlements;
- User involvement in training;
- Valuing user knowledge and experience in practitioners;
- Ensuring equal access to service users in its fullest sense;
- Developing effective and inclusive involvement in agencies and workforce.

These, taken together, provide a basis, from service users' perspectives, for consistent and positive practice across the different human-service roles and agencies. While issues of organisation, communication and coordination will also need to be addressed, this is more likely to be achieved if grounded in this way.

We can now look at each of these in turn. We begin with two key ideas and approaches which have been developed by service users and their movements. The first of these is the social model of disability. This was developed by the disabled people's movement but has subsequently been widened in both its meaning and application to provide a theoretical base for practice with much wider relevance.

Developing social/barriers-based models to underpin practice

The social model of disability represents a fundamental break from traditional, individualised, Western understandings of disability, which tend to be interpreted in personal 'tragedy' terms. The social model draws a distinction between the (perceived) impairment – intellectual, physical or sensory – which may affect the individual, and disability, the negative societal reaction to people seen as having such impairments. For the first time, the social model highlighted the oppression and discrimination experienced by disabled people (Oliver and Zarb, 1989; Oliver, 1996; Thomas, 2007). Since then, much work has been done to explore the nature of impairment as well as of disability, and to make better sense of the inter-relations of the two.

The social model makes clear the barriers faced by disabled and other people, restricting their lives and undermining their opportunities and quality of life. It has highlighted the way in which such traditional medicalised individual understandings have dominated public and policy understandings of disability, as well as professional responses to it and the inhibiting effects they have had on such agency and professional roles. A barrier or social model approach, including attitudinal, physical and communication barriers, is increasingly being seen as having relevance across a growing range of welfare policy users (Thomas, 2007). Certainly it provides a coherent and consistent model, which takes account of both personal and social factors, to inform human-service practice and agencies. It is likely to encourage more effective and helpful collaboration, underpinned by a shared model of understanding.

The philosophy of independent living

The philosophy of independent living was also originally inspired by the disabled people's movement. It follows from the social model of disability. It is based on a belief that disabled people should be enabled to live their lives on as equal terms as possible alongside non-disabled people. The philosophy of independent living turns traditional notions of independence on their head. It is not preoccupied with the individual, or narrow ideas of personal autonomy. It does not mean 'standing on your own two feet' or managing on your own. Instead of seeing the service user as having a defect or deficiency requiring care, it highlights the need to ensure them the support that they need to be autonomous and live their lives as fully as possible, on equal terms and interdependently with others (Morris, 1993). This support is not expected to come from family members required to be unpaid or 'informal carers'. It rejects the concept of care and replaces it with the idea of support. It sees independence as meaning autonomous decision-making rather than the physical capacity to carry out all activities of daily living unaided (Campbell and Oliver, 1996; Morris, 2004). Instead of people being assessed on the basis of what they can't do to qualify for 'care', under this model, support is provided to enable them to live their lives as fully as possible. There are two inter-related and key aspects to the philosophy of independent living. These are:

- Ensuring people the support that they need under their control to be able to live their lives as fully as they can, on as equal terms as possible, with non-disabled people;
- Equalising their access to mainstream policy and services, like housing, health, education and employment.

This emphasises the relevance of independent living as a value base across public policy, as well as specifically in relation to human services. In England, a governmental Independent Living Strategy with cross-departmental support signed up to these values (ODI, 2008), although again, it needs to be said that public services are still a long way from being organised and provided on a basis consistent with this.

Rights, responsibilities and entitlements

Human services have traditionally framed their users in terms of their *needs*. Such needs have tended to be defined by others on behalf of service users. Distinctions have also been drawn between 'needs' and 'wants', with wants taken to mean what service users might prefer, but not necessarily what policymakers and professionals regard as appropriate to provide for service users. Disabled people and other service users increasingly expressed their dissatisfaction with others defining their needs for them (Oliver and Barnes, 1998). While there has been a developing discussion from left of centre social policy writers arguing the value of 'need' as a formative concept, this is not a view that has generally been accepted by commentators coming from service-user movements (Doyal and Gough, 1991; Oliver, 1996).

Instead, the disabled people's and service-user movements have tended to frame their demands and objectives in terms of their rights, not needs, and requiring support and change, rather than care and welfare. They are concerned with the achievement of both their civil and human rights, collective as well as individual rights. To achieve these goals and values, service-user movements have developed new approaches to collective working. These place an emphasis on self-organisation – developing their own 'user-controlled' organisations – as well as on participation and people 'speaking for themselves'. But they also take account of people's feelings and needs for support in the process. To make this possible, they have increasingly highlighted ideas of inclusion and empowerment (Campbell and Oliver, 1996; Campbell, 1996).

Goals of achieving and safeguarding people's civil and human rights can be seen to offer a more accountable and less normative basis for human-service roles and services than the concept of need. They also highlight the need for particular care, consistency and accountability where such roles are concerned with restricting rights, as well as with supporting them.

User involvement in education and training

A continuing message from service users and their organisations over the years is that there are few more effective ways of changing and improving practice and service cultures than through involving service users in occupational education and training (Beresford, 1994). This has led to the widespread development of 'user-led training', 'user trainers' and 'training for user trainers'. Not only does this make it possible for workers to learn from people with direct experience of services and to find out more about what they want from services and how these can be most helpful for them, it also makes it possible for workers to relate to service users in positive, equal and active roles, rather than in the often passive and dependent role of patients or clients.

Service-user organisations have pressed for such involvement to extend through all aspects of training: from providing direct input in professional and in-service training, to being involved in developing course curricula, providing course materials and, indeed, selecting, evaluating and assessing courses and students. All these have become established in professional social work training and education. Other occupations, from allied health professions to the police, have also introduced user involvement into their training programmes. The challenge is to ensure that such involvement develops coherently and systematically within and across professions and occupations. What it makes possible and provides a stimulus for is consistency and coherence – both of values and aims, within and between them, encouraging collaboration from the bottom up, between both practitioners and agencies (Branfield, 2009; Branfield et al., 2007; Beresford, 2007; Levin, 2004).

Valuing user knowledge and experience in practitioners

One of the characteristics of traditional practice and agencies has been that they have been constructed top-down rather than bottom-up, drawing little on the understanding of their end users. There is often minimal overlap between service providers and service users, and this can work to the detriment of both. It does not make for improved understanding of service users, or encourage the most appropriate practice and service provision. User involvement in training offers some corrective to this. But service users and their organisations also argue the importance of encouraging the valuing of service-user experience and the recruitment of people with such experience to become workers in such services.

Clearly this would only apply where such experience did not clearly debar them from recruitment, as for example in the case of people with serious criminal convictions seeking to join the police, or child abusers being considered for work in child protection. They would also need to have the other necessary skills and qualities in addition to direct experience. Service users make clear that they see shared direct experience as a valuable quality in practitioners. The addition of a common strand of experience is clearly likely to encourage shared understanding, empathy and compassion between different occupations. Unfortunately, significant barriers to the inclusion of such experience still seem to exist (Snow, 2002) However, encouraging the recruitment of suitable workers with experience as service users is likely to provide an improved basis for common understanding, and shared principles and values, between different services and agencies.

Ensuring equal access to service users

Many forms of exclusion and bias continue to operate in services. The introduction of the disability equality duty, anti-disability discrimination and new equality legislation all signify this. Some groups face particular barriers in accessing services, or experience inferior treatment from them. Common standards of access and inclusion can be seen to be key if there is to be effective inter-agency and inter-professional practice. Key to this is the need to develop effective policies and practices for access to all agencies and occupations. In this way, it will be possible to ensure that they both operate inclusively, individually and together in relation to each other.

Developing effective and inclusive involvement in agencies and the workforce

Pressure and provisions for user involvement in public provision have mushroomed, particularly in human services like health and social care, in recent years. We have already seen how this has developed in professional and occupational education and training. But it has also taken root in a wide range of other spheres, including planning, management, standard setting, research and evaluation and practice development. Service users and their organisations complain that such involvement can often be tokenistic and patchy. Its impact has also varied between different professions and services. It continues, for example, to be underdeveloped in medical professions, contrasted with social work, while being particularly high profile in policy areas like social care and regeneration.

However, an effective strategic approach to user involvement can be expected to encourage common standards and consistent approaches, which can only help in inter-agency and inter-professional work. By connecting provision and practice closely and directly with the perspectives of service users, it makes possible greater coherence and consistency between them. This is rooted in the priorities of service users and the achievement of their rights and wants.

Conclusion

To conclude, if the idea and practice of participation are to be advanced effectively instead of being tokenistic, then they have to be taken seriously at all levels within and between organisations and services. A number of key components will be needed if this is to make possible effective user involvement, which can provide a basis for positive and improved inter-agency and inter-professional practice for the future. These will include:

- Building on service users' ideas, models and values;
- Being rights-based;
- Drawing on user-led education and co-learning;
- Valuing service user experience and knowledge;
- Ensuring access and inclusion.

Most important, service users and their organisations will routinely be regarded as part of the team that needs to work together. Improved collaboration and participation is not only about connecting with other professions and agencies. Crucially, it means seeing engaging with service users as key for both process and outcomes – means and ends.

Summary section

There is already much evidence and experience to build on to develop a participatory approach to support, service provision and inter-professional and inter-agency collaboration.

Professionals and agencies can draw on the new ideas and experiential knowledge of service users and their organisations

Service users and their organisations should be seen as new essential members of the team.

Key ways of taking forward effective user involvement are by:

- Developing social/barriers-based models to underpin practice;
- Drawing on the philosophy of independent living;
- Identifying rights, responsibilities and entitlements;
- Building user involvement in training;
- Valuing user knowledge and experience in practitioners;
- Ensuring equal access to service users in its fullest sense;
- Developing effective and inclusive involvement in agencies and the workforce.

Note

1 https://www.inclusionlondon.org.uk/directory/listing/shaping-our-lives/

References

Aspis, S. (1997), Self-Advocacy for People with Learning Difficulties; Does It Have a Future? *Disability & Society*, Vol. 12, No. 4, pp. 647–654.

Beresford, P. (1994), *Changing the Culture, Involving Service Users in Social Work Education*, London, Central Council of Education and Training in Social Work, Paper 32.2.

Beresford, P. (1999), Making Participation Possible: Movements of Disabled People and Psychiatric System Survivors, in T. Jordan and A. Lent (editors) *Storming the Millennium: The New Politics of Change*, London, Lawrence and Wishart, pp. 34–50.

Beresford, P. (2005), 'Service User': Regressive or Liberatory Terminology? Current Issues, *Disability & Society*, Vol. 20, No. 4, pp. 469–477.

Beresford, P. (2007), *The Changing Roles and Tasks of Social Work from Service Users' Perspectives: A Literature Informed Discussion Paper*, London, General Social Care Council, www.gscc.org.uk/NR/ . . . B915 . . . /SoLSUliteraturereviewreportMarch07.pdf, accessed 22 December 2009.

Beresford, P. and Croft, S. (1993), *Citizen Involvement: A Practical Guide for Change*, Basingstoke, Macmillan.

Beresford, P. and Harding, T. (editors) (1993), *A Challenge to Change: Practical Experiences of Building User Led Services*, London, National Institute for Social Work.

Branfield, F. (2009), *Developing User Involvement in Social Work Education*, Workforce Development Report 29, London, Social Care Institute for Excellence.

Branfield, F., Beresford, P. and Levin, E. (2007), *Common Aims: A Strategy to Support Service User Involvement in Social Work Education*, Position paper 7, London: SCIE.

Campbell, P. (1996), The History of the User Movement in the United Kingdom, in T. Heller, J. Reynolds, R. Gomm, R. Muston and S. Pattison (editors) *Mental Health Matters: A Reader*, Basingstoke, Macmillan, pp. 218–225.

Campbell, J. and Oliver, M. (1996), *Disability Politics: Understanding Our Past, Changing our Future*, Basingstoke, Macmillan.

Carter, T. and Beresford, P. (2000), *Age and Change: Models of Involvement for Older People*, York, York Publishing in Association with Joseph Rowntree Foundation.

Charlton, J.I. (1998), *Nothing about Us without Us: Disability, Oppression and Empowerment*, California, University of California Press.

Coleridge, P. (1993), *Disability, Liberation and Development*, Oxford, Oxfam in Association with Action on Disability and Development.

Doyal, L. and Gough, I. (1991), *A Theory of Human Need*, Basingstoke, Palgrave Macmillan.

Levin, E. (2004), *Involving Service Users and Carers in Social Work Education*, SCIE Guide 4, London, Social Care Institute for Excellence.

Meyer, J.E. and Timms, N. (1970), *The Client Speaks: Working Class Impressions of Casework*, London, Routledge.

Morris, J. (1993), *Independent Lives? Community Care and Disabled People*, Basingstoke, Macmillan.

Morris, J. (1996), *Encounters with Strangers: Feminism and Disability*, London, Women's Press.

Morris, J. (2004), Community Care: A Disempowering Framework, *Disability & Society*, Vol. 19, No. 5, pp. 427–442.

ODI (2008), *The Independent Living Strategy: A Cross Government Strategy about Independent Living for Disabled People*, London, Office for Disability Issues.

ODI (2008), *The Independent Living Strategy: A Cross Government Strategy about Independent Living for Disabled People*, London, Office for Disability Issues.

Oliver, M. (1993), *Social Work With Disabled People*, Basingstoke, Macmillan.

Oliver, M. (1996), *Understanding Disability: From Theory to Practice*, Basingstoke, Macmillan.

Oliver, M. and Barnes, C. (1998), *Disabled People and Social Policy: From Exclusion to Inclusion*, London, Longmans.

Oliver, M. and Zarb, G. (1989), The Politics of Disability: A New Approach, *Disability, Handicap and Society*, Vol. 4, No. 3, pp. 221–240.

Priestley, M. (1999), *Disability Politics and Community Care*, London, Jessica Kingsley.

Snow, R. (2002), *Stronger than Ever: Report of the First National Conference of Survivor Workers UK*, Stockport, Asylum.

Thomas, C. (2007), *Sociologies of Disability and Illness: Contested Ideas in Disability Studies and Medical Sociology*, Basingstoke, Palgrave Macmillan.

7 Participation in the context of service delivery

A comparison between the views held by older service recipients and service providers

Aud Elisabeth Witsø and Kjersti Vik

Introduction

The understanding of older adults' participation may be influenced by 'society'. There is, for example, an increasing emphasis on active and healthy aging and participation in policy documents (WHO, 2002, 2004, 2008a, 2008b; Meld. St. 29 (2012–2013)), as well as user involvement in service development and delivery (Meld. St. 26 (2014–2015)). At the same time, there is also substantial attention to fragility, and the need for help and care for older people (NOU, 2011: 11; EU, 2012). These apparent parallel discourses influence both the elderly and service providers. The views held by healthcare professionals towards adults are vital to the quality of service that older adults receive from them (Avers, 2014), including conditions for participation within and outside of the services. One may question if different perspectives on what constitutes participation represent a barrier to participation. The purpose of this chapter is to *compare the perspectives of service providers and older adults on participation in older adults in the context of receiving home-based services.*

Only a few studies have explored older adults' experiences and understandings of participation. Vik (2008) found that participation of older adults during home-based rehabilitation was understood as 'agency'. The older adults' wishes to be in control were viewed as a will to exert power. Participation included dynamic engagement, ranging from individual agency like choice, decision-making and acting in daily life, to letting life itself be the agent (Vik, 2008). Haak (2008) studied very old adults in a home context and found that the home was experienced as the place where participation as acting/doing and being took place. In the study, the very old adults experienced participation as performance-oriented and togetherness-oriented. Participation experienced as performance-oriented included engaging in the performance of activities for others, that is, meaning or doing something for others, and also getting personal satisfaction from performing. Participation experienced as togetherness-oriented included sharing experiences, being among others and connecting with the outside world. Being part of a larger context and being committed or devoted to something were other experiences of participation.

Participation among older adults who receive home-based services is influenced by the service systems and the service providers. Even though home-based service delivery is founded on the principles of user involvement and autonomy, studies have found that healthcare services can be experienced as barriers to participation, e.g. when participation is understood as being autonomous and being in control of one's daily life (Cardol et al., 2002; Haak, 2008; Vik, 2008). Some studies have shown that professionals have negative attitudes towards working with older adults and perceive them as vulnerable, sick, hopeless and dependent; and negative attitudes towards older adults are known to reduce the quality of care for aging individuals (Kydd & Wild, 2013; Kydd, Wild & Nelson, 2013).

Among barriers revealed in previous studies is the problem of interactions leading to feeling pressurised to concentrate on performing the most necessary daily activities rather than on participation (Vik, 2008), and services given on the providers' terms (McWilliam et al., 2001; Brown et al., 2006; McGarry, 2009). When professionals are more preoccupied with their own role in the relational aspects during service delivery than on the service recipients (as found by Olsson and Ingvad, 2001), this may take time and focus away from service recipients' preferred participation, and may thus form a barrier to participation. Studies have also found that the professionals' focus on interventions within the frame of available services may represent a barrier to revealing the real needs of the individuals (Vik & Eide, 2013a, 2013b).

However, empirical studies on this topic are still scarce, and little is published about the differences and similarities between how older adults experience participation in the context of receiving home-based services and the service providers' views. The aim of this chapter is therefore to compare and discuss the experience of participation in older adults receiving home-based services from the perspectives of home-based service providers and older adults. The findings result from the project 'Participation in older adults – in the context of receiving home-based services', which aimed at developing knowledge of how older adults receiving home-based services act and participate in everyday life, and how service providers work to support their participation. The project was financed by the Norwegian Research Council.

Methods

The studies which this chapter is based on had a qualitative design, with data derived from individual interviews with older adults and focus-group discussions with service providers. The participants in both studies were recruited by purposeful sampling as described by Charmaz (2006). The first study included qualitative in-depth interviews of ten older adults with varying age, gender, accommodation, social situations, level of service needs and health problems. The second study included six focus-group discussions with 30 service providers in home-based services. The participants varied in gender, age, work experience and education. Both studies were accomplished in mid-Norway: study 1 was in an urban municipality, while study 2 included two municipalities, one urban and one in a rural district. The main objective in the first study was to explore how older adults experienced participation in their everyday life in general, and in the context of receiving home-based services. In the second study, the main objective was to explore home-based service providers' perspectives on the participation of older adults when living at home and receiving home-based services. For further information on participants included in the studies, see Witsø, Eide & Vik (2012), Witsø (2013), Witsø, Vik & Ytterhus (2013), and Witsø, Ytterhus & Vik (2015).

Analysis

Analysis of data in both studies was based on a constant comparative method, inspired by constructivist grounded-theory methodology and coding principles (Strauss & Corbin, 1990; Charmaz, 2006). A key feature in the analysis process is that data collection and analysis are kept concurrent by initial and focused coding. Data were compared with data, codes with codes, and categories with data and codes. Writing memos was another analytic tool in the constant comparative process. This chapter is based on a comparison of the findings in both studies (Witsø, 2013).

In grounded-theory studies, analysis of data is closely related to the selection of participants and data collection. Processes of theoretical sampling, saturating and sorting are strategies for obtaining further selective data to refine and decide major categories. Consequently, and as a part of the ongoing analysis process in the main project, participants with greater service needs were selected and recruited during the data collection period. To exemplify, professionals described older service recipients as being lonely and in need of more social contact with service providers. Professionals experienced the service system, and the service delivery they were a part of represented a barrier to the older adults' participation in everyday life. Based on these and other findings, service providers were asked to recruit older adults they believed were lonely. The coding processes and procedures that led to the findings presented and discussed in this chapter are fully described in Witsø (2013).

Findings

Overall, participation was experienced by the older adults as a process of *keeping up dignity and pride*. They were concerned with getting themselves going in daily life. This was in accordance with the service providers' view, and they also highlighted the importance of older adults participating in their own life and carrying out tasks in everyday life. The older adults and the service providers shared an understanding of participation as doing. However, while the service providers talked about the older adults' participation as doing small tasks inside the house and in their immediate environments in everyday life, the older adults themselves expressed doing as a process of following everyday life routines, trying and striving to fend for themselves and adjusting to their changing capacity. The doing of tasks was emphasised by the professionals, while the older adults were process-oriented. The presentation of task- and process-oriented participation represents a synthesis of, and contrasting perspective on, older adults' participation among service providers and older adults, respectively.

Process- and task-oriented participation

Process-oriented participation was experienced by the older adults as value-based, a process reaching beyond having tasks carried out, and generally concerned the maintenance of dignity and pride.

As well as getting themselves going in everyday life, the older adults were concerned about keeping up roles and activities at home, in the neighbourhood and in their family. These processes embraced how the older adults concentrated on being an agent in day-to-day life. The older adults seemed to accept, but at the same time act on, their unstable capacity and changes, in order to keep up a meaningful day-to-day life. Understanding older adults' participation as agency turned out to embrace the whole process of living everyday life, including practical, emotional and intellectual dimensions of participation, illuminating how the older adults engaged in order to fend for themselves. Receiving limited help in a concrete situation of daily life activities could represent a practical dimension or strategy of participation in the sense of having something done in order to do something else (e.g. having one's back washed and receiving help with a bra before completing dressing on one's own). Feelings such as gratitude or indulgence, depending upon the situation, could represent both emotional and intellectual dimensions of this participation with the service providers in the sense of being a way to feel and reflect on the situation. The inclusion of home-based services in everyday life could thus represent ways of acting on and adapting to a change in capacity in everyday life; this incorporation could also represent an integration of the practical, emotional and intellectual dimensions of participation.

The 'practical' dimension of participation covered the older adults' handling, organising, reorganising, changing, structuring or restructuring their participation in everyday life. Thus, this dimension included task-oriented participation, too. The 'emotional' dimension of participation embraced the older adults' feelings and their expression of feelings relating to, and in order to manage, the participation that was of special importance to them. The dimension of 'intellectual' participation embraced thinking, planning, negotiating, making choices and reflecting in relation to participation and other activities. The integration of practical, emotional and intellectual dimensions of participation included understanding participation most of all as process-oriented. The older adults applied different strategies in creative and flexible ways in order to continue to be agents. An example from the first study was how an old man, who lived with increasing pain in his arms, maintained valued participation, such as going food shopping. By making practical arrangements like shopping just a little at a time and relatively often, he avoided situations of helplessness. By asking for help at the food store, he could also compensate for functional decline. Thus, his participation could exemplify both an integration of intellectual and practical aspects of participation.

Compared to the older adults' understanding and perspectives on participation in everyday life, the perspectives of service providers were more limited. They focused on participation as carrying out tasks, including attending to minor matters inside the house, like doing primary daily life activities and occupations like watching TV, listening to the radio or doing crosswords. Interestingly, they did not relate older adults' participation to leisure or cultural activities like going to the theatre; and participation like spending time with and visiting family and friends was barely mentioned. Although service providers overall had a practical and task-oriented understanding of participation in the older adults, the dimension of intellectually oriented participation found among the older adults was also found in service providers' understanding of how older adults kept control during interaction in service delivery. The service providers related the properties of keeping control to inclusion in decision-making. Interestingly, these dimensions of participation turned out to be less emphasised by the older adults. Service providers talked about including the older adults in decision-making in their everyday life, and were concerned about their duty to enhance decision-making among clients. However, the older adults' participation was characterised both by balancing agency in their encounters with the service providers and considering themselves to be natural agents in their daily life.

Contrasting perspectives on social participation

Although the perspectives on older adults' social participation were more process- than task-oriented in both service providers and older adults, their perspectives included several interesting contrasts. While the older adults emphasised the importance of family and neighbours for their opportunities for participation, the service providers were more concerned about the importance of their own role. Even though the older adults considered themselves to be managing well and adapting to their situation, they were often seen by the service providers as lonely and in need of care, social contact and social connection with service providers. Service providers believed the older adults were passively waiting for service providers to come, and were concerned with what they experienced as the service recipients' lack of participation and engagement in everyday life. When asked about what the older adults needed most of all, service providers felt that more time for social contact in service delivery constituted the most urgent need. They expressed a concern for the lack of continuity and time in service provision and service delivery, and believed they and the service organisation represented barriers to older adults' social participation with service providers in everyday life.

Interestingly, the older adults did not perceive themselves as either lonely or passive recipients of services. However, they could be bored. They took home-based services into their ongoing life in several ways. Service delivery represented, e.g. a source of small talk, an activity they highly appreciated. In addition, contact with the service providers meant encounters with people of different ages and cultural backgrounds, and therefore provided an appreciated link to society. However, although they were mostly content with both services and service delivery, they experienced time delays and lack of information about delays that could represent barriers to planned participation beyond home. Another experienced barrier to their participation was when service providers lacked the initiative or confidence to carry through the routines of service delivery.

The older adults highly valued their social participation with family, friends and neighbours, and actively sustained their place in this by combining independence, dependence and social contact. Social participation with family included processes of problem-solving together. We found that when problems with maintaining independence arose, the older adults discussed the problem in terms of how to solve it best together with, for example, the family member, rather than in terms of asking the family member to take responsibility for the troublesome task. It seemed that the two parties resolved obstacles in a manner that maintained the older adults' participation and agency. Thus, problem-solving could represent the practical, emotional and intellectual dimensions of participation. For example, one of the female participants had a son who offered to do the regular shopping on Saturdays for her. However, she felt it was important to keep up her role as a competent housewife, even though she needed a lift to the store. This way of organising everyday life could thus represent a practical dimension of participation. The participant wanted to see and feel the products in order to judge and decide if they were of the quality she preferred, which could represent an intellectual dimension of participation. Finally, going to the shops together with her son and experiencing his support could represent both a feeling of belonging and gratitude, and could thus represent the emotional dimension of participation. Furthermore, the fact that the participant did not hand the task over altogether could also contribute to a feeling of equivalence and continuity, and of taking her place as an equal family member, representing both the emotional and intellectual dimensions of participation.

Discussion

The distinction between task-oriented and process-oriented participation was identified as a key finding, representing contrasting perspectives on older adults' participation in service providers and older adults, respectively. Findings illuminated participation in everyday life being experienced by the older adults as a value-based process, overall concerning the maintenance of dignity and pride. This process demonstrated how the older adults concentrated on being agents in order to fend for themselves and to live their ongoing life. Process-oriented participation was identified as the integration of emotional, intellectual and practical dimensions of meeting everyday life challenges. We argue that these dimensions may serve to illustrate the complex and dynamic relation between the participation, environment and personal factor domains in the International Classification of Functioning, Disability and Health (ICF). The ICF model points at important relations between the domains – but in order to capture what this means to the individual, it is important to include the subjective experiences of individuals involved.

The variety of practical, intellectual and emotional strategies in the older adults could be understood as resources that the older adults used in the process of selecting valued participation, adaptation and compensation for changing capacity and loss of functions (Baltes & Baltes, 1990). These findings may also illuminate those in a study by Nicholson et al. (2013), which looked at the experiences of living at home with frailty in old age. This study argues that older adults bring creativity to bear on loss in order to live with changing capacity in their everyday life at home, which challenges the negative terms in which frailty in old age is viewed in society. Nicholson et al. (2013) conclude that, for frail older people, valuing the daily rituals that anchor their experience and facilitating creative connections are vital if they are to retain capacity and quality of life whilst being frail.

Compared to a process-orientated understanding, the service providers' perspectives on older adults' participation in everyday life seemed to include a more limited and task-oriented understanding. One way to understand the service providers' task orientation could be in light of the organisation of services. Findings showed that service providers felt they were marked by standardisation and strictly time-limited services, and hence represented barriers to the older adults' participation in daily life. The task-oriented perspective in the service providers could be explained by their short meetings and interactions with the older adults. Consequently, service providers probably had limited opportunities to observe, capture or understand older adults' participation beyond the observable tasks carried out in situations of service delivery. In addition, plausible reasons for task orientation in the service providers could be related to the foundation, assignment and assessment of services as well as organisation of the services. Previous research has also shown that service providers experience organisational factors as barriers to older adults' participation in everyday life (McGarry, 2009; Vik & Eide, 2013a, 2013b).

A second finding is the interesting contrast among service providers' and older adults' understandings of older adults' social participation in everyday life. The older adults were, in general, content with their social life, and they highly valued social participation with family, friends and neighbours.

This is in line with the findings of other researchers who have emphasised the importance of family and neighbours in the lives of older adults (Duner & Nordström, 2007; Larsson, Haglund & Hagberg, 2009; Vik, Nygård & Lilja, 2009). Although the service providers were more task- than process-oriented, they did indeed view socialising as an important need in the older adults. Interestingly, the service providers seemed to define their own role in the life of older service recipients as crucial for their social participation. The professionals viewed the older adults as passive and in need of social contact and connection with the service providers. It is important to note that when observing the older adults' strategies out of context, the service providers might experience the aforementioned examples from the findings as expressions of unwanted strife and struggle in, or barriers to, the older adults' participation. Service providers' experiences of professional values like care and user involvement, which are threatened because of time limits to visits, could represent reasons why they seemed to be concerned with the importance of, and need for, socialising. Some studies have found that older adults desire a close relationship with nurses in home-based services (McGarry, 2009; Turpin, McWilliam & Ward-Griffin, 2012). However, the older adults in this study expressed contentment with the service providers' short visits, not expecting the service providers to stay long. These different findings could possibly mirror a shared experience among the service providers and the older adults within a service system that is very strict on standardised services and time limitations. One reason for this finding could be that the older adults did not want to be a burden to the service providers. On the other hand, research has documented that older adults in Scandinavia are less lonely compared to those in other European countries (Hansen & Slagsvold, 2015).

Service recipients may see that the service system places great pressure on the service providers, so the older adults' lower expectations of close interaction could be an expression of their sympathy with the service providers. In line with the service providers' perspectives, the older adults appreciated the small-talk dimension of participation in service delivery. However, chatting to the service providers was mostly related to the everyday level of social interaction and hospitality. They seemed to relate private conversation and socialising mostly to family, friends and neighbours. One interpretation of this finding could be that the small-talk dimension should be situated in relation to its influence on older adults' general well-being, their self-presentation, and their identity as equal human beings and their linkage to society (Vik, Nygård & Lilja, 2009). One reason why the older adults accepted that the service providers just did the necessary tasks and then left could be a need to resist unwanted intimacy or aspects of surveillance via small talk, and to keep conversation on an everyday level. Additionally, the drive to fend for themselves could draw some lines between them and the service providers in the sense of preserving privacy, and perhaps resisting sharing supplementary information about their lives with the service providers beyond the short meetings during service delivery. The findings, rather, indicate that the older adults' experiences reached beyond small talk as an expression of warm and close relationships. Small talk with the service providers represented access to variety in people, age, gender and culture, and was a way of connecting them with the rest of society. The diversities of the service providers represented access to the wider society, and thus represented ways of participating in society. The interface with the service providers represented opportunities for presenting their own experiences and themselves, and could thus represent a way to practice equality. These findings may support research that has found that older adults' participation is closely related to a sense of belonging in society (Haak et al., 2007; Vik et al., 2008) and to activities at home (Haak et al., 2007).

Finally, one may question whether the service providers' understanding reflects a common perception among the general public that older adults are lonely. A recent study indicates that if older adults are viewed in this way, they also risk becoming more passive (Boduroglu et al., 2006). Pikhartova, Bowling and Victor (2016) argue that the linking of loneliness with individuals' beliefs and expectations of what old age will be like suggests that, potentially, mass campaigns to change these may be more effective in combating loneliness than the befriending services frequently offered.

A third finding is that service providers experienced the older adults as passive recipients of services and expressed a need for involving the older adults in decision-making, while the older adults were more concerned with balancing agency at the interface with service providers. This finding expands upon the participation in service delivery that reaches beyond the socialising aspects discussed above. The service providers' understanding of participation as decision-making in service delivery coincides with the terms used in Norwegian policy documents and legislation: user participation, user involvement (St. Meld. nr. 47, 2008–2009) and user influence (https://lovdata.no/dokument/NL/lov/2011–06–24–29, Act of National Health). Consequently, a strong focus on these aspects of participation in political documents, legislation and organisation of welfare services may contribute to explaining the wish of service providers to practice and facilitate participation in the sense of involvement in decision-making. Findings in this study could indicate that the participants lived their everyday life without experiences of being disempowered by the service system or the service providers. Although the older adults' experiences overall included a more complex and process-oriented understanding of participation in their everyday life, when it came to service delivery, they preferred service providers to accomplish the tasks they came for in appropriate, timely and skilled ways, and in accordance with the preferences of the older adults. This could be understood as an appreciation of task-oriented service delivery.

Conclusion

The diversity in perspectives of task- and process-oriented service delivery, and social participation, as illuminated in this chapter may form a key to understanding why service providers' intentions do not always lead to user involvement and autonomy, and also why the result sometimes is the opposite. Service providers and service systems represent important environmental factors in the lives of older service recipients. Our findings indicate that professionals and service delivery need to pay more attention to different aspects of participation. Individualisation of services and the person-centred approach in service delivery claim insight into the service recipients' perspective of their everyday life, values and social life. Peoples' experiences and processes of participation – like choice, satisfaction and importance – are crucial to capture the subjective experience of participation in order to develop and individualise services.

The older adults in this study seemed to be content with their social participation in everyday life. Naturally, this could be explained by socioeconomic, social capital and cultural aspects as well as by a wish not to be a burden to family or to the home-based services. In line with these arguments, it is not our intent to minimise or downplay the situation in which vulnerable older adults live. Differing understandings between service providers and service users may create conflicting interests, and also result in service delivery failing to meet the needs or wishes of the service users.

In order to enhance participation in service delivery, it is important that service providers are aware of the fact that participation is contextual and that the understanding of participation may vary among service providers and service recipients. To support participation in older adults depending on home-based services, it is important to recognise the complexity of dignity and pride, the multiple expressions and strategies of being and staying worthy.

References

Avers, D. (2014). Infusing an optimal aging paradigm into an entry-level geriatrics course. *Journal of Physical Therapy Education*. 28(2), 22–34.

Baltes, P.B., & Baltes, M.M. (1990). "Psychological perspectives on successful aging: The model of selective optimization with compensation," in *Successful aging: perspectives from the behavioural sciences*, P B. Baltes and M.M. Baltes, Eds., pp. 1–35, Cambridge University Press, Cambridge, UK.

Boduroglu, A., Yoon, C., Luo, T., & Park, D.C. (2006). Age-related stereotypes; a comparison of American and Chinese culture. *Gerontology*. 52, 324–323.

Brown, D., McWilliams, C., & Ward-Griffin, C. (2006). Issues and innovations in nursing practice. Client-centered empowering partnering in nursing. *Journal of Advanced Nursing*. 53, 160–168.

Cardol, M., de Jong, B.A., & Ward, C.D. (2002). On autonomy and participation in rehabilitation. *Disability and Rehabilitation*. 24(18), 970–974.

Charmaz, K. (2006). *Constructing grounded theory: A practical guide through qualitative analysis*. Sage Publications, London, England.

Duner, A., & Nordström, M. (2005). Intentions and strategies among elderly people: Coping in everyday life. *Journal of Aging Studies*. 19, 437–451.

Duner, A., & Nordström, M. (2007). The roles and functions of the informal support networks of older people who receive formal support: A Swedish qualitative study. *Ageing & Society*. 27(1), 67–85.

EU (2012). The 2012 Ageing Report. [Accessed April 22, 2013]; Available at: http://ec.europa.eu/economy_finance/publications/european_economy/2012/pdf/ee-2012–2_en.pdf.

Haak, M. (2008). Participation and independence in old age. Aspects of home and neighbourhood environments. Doctoral Thesis. Department of Health Sciences, Division of Occupational Therapy and Gerontology. Lund University.

Haak, M., Fange, A., Iwarsson, S., Dahlin, S. (2007). Home as a signification of independence and autonomy: Experiences among very old Swedish people. *Scandinavian Journal of Occupational Therapy*. 14, 16–24.

Hansen, T., & Slagsvold, B. (2015). Late-life loneliness in 11 European countries: results from the generations and gender survey. *Social Indicator Research*, 1–20. Available at: https://lovdata.no/dokument/NL/lov/2011–06–24–29; Lov om folkehelsearbeid/Act of national Health. Helse og omsorgsdepartementet.

Kydd, A., & Wild, D. (2013). Attitudes towards caring for older people: Literature review and methodology. *Nursing Older People*. 25(3), 22–27.

Kydd, A., Wild, D., & Nelson, S. (2013). Attitudes towards caring for older people: Findings and recommendations for practice. *Nursing Older People*. 25(4), 21–28.

Larsson, Å., Haglund, L., & Hagberg, J-E. (2009). Doing everyday life-experiences of the oldest old. *Scandinavian Journal of Occupational Therapy*. 16, 99–110.

McGarry, J. (2009). Defining roles, relationships, boundaries and participation between elderly people and nurses within the home: An ethnographic study. *Health and Social Care in the Community*. 17(1), 83–91.

Meld. St. (White Paper) nr. 47, (2008–2009). Samhandlingsreformen. Rett behandling – på rett sted – til rett tid. Meld. St. (White Paper) 26 (2014–2015) Fremtidens primærhelsetjeneste – nærhet og helhet.

Meld. St. (White Paper) nr. 29, (2012–2013). Morgendagens omsorg.

Nicholson, C., Meyer, J., Flatley, M., & Holman, C. (2013). The experience of living at home with frailty in old age: a psychosocial qualitative study. *International Journal of Nursing Studies*. 50(9), 1172–1179.

NOU/Official Norwegian Report (2011:11). Innovasjon I Omsorg: Innovation in Care.

Olsson, E., & Ingvad, B. (2001). The emotional climate of care-giving in home-care services. *Health & Social Care in the Community*. 9, 454–463.

Pikhartova, J., Bowling, A., & Victor, C. (2016). Is loneliness in later life a self-fulfilling prophecy? *Ageing & Mental Health*. 20(5), 543–549.

Strauss, A., and Corbin, J. (1990). *Basics of qualitative research*. Vol. 15. Newbury Park, CA: Sage.

Turpin, L., McWilliam, C., & Ward-Griffin, C. (2012). The meaning of a positive client-nurse relationship for senior home care clients with chronic disease. *Canadian Journal on Aging*. 31(4), 457–469.

Vik, K. (2008). Older adults' participation in occupation in the context of home-based rehabilitation. Thesis for Doctoral Degree. Karolinska Institutet.

Vik, K., & Eide, A.H. (2011a). The exhausting dilemmas faced by home-care service providers when enhancing participation among older adults receiving home care. *Scandinavian Journal of Caring Sciences*. 2012, 26(3), 528–536.

Vik, K., & Eide, A. (2011b). Older adults that receive home-based services, on the verge of passivity; the perspectives of service providers. *International Journal of Older People Nursing*. 8(2), 123–130.

Vik, K., Josephsson, S., Borell, L., & Nygård, L. (2008). Agency and engagement: Older adults' experiences of participation in occupation during home-based rehabilitation. *Canadian Journal of Occupational Therapy*. 75, 262–271.

Vik, K., Nygård, L., & Lilja, M. (2009). Encountering staff in the home: three older adults' experience during six months of home-based rehabilitation. *Disability and Rehabilitation*. 31, 619–629.

WHO. (2002). *Active ageing: A policy framework*. WHO, Geneva.

WHO. (2004). *Towards age-friendly primary health care*. WHO, Geneva.

WHO. (2008a). *Demystifying the myths of ageing*. WHO, Geneva.

WHO. (2008b). *The solid facts. Home care in Europe*. WHO, Geneva.

Witsø, A.E. (2013). Participation in older adults – in the context of receiving home-based services. Doctoral Thesis. NTNU – Trondheim.

Witsø, A.E., Eide, A., & Vik, K. (2012). Professional carers' perspectives on participation for older adults living in place. *Disability and Rehabilitation*. 33(7), 557–568.

Witsø, A.E., Vik, K., & Ytterhus, B. (2013). Participation in older homecare recipients: A value-based process. *Activities, Adaptation & Aging*. 36(4), 297–316.

Witsø, A.E., Ytterhus, B., & Vik, K. (2015). Taking home-based services into everyday life. *Scandinavian Journal of Disability Research*. 17(1), 46–51.

8 Participation at the interface with health and welfare services

Lisbeth Kvam, Heidi Pedersen and Aud Elisabeth Witsø

The priorities of equal rights to work, user involvement and universal design are examples of how intentions of participation in society influence working methods within the service systems. The interface between individuals and service systems has great influence on the legitimacy and efficiency of the welfare state. Recent research has studied patient participation and user involvement in the interface with professionals, e.g. patients and medical doctors (Graffigna, 2015; Thygeson, Morrisey & Ulstad, 2010), patients and nurses (McGarry, 2009; McCormack, Karlsson, Dewing & Lerdal, 2010), and clients and social workers (Slettebø, Brotkorp & Dalen, 2012). Findings across these studies show that promoting participation for individuals who receive services depends on the professionals and the system in which they are embedded, and how they interact with and adapt to patients and users. The International Classification of Functioning, Disability and Health (ICF) model may be suitable to illustrate the interaction between the service system and the service recipients. A transactional perspective may be useful to add to the ICF model, as it can contribute to explaining the interactions between the different domains in the ICF. Thus, in this chapter we will apply a transactional perspective to illuminate how participation can be understood in service delivery contexts. We will do this by exploring how three women experience participation across different life situations and their interface with different services within the health and welfare system. This is important, as central political ambitions of participation are shaped at the interface between individuals and service providers.

In occupational science, the transactional perspective, which stems from the work of the American philosopher and pragmatist John Dewey, has been applied to overcome the dominant view of occupation and participation as an individualised act (Cutchin, 2004; Cutchin & Dickie, 2012; Dickie, Cutchin & Humphry, 2006). One aim is to recast the thinking about occupation and participation to overcome the limitations of decontextualised, linear and mechanistic theories in order to counter the criticism that welfare services ignore the emergent character of human life (Cutchin & Dickie, 2012). From a transactional perspective, everyday problems, goals and solutions are continuously changing. Recognising the ongoing and emergent character of service recipients' lives may illuminate implications for service provision (Rosenberg & Johansson, 2012). Failing to recognise the constant redefinition of goals, problems and solutions can lead to wasted efforts and resources as well as failed interventions (Heywood, 2004). Transactions between individuals and environments are viewed as functional and continuously changing, and transactions are therefore continuously co-ordinated or re-co-ordinated by individuals in their lives (Cutchin, 2007). The transactional perspective may bring to the forefront where, when and how actors within the health and welfare sector and their contexts are connected in ongoing processes (Rosenberg & Johansson, 2012), and help to understand how the service systems can be designed and provided to adequately support participation for service recipients and clients in their everyday lives.

Service recipients and professionals may have different understandings of participation (Witsø, Eide & Vik, 2011). However, it is often the professionals' understandings of participation that give direction to intervention or care (Imrie, 2004; McGarry, 2009). Several studies have explored the subjective experience of participation and found that there is a close link between participation and context (Borell, Asaba, Rosenberg, Schultz & Townsend, 2006; Hammel, Magasi, Heinemann, Whiteneck, Bogner & Rodriguez, 2008; Kvam, Eide & Vik, 2013; Vik, Nygård, Borell & Josephsson, 2008; Witsø, Ytterhus & Vik, 2012). Some have found that participation is understood as a cluster of values (Borell et al., 2006; Hammel et al., 2008). In a study of autonomy and participation in rehabilitation, Cardol, De Jong and Ward (2002) found that autonomy is a prerequisite for participation, but that autonomy does not necessarily mean the same as independence or being independent of help from the health and welfare systems. Witsø, Ytterhus and Vik (2012) found that older adults receiving home-based services understood participation as a process of keeping up dignity and pride. Together, these studies have contributed to the exploration and illumination of subjective dimensions of the concept of participation. In this chapter, we will explore different situational aspects of participation by applying a transactional perspective, in the context of receiving different welfare services.

Method

Design and sample

This is a case study of three in-depth interviews with women from three separate and original studies (Kvam, Eide & Vik, 2013; Pedersen et al., 2011; Witsø, Ytterhus & Vik, 2015). The aim in all of the three original studies was to explore the concept of participation and/or interaction with welfare services. We chose case study methodology in the present study because it can generate rich, detailed and varied information about the informants' experience of interaction (Yin, 2003). In all three original studies, the samples were strategic and comprised ten to twelve semi-structured interviews. The interviews chosen were of three women of different ages, in different life situations, receiving different kinds of welfare services due to reduced function. One of the goals with case studies is to obtain knowledge that is transferable to other situations or cases (Yin, 2003). A strength of the present study is that by merging three interviews originating from different studies into one case, we are able to provide data that may reveal various dimensions of participation in the interface with the welfare service in general. An even broader data sample could have shown other aspects of 'participation in the interface with welfare services'. However, the data used are sufficient to analyse thematic similarities and differences within the case.

About the informants and their context

Lena was self-employed and around fifty years of age. She was interviewed in an office at the Norwegian Labour and Welfare Administration (NAV). She had completed vocational rehabilitation and applied for disability pension subsequent to the rehabilitation. At the time of the interview, her application for benefit was under consideration. She was in contact with many professionals: her medical doctor (general practitioner or GP), chiropractor, social caseworker at NAV, vocational rehabilitation professionals, and a medical specialist in back pain.

Berit had a higher medical education and was in her forties. She was interviewed at the premises of a multidisciplinary vocational rehabilitation programme that she attended. She attempted to return to work after a long period of sick leave. Her contacts with the welfare system were her GP, the social caseworker at NAV, and professionals at the rehabilitation institution.

Kari was in her seventies. She was interviewed in her own apartment and received municipal home-care services four hours per day. Her home care included help with personal care and nursing, getting dressed, a safety alarm, cooking, help with activities in the senior residence, and transport to the day centre.

Common to all the women were chronic health problems and regular interaction with different parts of the welfare services.

Collecting data

In the original studies, the participants were asked to describe their experiences with participation at the interface with welfare services and how they understood participation in this setting. The interviews lasted for about 1.5–2 hours. They were tape recorded and transcribed. Two of the studies were approved by Norwegian Social Science Data Services (NSD), and one by the Regional Ethical Research Committee (REK).

Analysis

The data consisted of about sixty pages of text. It was analysed by a constant comparative method (Charmaz, 2006). This approach gives systematic, but still flexible, guidelines for collecting and analysing qualitative data. The approach represents a process consisting of both initial open coding and focused coding, and writing supplementary memos. The approach is also based on a social constructivist philosophy of science (Charmaz, 2006), which emphasises the informants' ideas, experience and knowledge, and the interactive part of data collection and analysis – which means that categories and concepts grow out of the researcher's interaction with the field. We acknowledge that our interactions with the field and thereby the data material is under the influence of the authors' previous experiences and contacts with different parts of the welfare services. However, more important is that each of the authors had analysed the data from their 'own' original study before. To counteract possible bias from earlier findings, we co-operated on the analysis and discussed every step thoroughly.

Initially, each author coded the data, and then did it again with the others. Second, we selected some of the data for the purpose of more detailed analysis. We compared codes and highlighted those that dealt with participation at the interface with welfare services. Relevant themes in the text were compared to the total set of data. In connection with the initial coding, one of the researchers wrote detailed memos based on emerging discussions between the researchers. Then more structured memos where written in our analysis meetings.

The next step, focused coding, was also done collaboratively. A comparison of initial coding, data with data, codes with detailed memos and sorting was accomplished, and new codes were discussed. Authors compared dimensions of each focused code and the relation between codes before the final decision on a code was made. After repeated comparisons of codes and the connection between them, we ended up with 'goal-oriented participation at the interface of welfare services – having one's own agenda' as a core category. Furthermore, two themes appeared from the data: participation as 'active' and 'passive' strategies for participation. Both themes were about adaptation to the welfare services. The data were detailed enough to shed light on both because of their coinciding dimensions: to receive or to gain control, and how the informants present themselves.

Results

The core category 'goal-oriented participation' describes how the informants interacted with the welfare services and how they achieved the results they wanted. Although the women had different objectives, the principal goal for all three seemed to be to achieve and uphold the best possible way of living their everyday lives. Kari wanted to maintain the care she received from the home-based service. Lena perceived herself as having lost her ability to work, and was therefore aiming at being granted disability benefit. Berit, on the other hand, was conducting vocational rehabilitation and striving for an adapted workplace so that she could work despite her chronic pain problems. The informants used different strategies of adaptation to either uphold or gain control of their own situation, and they presented themselves in accordance with their choice of strategy.

Participation as active adaptation

The main characteristic of active adaptation was to make decisions that appeared to be autonomous. Thus, the decisions did not seem to be guided by expectations and norms within the service. This can be illustrated by Berit's story of her decision on when and how to be referred to get help to reach her goal of returning to work:

> [S]o I've thought about it now and then, but didn't feel the time was right because I only needed help to achieve the last step (to find a suitable workplace). Everything else I felt I could manage myself. So I asked to be referred to the rehabilitation institution myself.

The quote also shows that participation can be understood as being in charge of obtaining the help one needs. Thus, it demonstrated participation as making decisions about getting help, to have found a solution oneself, and to be able to act in accordance with the decision.

Moreover, participation as active adaptation was recognised as experiencing a common understanding, trust and co-operation at the interaction with the welfare service. Lena and her GP worked together in outlining the treatment. Lena's narrative showed that the trust and co-operation between her and the health professionals were important in order for her to be able to make the right choices to improve her health and everyday life. She said:

> My GP and the specialist in lower back pain are very thorough and that builds a feeling of trust. The back specialist said I have a hollow back and that makes it difficult to stand and have pressure on it. What I can do to make my everyday life better is exercise to build up the muscles in my back.

This was an example of how active participation in interaction with the service system resulted in making Lena able to improve her own health. The collaboration with competent persons she trusted facilitated her health-promoting behaviour. It was not a matter of submission to treatment; rather, it emphasised the importance of negotiation and choosing to work together with health professionals to reach the aim of living as she wished.

Kari was also acting in ways that fell within the active sub-category. She used her safety alarm to call the home-based services. Kari experienced a mutual understanding that she could not do anything by herself because of her dizziness. She adapted to the service system by using the safety alarm when she needed help, at the same time as being very cautious not to use the alarm unnecessarily. There was an important presumption of trust in this interaction, as Kari said:

> because everybody wants to do what is best for me.

Participation as active adaptation was linked to representation of self and control of the situation. When active adaptation was apparent, the actions were mostly described as being in accordance with norms in the specific context. Berit said:

> I don't want to be seen as weak and ill. I want to be seen as healthy and independent. It has been difficult to show that side of me that needs help and is miserable.

However, there were difficult contradictions with regard to presenting oneself as an actively participating person and at the same time being in need of help. On the one hand, it was important to appear as a resourceful person that was able to return to work despite chronic pain. On the other, it was necessary to expose the need for help to be able to realise the goal of returning to work. There was a conflict between the fear of being thrown into something that she could not handle and her desire to demonstrate her ability to work. The fear stemmed from previous experience: the interaction with the welfare service could be humiliating when exposing a need for help without being granted the help.

The analysis also showed that presentation of oneself was connected to gaining or maintaining control. Hence, the presentation mirrored the participants' perceptions of the service system and their goals of achievement. An example of this was Lena, who did not believe that she would return to work. The NAV insisted on testing her workability, and this limited her own initiative. Thus, she tried to control the outcome by adapted participation. In contrast, we saw that other contexts and goals could mobilise new engagement. This can be illustrated by Lena's strategy to take control of the treatment for her hypertension:

> We started with the hypertension. He [GP] wanted to put me on medication but I said that I would wait and see how exercise could help. Maybe the exercise would lower my blood pressure.

The quote shows an example where Lena makes choices and exercises control with regard to treatment. Her presentation when substantiating her need for a disability pension took on a quite different form. Even though the thought of receiving a disability pension made her uncomfortable, she had detailed narratives describing health problems that affected her workability negatively. It seemed like it was important to her to present herself in a way that left no doubt about her goal being legitimate. She appeared reflective and conscious of what was best for her. However, as we saw with Berit, Lena's interaction with the service system was experienced as contradictory due to the conflicting goals of the individual and the service system. There was clearly a tension between, on the one hand, being in need of help and fulfilling the expectations of the particular part of the service system and requirements of the law, and on the other hand, being in control of the situation.

Participation as passive adaptation

The passive adaptation strategies varied. However, the common characteristic seemed to centre on satisfying the service system, even though this strategy sometimes did not mirror the participants' perception of what was best for them. To some extent, passive participation was a result of a wish to meet the requirements of the system, even though it had negative repercussions on the individual. Lena did, for example, participate in a rehabilitation programme, even though she did not have any faith in a positive outcome:

> So I attended a meeting and talked to the social security officer and I filled out some forms and things. She said she didn't know when I had to attend

the rehabilitation, but that I had to go through with it. I had to undergo the rehabilitation. Oh well, I have to do it then, I thought. (. . .) You know, laws are laws and rules are rules.

Participation as passive adaptation was also reflected in the way Lena described the decisions made:

NAV wanted me to attend a course in stress management, and they thought that was a suitable solution for me.

Thus, the wish to adapt to the service system might result in giving in to pre-scribed remedies, even when these were perceived to be useless. Another aspect of passive participation is that the demands of the service system can lead to a worsening of health problems. This happened to Lena after she had been through rehabilitation:

[S]o the rehabilitation really contributed to the worsening of my problems with standing up. The pain in my groin just escalated. . ... I am also troubled with inflammations, which have increased after attending the rehabilitation program.

Berit's health problems had also increased after she repeatedly went back to work too soon after sick leave, but this was not a result of a direct adaptation to the ser-vice system, as was the case with Lena. However, indirectly it could be the result of a lack of trust in the system, which resulted in trying too hard, with negative consequences, just to avoid having to ask for help and risk rejection:

I worked too much and then collapsed totally for 2 weeks, then I worked too much again, and so it went on. It was an uphill struggle. . ... I postponed ask-ing for help and felt reluctant . . . I was not able to ask for help.

Both Lena and Berit fulfilled the expectations of the service system at a cost to their own health and well-being. Kari's passive participation was slightly differ-ent. She had the impression that the home-based service wanted to help her, and that the service system was concerned with her health. She said:

I'm not allowed to walk by myself due to my dizziness. You see, they are really worried about me falling.

Kari passively left it to the service to decide that she was not allowed to walk when she was by herself, even though she could. Her influence over her every-day life appeared limited and strictly regulated. This strategy might, however, be interpreted as a mix of active and passive participation. Giving away control was Kari's choice (active); on the other hand, doing what she was told might weaken her ability to walk in the long run (passive).

Another aspect of passive participation might be the participants' tendency to adapt to the service system because they understood the service providers' situation. As Lena said:

> I've done everything they've asked me to do. There is good chemistry between us. It has nothing to do with the social security officer. I understand that she wants to do her job right in every possible way.

We see from this that the participants partly disagreed with what they had to go through, and they even believed that the actions were negative for them, or the system, in the end. They nevertheless chose to fall into line because they felt that the 'system' required both them and the helpers to do so.

Personal goals and the requirements of the service system

The analysis showed that participation as adaptation to the service system with either active or passive participation might be strongly linked to how one presents oneself. Kari presented herself as someone who needed care. Berit, on the other hand, found it hard to ask for help, and as a result worked too much, hoping that the service system would eventually recognise her need for help.

Another dimension in the space between active and passive participation was the participants' wish to appear agreeable in the interaction with the service providers. For example, acting in a certain way to uphold or gain a wanted goal might be understood as active participation. In contrast, acting in a certain way to avoid unpleasant interaction with the service system might be seen as passive participation. An example was Kari, who did not want the home-based service to think of her as complaining. It was important to her that the helpers did not get the impression that she misused her safety alarm. She said:

> They don't think that I use it too much. I am relieved to hear that, because then I don't feel that I'm nagging them.

Being in contact with the service system seemed to trigger participation on a mental level, as a process of consciousness-raising. The process was about reflecting on how to act and to gain control over the situation and the outcome – to live as well as possible. The participants' interaction with the system seemed to influence the way they thought about themselves and their situation. The data analysis revealed the reflective processes in different contexts. Berit reflected as follows with regard to applying for further rehabilitation:

> I've been here five weeks now, and I've come to the conclusion that I'm going to apply for a further six weeks. I felt ambivalent about applying, because I know I have to take it slowly. I'm afraid to be thrown into something that I'm not ready for.

Lena had gone through a process, and had learned to think ahead and acknowledge that she needed a disability pension:

> So, we don't know about tomorrow. The doctor told me that I have to think ahead. How will the future look? He has a great point. So it has been a process to accept that one is in need of a disability pension. I don't think it's pleasant. I've had a reaction, I have to say.

Kari also expressed ambivalence about relinquishing her independence and leaving the helpers to do almost everything for her. She said:

> It's sad in a way (having left everything to others to deal with), but in a way it's also nice to let go and . . . the safety alarm means everything.

It seemed like the safety and control she experienced as a result of the help she got compensated for the loss of independence.

Discussion

In this case study of three women, we have explored different aspects of participation in the context of receiving welfare services. The women's participation in interaction with the welfare system seemed to be goal-oriented. Goal orientation is often viewed in a psychological perspective as a dimension of motivation, and connected to the willingness to change as well as the desire for, and dedicated pursuit of, something (van Hal, Meershoek, Nijhuis & Horstman, 2013). Primarily, participation has been seen as an individual issue, and not a matter of motivation and goal orientation being constructed in interaction between the individual and the environment. Our findings show that participation strategies were modified in an ongoing process of transactions between the goals of the individual and the goals of the welfare system in particular, as well as in changing contexts. It is important to note this, because people who receive services are likely to be granted different kinds of intervention and help depending on how the professionals understand their motivation or goals, as congruent with, or differing from, the goals of the particular service (Nair, 2003). In a transactional perspective, this understanding of goal orientation is relevant because it provides the opportunity to capture important dimensions of how individual participation strategies are influenced by the goals and working methods of the welfare service.

When the goal for the women in the present study was to achieve help from the public welfare system, the presentation of the self by the informants was in accordance with their goals. This reveals the informants' social competence and ability to *actively modify* their social surroundings (Cutchin & Dickie, 2012).

The active-passive participation 'dichotomy' found in the present study is not new. Molin (2004) has previously presented participation as a concept of dimensions, including personal, social, active and passive dimensions. Our findings suggest that active and passive aspects of participation can be intertwined, varied and adjusted, depending on the way the service providers and the service recipient interact, how they understand the situation, including problems and solutions, trust, earlier experiences and values.

A constant co-ordination of the relationship between the environment and the person was shown through the active/passive dimensions, and by understanding the dimensions of the service providers' needs. According to Cutchin and Dickie (2012), this co-ordination is both subtle and unrealised, but our findings have contributed to a more explicit revelation of such coordination and transactions. The three women kept changing between active and passive participation strategies, which can be viewed as a transaction via the dynamic restructuring of relationships of person and situation (Cutchin & Dickie, 2012). The transactions did not always represent processes of optimal participation, including a perfect fit between the individual's reality (how activities and roles are actually realised) and expectations of how activities and roles should be accomplished (Rochette, Korner-Bitensky & Levasseur, 2006). Nevertheless, the transactions represented processes of how the individuals made sense of their own situation and how they acted and adapted to the welfare services in the short and long term. Thus, the passive and active participation strategies could be understood as transactions, experienced as functional there and then – and sometimes in order to reach a future goal.

The informants showed active behaviour in one situation, and seemed to be inactive in other situations. This is, of course, normal; but interestingly, the activity seemed to depend on their experiences of situated competence in the professionals – hence, the importance of trust and of professionals trying to seek a common understanding in relation to users (Reed and Hocking, 2012). In a transactional perspective, people see the future through earlier experiences, and modify their behaviour when new learning arises. Knowledge is based on transactional experiences in the world. Some studies have shown that the professionals' relational qualities, recognition of users' experience-based knowledge, and training on user interaction are important in order to achieve good quality in individualised service delivery. Thus, personal qualification is a prerequisite to raising user interaction in relations where the power belongs to the professional (Slettebø et al., 2012).

In a study by Slettebø et al. (2012), users customised their behaviour not to provoke or to act against the rules of the welfare system. They also sometimes did this in loyalty to their helping professionals. However, to succeed with user involvement, both the users and the professionals must experience positive outcomes from interacting – and partnership was promoted as a better concept than user interaction. Stories from the informants in the present study revealed that both the service users and the professionals acted according to the rules of the welfare service, despite a lack of belief in the system's solutions and measures. Hence, social aspects seem to be highly conducive to how we behave. Adjustment to the welfare system may seem natural and adequate at an individual level. However, the adjustment may be challenging at the interface between the individual and the service system because of the different reasons for the adjustment. These reasons could be the individual's personality, previous experiences, health issues, environmental aspects like attitudes or expectations, or coming up against the service system's perspective on solutions to problems in people's lives sometimes presented in terms of 'what we have is what they get'. This reduces the person to a client and contributes to a mismatch in the process of reaching either individual or service system goals.

In summary, this chapter has shown that participation is influenced by, and intertwined with, environmental, health and personal factors, in changing constellations and transactions. Service providers should interact with service recipients in ways that uncover transactional aspects which influence the working relationship and the chosen solutions. Our findings point to acknowledging the importance of understanding participation as a value based at the individual level. This is in line with several studies exploring the concept of participation in different contexts (Hammel et al., 2008; Kvam et al., 2013; Witsø et al., 2012). However, if the starting point of the service system is that 'this is what we have', it could result in starting at the wrong end, and as such represents an instrumental approach. It is important to talk about individuals' values and what they consider important; what *can* be done – not only focus on what *must* be done or change.

References

Borell, L., Asaba, E., Rosenberg, L., Schultz, M.L., & Townsend, E. (2006). Exploring experiences of participation among individuals living with chronic pain. *Scandinavian Journal of Occupational Therapy*, 13: 76–85.

Cardol, M., De Jong. B.A., & Ward, C.D. (2002). On autonomy and participation in rehabilitation. *Disability and Rehabilitation*, 24(18): 970–974.

Charmaz, K. (2006). *Constructing grounded theory: A practical guide through qualitative research*. London: Sage.

Cutchin, M.P. (2004). Using Deweyan philosophy to rename and reframe adaptation-to-environment. *The American Journal of Occupational Therapy*, 58: 303–312.

Cutchin, M. (2007). From society to self (and back) through place: Habit in transactional context. *Occupation, Partcipation and Health*, 27(1): 509–598.

Cutchin, M.P., & Dickie, V. (2012). Transactional perspectives on occupations; an introduction and rationale. In: Cutchin, M.P., & Dickie, V. (ed). *Transactional perspectives on occupations*. The Netherlands: Springer: 303–312.

Dickie, V., Cutchin, M.P., & Humphry, R. (2006). Occupation as transactional experience: A critique of individualism in occupational science. *Journal of Occupational Science*, 13(1): 83–93.

Graffigna, S.B.G. (2015). Patient engagement in healthcare: Pathways for effective medical decision making. *Neuropsychological Trends*, 17: 53.

Hammel, J., Magasi, S., Heinemann, A., Whiteneck, G., Bogner, J., & Rodriguez, E. (2008). What does participation mean? An insider perspective from people with disabilities. *Disability and Rehabilitation*, 30(19): 1445–1460.

Heywood, F. (2004). The health outcomes of housing adaptions. *Disability & Society*, 19(2): 129–143.

Imrie, R. (2004). Demystifying disability: A review of the international classification of functioning. *Disability and Health Sociology of Health & Illness*, 26(3): 287–305.

Kvam, L., Eide, A.H., & Vik, K. (2013). Understanding experiences of participation among men and women with chronic musculoskeletal pain in vocational rehabilitation. *Work*, 45(2): 161–174.

McCormack, B., Karlsson, B., Dewing, J., & Lerdal, A. (2010). Exploring person-centredness: A qualitative meta-synthesis of four studies. *Scandinavian Journal of Caring Sciences*, 24(3): 620–634.

McGarry, J. (2009). Defining roles, relationships, boundaries and participation between elderly people and nurses within the home: An ethnographic study. *Health & Social Care in the Community*, 17(1): 83–91.

Molin, M. (2004). Delaktighet inom handikappområdet–en begreppsanalys. In: Gustavsson, A. (red). *Delaktighetens språk*. Lund: Studentlitteratur: 61–80.

Nair, K.P.S. (2003). Life goals: The concept and its relevance to rehabilitation. *Clinical Rehabilitation*, 17(2): 192–202.

Pedersen, H., Aasback, A., Alseth, A.K., Martinsen, E., & Nyland, J.O. (2011). *Arbeidsevnevurdering i NAV – Brukerorientert prosess eller ren prosedyre*. Research Report. NTNU Samfunnsforskning AS.

Reed, K., & C. Hocking (2012). Resituating the meaning of occupation: A transactional perspective. In: Cutchin, M.P., & Dickie, V. (ed). *Transactional perspectives on occupations*. The Netherlands: Springer: 39–50.

Rochette, A., Korner-Bitensky, N., & Levasseur, M. (2006). 'Optimal' participation: A reflective look. *Disability and Rehabilitation*, 28(19): 1231–1235.

Rosenberg, L., & Johansson, K. (2012). Where the transactions happen: The unit of analysis when applying a transactional perspective. In: Cutchin, M.P., & Dickie, V. (ed). *Transactional perspectives on occupations*. The Netherlands: Springer: 147–156.

Slettebø, T., Brotkorp, E., & Dalen, H. (2012). Brukernes erfaringer og syn på kollektiv brukermedvirkning. *Fontene Forskning*, 1(12): 43–55.

Thygeson, M., Morrisey, L., & Ulstad, V. (2010). Adaptive leadership and the practice of medicine: A complexity-based approach to reframing the doctor–patient relationship. *Journal of Evaluation in Clinical Practice*, 16: 1009–1015.

Van Hal, L., Meershoek, A., Nijhuis, F., & Horstman, K. (2013). A sociological perspective on "the unmotivated client": Public accountability and professional work methods in vocational rehabilitation. *Disability & Rehabilitation*, 35(10): 809–818.

Vik, K., Nygård, L., Borell, L., & Josephsson, S. (2008). Agency and engagement: Older adults' experiences of participation in occupation during home-based rehabilitation. *Canadian Journal of Occupational Therapy*, 75: 5262–5271.

Witsø, A.E., Eide, A.H., & Vik, K. (2011). Professional carers' perspectives on participation for older adults living in place. *Disability and Rehabilitation*, 33(7): 557–568.

Witsø, A.E., Ytterhus, B., & Vik, K. (2012). Participation in older home care recipients: A value-based process. *Activities, Adaptation & Aging*, 36(4): 297–316.

Witsø, A.E., Ytterhus, B., & Vik, K. (2015). Taking home-based services into everyday life; older adults' participation with service providers in the context of receiving home-based services. *Scandinavian Journal of Disability Research*, 17(1): 46–61.

Yin, R.K. (2003). *Case study research: Design and methods* (3rd ed.). Thousand Oaks, CA: Sage.

9 The ICF and collaboration about participation

Ebba Langum Bredland and Kjersti Vik

Rehabilitation towards participation in society

The United Nations (UN) adopted the Standard Rules on the Equalisation of Opportunities for Persons with Disabilities in 1993 (UN 1993). The purpose of the Standard Rules was to ensure that people with disabilities would achieve the same rights and obligations as others, and allow them to participate fully in society. The Standard Rules dealt not only with the medical aspects of rehabilitation, but also the social aspects: the right of disabled people to participate in their own context in society.

In recent years, being part of and participating in society on a par with others have been highlighted as important goals in rehabilitation for children also (Anaby et al. 2013; Law et al. 2015). A number of authors argue that rehabilitation should promote social participation and pay more attention to psychological and environmental aspects in rehabilitation (Bredland, Linge & Vik 2011; Wade 2012). However, the participation aspects have been less pronounced in both theory and practice, and the service will vary from treating impaired body structures/functions to improving participation in daily life (Stucki, Ewert & Cieza 2002; WHO 2002).

The International Classification of Functioning, Disability and Health (ICF) integrates the medical and the social perspectives (WHO 2002), and the model can therefore be used to combine these two perspectives to give a better understanding of the rehabilitation process. While providing a framework for the description of health and health-related states from two different perspectives, the model can also be helpful in visualising the interaction of factors influencing a rehabilitation process, and particularly the role that contextual factors (i.e. *environmental and personal factors*) play in the process (WHO 2002).

The story of Daniel will be introduced to illuminate how the ICF model may serve as a tool for a discussion of collaboration in rehabilitation. The case of Daniel is a clinical example from the first author's experience working as a physiotherapist in a municipality.

Daniel's case and application of the ICF

Daniel was born with a serious heart defect in a part of Norway where no specialist healthcare services were available to treat his condition. He therefore had to

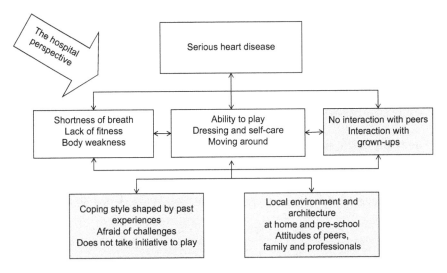

Figure 9.1 The hospital perspective (mainly on *disease and body functions and structures*)

travel to a specialist hospital in another part of the country to receive surgery and the necessary medical treatment.

During the first four years of his life, Daniel was seriously ill, and he spent most of his time in and out of hospital, both his local hospital and the specialist one. His family experienced long periods of uncertainty and periods of crisis because of Daniel's health condition.

Looking at the ICF model, the *health condition and body functions and structures* were the main issues during these four years. The most important goal was to ensure the survival of the patient, to treat the heart problem and to offer medical treatment. Daniel was dependent on a biomedical perspective to solve his main problem – a dysfunctional heart.

At the age of four and a half, his heart condition was cured after many difficult but successful operations. The specialist hospital with their high-quality expertise had been able to treat his heart problem. However, since he needed to improve his general condition, with an emphasis on building up his heart/lung capacity and to strengthen his muscles (*body functions and structures*), he was referred to a rehabilitation team in his municipality.

Coming home

Daniel returned home with a well-functioning heart and ready to start an ordinary life in his municipality. He no longer needed to take special precautions. Representatives from the rehabilitation team, which in Daniel's case meant a health visitor and a physiotherapist, visited Daniel and his family. They met a four-and-a-half-year-old boy who was more timid and afraid to meet new people than most boys of the same age. He had started to attend the local preschool and was transported there in a pushchair. As Daniel had been a patient all his life, he had not been used to living like other children, and he was not used to participating in activities along with his peers. According to his parents, he had no friends and he was afraid of, and withdrew from, new situations. Because of Daniel's needs and challenges, the professionals, together with the parents, decided to form a multi-disciplinary rehabilitation team.

The team in the municipality

Daniel's team consisted of Daniel's parents as well as staff from the preschool and health professions, such as a physiotherapist and health visitor, representing professionals with different types of knowledge. They started with collecting information.

The parents

Daniel's parents admitted they had been constantly worried during the first four years of their son's life. They had travelled to and from hospitals and had spent long periods in different and unfamiliar environments because of Daniel's illness. According to his parents, he had experienced pain after each operation, and had long periods of not feeling well. He was known in the neighbourhood (*environment*) as the 'heart boy'.

Daniel's parents did not have any other children. Over the years, they had got used to his role as a patient and they had often been afraid of losing him. The norm for them was to continue to protect and take care of him in the same way as they had always done. They had been taught to watch out for signs like blue lips or heavy breathing (*body structure and function*), and to always take precautions. Now their greatest wish for Daniel was that he could have some friends to play with (*participation*) and live like other children of his age.

The preschool

At this point, preschool was considered important to Daniel. However, the staff at the preschool said they were concerned that Daniel did not quite fit in. He did not seem to know how to play with other children and how to participate in games. The preschool staff also admitted that they felt uncertain about his medical condition. Big scars on his chest reminded them about what he had been through, and they were afraid to do anything wrong that could harm him. Therefore, he was treated more carefully than the other children. Daniel was used to getting help as soon as he failed to accomplish what he wanted, and he was not used to making any effort. He preferred to play with adults or on his own; he seemed to continue to be Daniel 'the heart boy'.

The physiotherapist

Daniel's physical fitness was not on the level of his peers. He had difficulties walking the same distance as the other children, and he easily got tired and gave up. Walking upstairs was hard for him, and he was far behind the other children as far as physical strength was concerned. However, the physiotherapist's main concern was that Daniel was used to being on his own, not playing or having social interaction with the other children. Thus, he was not getting physical activity the natural way. While the other children spent a lot of time playing together on their tricycles, on the swing or the seesaw, Daniel was sitting alone in the sandpit not being physically active.

Conclusions in the municipality

The big wish from Daniel's parents was that he should have friends and play with other children (*participation*). Therefore, the team first wanted to work on how Daniel could learn to participate with and be a part of the group of children, and how to play and socialise with them. They assumed that the continuous medical treatment during the first years of his life somehow had given him side effects that affected his social life. He had not had the opportunity to develop socially like his peers. Now he needed to develop skills to learn how to participate in social activities, like waiting his turn, queuing up and playing with others. The team also suggested that Daniel gradually had to make a greater effort in achieving what he wanted, for instance not receiving help immediately, like he was used to.

Second, his lack of physical fitness made him suffer from breathing problems and fatigue. According to the experts at the hospital, these symptoms were no longer due to the heart disease, but rather a result of Daniel's inactivity. The physiotherapist argued that if he started to enjoy playing with other children, he should be able to get his daily physical activity in a natural way without separating him from the other children in order to carry out special exercises. Consequently, the team agreed that the best way to approach his general lack of fitness was to encourage him to be physically active every day at preschool. In the beginning, Daniel started to play with one child, assisted by a preschool teacher, and then gradually other children were introduced. In this way, he would both improve his fitness and get used to socialising with other children.

Third, Daniel's parents said that they needed time to get used to not worrying about Daniel. They said they needed assistance to master the situation better and to know how they could encourage Daniel to be more active.

According to the ICF, the team in the municipality had started to focus on the social aspects (*personal and environmental factors, activity and participation*). This approach to assisting Daniel with living an ordinary life, where he could participate naturally with his environment, was in line with research about improving participation for children with disability (Anaby et al. 2013; Law et al. 2015). Thus, the main goal was now to assist Daniel to function socially with other children. The people close to him had to encourage *participation* in his daily activities.

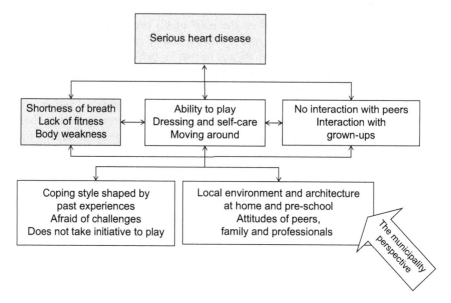

Figure 9.2 The municipality perspective (mainly on *personal and environmental factors, activity and participation*)

Interventions

As the main goal for Daniel now was to live like an ordinary boy (*participation*), the emphasis was on his resources and his opportunities to participate and play with other children. His parents, along with the preschool staff, the health visitor and the physiotherapist, made a plan for Daniel's progression, both at home and in the preschool. The physiotherapist and the preschool teacher jointly produced a play programme designed to promote physical activity together with the other children.

Daniel gradually learned to play and become physically active along with the other children. Sometimes he started breathing heavily when playing, but the physiotherapist assured the preschool teachers this was only because he was not used to physical activity. They had to get used to the fact that the heavy breathing was not a sign of danger anymore and might even be good for him. Daniel also had to be reassured and to get used to this special feeling; it was not a sign of danger, it was a sign of his heart working – a normal sign of him using his body (*body functions*).

His parents had asked for guidance in order to be more aware of what Daniel could master, rather than what he could not. In the beginning, the physiotherapist stayed with them and explained what was happening to his body when he was active, including all the normal reactions such as change of breathing or the colour in his face. His parents had to be assisted in allowing him to be on his own little by little (*environmental factors and participation*). From the start, it was difficult for them to leave him to play with other children, even for a short period of time. They needed to gradually grant him the same freedom and responsibility as other children. Another change was to let him walk more on his own instead of transporting him in the pushchair. Daniel had been teased by the other children – only babies were wheeled around in pushchairs.

Step by step, Daniel let go of the patient role, and both he and his parents dared to let him explore the world on his own. He was now ready to take part in new activities and was able to play with other children without having adults around him all the time. Another positive development was that his parents now said they dared to allow him an increasing degree of freedom. The main focus was now on social rehabilitation (*environmental and personal factors, participation and activity*).

Medical checkup and collaboration with the hospital

After six months at home, Daniel returned to the specialist hospital for his half-yearly assessment. The checkup went to everyone's satisfaction, until the doctor asked the family what type of medical follow-up they had at home and specifically how Daniel was getting on with the physiotherapy. The parents replied that for the time being, he did not have any regular physiotherapy. This was questioned by the doctor, since the hospital had referred him for physiotherapy. The parents did not have an answer to this and started to worry again, and were afraid that they had failed in the follow-up of their son.

When they returned home, they told the municipality team that the hospital assessment had made them feel worried and uncertain again. They asked themselves if they could really trust the multidisciplinary team. As they had understood it, according to the doctor at the hospital, Daniel had been treated the wrong way. He should have had physiotherapy treatment every week.

At this point, the story illustrates how the different service levels have different perceptions of goals in the rehabilitation process, and these influence which issues are emphasised in collaborations between the client, their next of kin and the professionals. These differences can lead to difficulties in collaboration.

Discussion

Three main issues will be discussed from this case where participation is the main component: first, the importance of different types of knowledge in the rehabilitation process; second, the challenge from the individual client's point of view to understand the different perspectives among the service levels; and third, the challenge to achieve good collaboration and co-ordination between the service levels.

Different knowledge

By making use of the ICF model, we can see that different types of knowledge are necessary within the different components, for example medical knowledge about *disease and body function and structure*; pedagogic knowledge about *activity*, for example in instructing daily activities and communication; and motivation

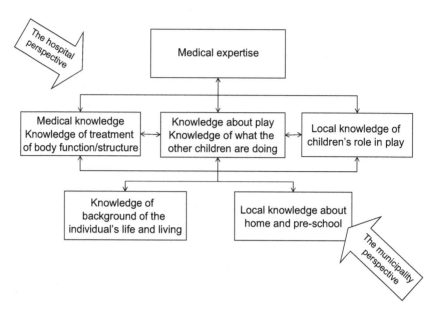

Figure 9.3 Different knowledge

and local knowledge within *participation and environment*. It is crucial that all professionals, both at the hospital and in the municipality, recognise the need for this wide diversity of knowledge during a rehabilitation process.

There is a reason for having different service levels. The medical world, on the one hand, seems to need its professions to work closely together, and somewhat secluded from society, in order to develop disease-specific high competence. Traditionally, this medical paradigm has also been dominant in rehabilitation services and is still considered to be the paramount type of knowledge. Expertise on participation and environment, on the other hand, brings professions closer to where people live their everyday lives and requires another kind of knowledge (Bredland et al. 2011). However, this latter type of knowledge seems to have been neglected within the medical paradigm. Giving more attention to this kind of everyday knowledge has the potential for the further development of rehabilitation services. This implies that the professionals in the municipality themselves will acknowledge their responsibility for developing this new and different type of knowledge (*participation, personal and environmental factors*) and interventions needed to promote participation for individuals in order for them to be able to get back to an ordinary life.

Rehabilitation services for children have a particular challenge. King et al. (2003) describe how everyday activities are vital for children's development, both in terms of quality of life and future life outcomes. Scherer and Discowden (2008) also argued for increased attention to *personal and environmental factors* in rehabilitation programmes. We argue that such an approach offers the greatest possibilities of success for the services at the municipality level. This means that the professions involved in everyday life need to appreciate and develop more knowledge on these issues. The revival of the municipality/local community as the level of intervention in rehabilitation is an international trend (Anaby et al. 2013; King et al. 2003; Law et al. 2015). As illustrated in the ICF, it is natural that the attention should shift from a medical to a social and environmental perspective in the rehabilitation process (see Figure 9.4). However, this shift may still be difficult to achieve because of the dominance of a medical paradigm and/ or because the expectation from the hospital level often is a continued medical approach. The municipality will often follow up the medical referral from the hospital, since the medical paradigm is so dominant in the health service as a whole, and this could undermine the trust in their everyday knowledge of participation and environment. There seems to be a power imbalance, as described by Clapton and Kendall (2002), including among different types of knowledge.

By using the ICF model as illustrated, the need for sharing knowledge can be better understood. Hospitals have specialist knowledge of *disease and body function and structure*, while the municipality has specialist knowledge of *participation, personal and environmental factors*. However, this implies that the professionals in hospitals should give attention to and acknowledge the responsibility, expertise and ability of the municipal level to work differently from the team in the hospital. In a rehabilitation process, the municipality probably has the best chance of promoting participation in society because they are near to where the patients live their lives.

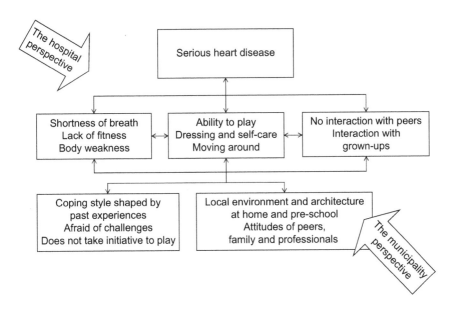

Figure 9.4 Both perspectives are necessary

Challenges from the individual client's point of view

During a rehabilitation process, the client and his or her family may have problems with understanding the different types of knowledge and ways of reasoning, and why **both** levels are important in rehabilitation. For the patients and their families, this shift between levels may create uncertainty.

In Daniel's case, the clients/parents had, over the years, got used to feeling safe with the hospital's medical knowledge (*disease and body functions and structure*) – after all, they are the experts on complicated medical conditions. What experts say is often perceived as correct, and the most important thing. A side effect of this trust in medical knowledge is that the patient and, as illustrated in Daniel's case, the parents, can lose confidence in both the professionals in the municipality and in their own judgement. Early in the process, the family had to listen to the medical experts and do what they were told, such as working with a physiotherapist in order to improve mobility and physical fitness. Later in the process, the family's preferences and their daily life expertise also became important. During this stage of the rehabilitation process, the client should perhaps be asked to pay attention to the shift in focus. This would help them to understand the new perspective, and to appreciate the reason why it is done and the different types of approach in the process. For example, for Daniel as well as for other clients, there are many ways of being physically active in everyday life, and it is not just exercise that matters (Bredland, Magnus & Vik 2015). The professionals, together with the individuals and sometimes the family, must be encouraged to find measures that suit their family and their environment to reach their goal for (in Daniel's case) their child.

In our experience and practice, using the ICF model to explain the different perspectives of the different phases in the rehabilitation process and why they are all important, but at different stages in the process, has proven to be useful in increasing the awareness and capability of the patient and/or the family.

Collaboration between service levels

Different service levels – the municipalities and hospitals – are necessary, and the different roles and responsibilities involved in the provision of rehabilitation services need to be appreciated. The specialist hospitals, with their teams of different professions, are experts on *disease and health conditions*. Their expertise on *body functions and structure* is necessary in order to solve the patient's problem through medical assessment and treatment. The doctors, nurses and physiotherapists at the hospital have the best knowledge about the patient's medical problem, and thus represent the medical expertise. However, in Daniel's case, they seem to have extended their expertise to the treatment in the municipality. Their referral indicated that the best way to solve the problem would be by further medical treatment, namely physiotherapy exercises directed towards his heart/lung disease and its consequences. The case study presented above revealed minimal collaboration between the hospital and the municipality beyond the hospital prescribing further medical treatment.

The expertise at the municipal level comprises a more mixed professional background. Their role is to tailor rehabilitation to patients in the context of their normal daily lives. The expertise of the professional health workers in the municipality is a mix of their medical and therapeutic background on the one hand; and their knowledge of everyday life in that specific municipality, and the culture and the opportunities for and barriers to participation on the other hand. They are the *participation and environmental* experts in the municipality where the patient and the family live. A rehabilitation team in the municipality has, together with the client and their next of kin, knowledge and expertise on *environmental and personal factors*. The professionals' challenge is to use this knowledge to assist the individual to become integrated in society, helping and motivating him or her to stop being a patient in order to be able to live an ordinary life in the local environment. In Daniel's case, his heart condition had healed, and they felt that Daniel's heart/lung problem would improve when he started playing and being one of the other children. Research has also documented that people undergoing rehabilitation after a stroke (Lund et al., 2013) and older adults (Witsø, Vik & Ytterhus, 2012) are more focused on living their ordinary daily life than concentrating on their illness or disability.

The ICF integrates the medical and social models into one bio-psychosocial model, and this gives both service levels the opportunity to envisage the whole rehabilitation process. Perhaps this will resolve the debate about which of the service levels has the best competence to define and solve the client's problems – the expert hospital team or the team in the municipality – and to acknowledge that each level can be of great importance, depending on how far into the rehabilitation process the person is. As illustrated in Daniel's case, early on in a rehabilitation process, the specialist hospital will often be vital for survival; they are in charge and they know the best course of action in the acute phase. Later, when the medical condition has been treated, the definition of 'expertise' and knowing who the 'expert' is becomes more blurred. There are many challenges during the period when the client is in transition between the two service levels, i.e. when the focus is changing from *body* and *activity* to *participation and environment*.

Daniel's main problem during that time was inactivity, a side effect of having been a patient all his life. By using the medical model and having the prescribed heart/lung physiotherapy, Daniel would most probably have achieved the physical ability to play with other children. On the other hand, he most probably would not have the courage to play with them (*personal factors*), physical ability not being enough. Seen from the perspective of the municipal health and rehabilitation workers, the boy's main goal was now to get out of the patient role and to build up his capacity to dare to try new activities. From their point of view, this could be achieved if everyone around Daniel worked together towards the goal of getting him to *participate* on a par with other children in the same activities as children his age and in his own environment (Scherer & Discowden 2008).

Since the different perceptions of goals between the specialist healthcare services in the hospitals and municipalities can cause conflict, and create an atmosphere of resistance and lack of communication at the time when the focus shifts from medical to participation, both levels need to be aware of and discuss this transition.

The municipality in this story saw the need for Daniel to develop functioning in daily life, and their focus was on preventing a disabling outcome of the interactions between health conditions and contextual factors (Scherer & Discowden 2008). In collaboration with Daniel's parents, the preschool teachers started to work on the social aspects of his rehabilitation process and played down a continuation of the patient role. Continuing to focus on medical problems may foster more patients; and for Daniel, as for other clients, shedding the persistent sickness-role behaviour that many, particularly in a closed clinical environment, are taught and have learned, is of vital importance to promote participation (Smith 2002).

The problems with collaboration and co-ordination across service levels can appear to be caused by the different professional foci. The power imbalance, with the medical expertise as dominant, impacts directly on the perception of who has the most important knowledge. Clapton and Kendall (2002) claim that power imbalances are inevitable, and that power is unevenly distributed in all relationships. This imbalance can be used positively or negatively, often unintentionally. Considerable attention has been paid to the power imbalance in rehabilitation between professionals and patients, and all the difficulties that can arise from that (Cardol et al. 2002; Clapton & Kendall 2002; Normann et al. 2004). However, this same power imbalance can be an issue between the service levels due to their different types of knowledge and the perceived value of different types of knowledge and expertise.

Conclusion

Collaboration and co-ordination are of great importance in rehabilitation and can often be difficult, especially with two different service levels that have different cultures and different types of knowledge and focus of attention. The collaboration and co-ordination should be built on understanding and mutual respect to assist the patient in the best way. By using the ICF systematically in this process, the two levels can get a better understanding of the fact that they need each other's competence for the benefit of the patient.

The hospital has a crucial job as long as the medical condition (*the disease and the body functions and structures*) is not under control. However, at some point when control has been achieved, a new approach is needed. This is when the municipality will have the most important part to play, in working with the local challenges (*participation, environmental and personal factors*). In order to give the person in the rehabilitation process the very best support and assistance to enable them to carry on with their life in an effective way, it is essential for the two teams to collaborate and co-ordinate their work. In that way, the person will have the best expertise for all the elements in the ICF model at the right time, and the two service levels will work together with mutual respect and understanding so that the person can feel safe and confident. Using the ICF across service levels as a framework to organise communication in a structured, meaningful and easily accessible way can promote an understanding of collaboration and co-ordination in the rehabilitation process. The ICF represents a potential common language that may well be an instrument which is conducive to meeting the challenges linked to collaboration between service levels and professionals, and between professionals and patients.

> When the family returned home, the municipal team used the ICF model to discuss the importance of giving children with conditions such as Daniel's interventions that were tailored for them. This gave the parents more confidence, both in themselves and in the municipal team. Before Daniel's next checkup, the team also discussed the intervention for Daniel with the 'experts' at the hospital. By looking at the ICF, both parties agreed that they had different roles in the rehabilitation process, both for Daniel and other children.

References

Anaby D, Hand C, Bradley L, DiRezze B, Forhan M, DiGiacomo A & Law M. The effect of the environment on participation of children and youth with disabilities: A scoping review. *Disability and Rehabilitation.* 2013, 35(19), 1589–1598. doi: 10.3109/09638288.2012.748840.

Bredland EL, Linge OA & Vik K. *Det handler om verdighet og deltagelse.* Oslo: Gyldendal Akademisk; 2011.

Bredland EL, Magnus E & Vik K. Physical activity patterns in older men. *Physical & Occupational Therapy in Geriatrics.* 2015, 33(1), 87–102.

Cardol M, De Jong BA & Ward CD. Clinical commentary: On autonomy and participation in rehabilitation. *Disability and Rehabilitation.* 2002, 24(18), 970–974.

Clapton J & Kendall E. Clinical commentary: Autonomy and participation in rehabilitation: Time for a new paradigm? *Disability and Rehabilitation.* 2002, 24(18), 987–991.

King G, Law M, King S, Rosenbaum P, Kertoy MK & Young NL. A conceptual model of the factors affecting the recreation and leisure participation of children with disabilities. *Physical & Occupational Therapy in Pediatrics.* 2003, 23(1), 63–90.

Law M, Anaby D, Imms C, Teplicky R & Turner L. Improving the participation of youth with physical disabilities in community activities: An interrupted time series design. *Australian Occupational Therapy Journal.* 2015, 62(2), 105–115.

Lund A, Mangset M, Wyller TB & Sveen U. Occupational transaction after stroke constructed as threat and balance. *Journal of Occupational Science.* 2013, 22(2), 146–159. doi:10.1080/14427591.2013.770363.

Normann T, Sandvin JT & Thommesen H. *A holistic approach to rehabilitation.* Oslo: Kommuneforlaget; 2004.

Scherer MJ & Discowden MA. Organizing future research and intervention efforts on the impact and effects of gender differences on disability and rehabilitation: The usefulness of ICF. *Disability and Rehabilitation.* 2008, 30(3), 161–165.

Smith DS. Clinical commentary: Autonomy and participation in rehabilitation. *Disability and Rehability.* 2002, 24(18), 999–1000.

Stucki G, Ewert T, & Cieza A. Value and application of the ICF in rehabilitation medicine. *Disability and Rehabilitation.* 2002, 24(17), 932–938.

United Nations. *Standard rules on the equalization of opportunities for persons with disabilities; 1993 A/RES/48/96.* New York.

Wade, D. Rehabilitation – a new approach. Overview and part one: The problems. *Clinical Rehabilitation.* 2015, 29(11), 1041–1050.

Witsø AE, Vik K, & Ytterhus B. Participation in older home care recipients: A value-based Process. *Activites, Adaptation & Aging.* 2012, 36(4), 297–316.

World Health Organization. *Towards a common language for functioning, disability and health: ICF.* Geneva, Switzerland: World Health Organization; 2002.

10 Parents' participation in child welfare investigation processes

Turid Midjo

Introduction

Participation is a key concept in social trends toward democratisation as well as in realising citizen rights within the fields of health and welfare. User participation is highly valued as a strategy to ensure user perspectives in policies as well as in promoting individual health and social well-being through opportunities to influence ongoing processes and decisions of importance to one's life (see Eide et al. this volume, Chapter 1). As such, the trend may also be seen as a shift in positioning service users from passive informants and recipients to competent and active actors. Although a widespread and valued concept, participation is criticised as vaguely defined and differently framed (see Eide et al. this volume, Chapter 1). The participation discourse might, however, be seen as reflecting the complexity of a concept that refers to an interactional phenomenon that takes different forms in different contexts. This chapter deals with participation as a situated interactional phenomenon, by exploring parents' participation within the context of child welfare investigations in Norway.

The role of parents as service users within child welfare in Scandinavian countries differs from traditional user roles in welfare service systems in that the child is understood as the primary client, and the parents as collaboration partners. The collaboration frame refers to an underlying view of a common interest between the state (child welfare) and the parents in creating good care based on children's interest and needs (Gilbert et al. 2011). This community creates a basis for a family approach to child welfare, where priority is given to support before more serious measures are considered, and that parents, as responsible for their child's 'best interest', enter into collaboration with child welfare services (Gilbert et al. 2011; Khoo et al. 2002). In line with this approach, assistant measures in Norwegian child welfare are in principle voluntary, meaning that decisions and implementation depend on parents' consent at the end of the investigation. Although having a common interest in realising the child's best interests, parents and child welfare professionals might disagree about the investigation and whether the child and the family need some form of support. It then becomes a matter of urgency for the child welfare services to develop a participatory relationship with the parents throughout the investigation process in order to create a basis for a common understanding of the child's situation and need for assistance. This might be a challenging task for both parties, as parents must accept being involved in an investigation process even if they disagree with any concerns about their child. It is important to know more about how participation processes might enfold when people are more or less forced to participate, as seen in most child welfare investigation cases where parents have not asked for support.

Parents' participation in child welfare investigations is governed by their positions as citizens with civil rights to influence decisions affecting them, but also by their role as parents, whose experience, knowledge and opinions about their children's everyday life and challenges are valuable to professional assessments and decisions. Parents are, however, not just passive informants. The search for agreement regarding the children's situation as well as possible need for support implies that parents have to get involved in a shared knowledge-construction process with the professionals. Their position as influencing actors in this co-production process is, however, unclear due to differences in institutional positions that give parents and professionals different knowledge and decision power (Midjo 2010). The role of service users and the power relations between professionals and users are generally defined as key factors in developing participation practices. In child welfare investigations, the development of participatory practices is even more challenging, as parents are not just service users, but also themselves subjects of the investigation. This might influence their moral status and position as knowing actors in relation to their children (Midjo 2010). To have their perspectives and knowledge recognised when exploring and defining children's life situation might depend on which parent position is actualised during the investigation process.

Although parents' participation is seen as feasible and desirable in child welfare processes, there is a question about the outcome. This is because the position available for parents and the opportunities to exercise power by professionals against the wishes of parents might present barriers to the development of positive participatory practices (Broadhurst & Holt 2010; Midjo 2010; Sheppard 2005). When looking at the development and use of participatory models and methods in child welfare, partnership models based on the 'ladder' concept (Arnstein 1969) seems to have had an influencing position (Darlington et al. 2010; Healey & Darlington 2009; Slettebø 2013). The implication of this approach is that participation easily gets framed as a normative concept, focusing on a particularly valued outcome. To make visible the complexity and challenges of participation as a process, there is a need for more detailed attention to what is going on in interactions between professionals and users (Forrester et al. 2008). By taking a micro-analytical perspective on the interaction between parents and professionals in the first meeting of the child welfare investigations, this chapter explores how participation is not only a result, but just as much a situated process influenced by the context, the interactional activities that have to be realised, and the actors' positions or role performance in managing and coping with the interactional activities.

Analysis strategy

The analysis adopts a discourse perspective that gives attention to the details of institutional talk as well as how this talk is influenced by the context (Midjo 2010). Drawing on positioning theory, the analysis explores the dynamic between what participants say and what the saying does (van Langenhove & Harré, 1999). Positioning refers to an inherent feature of the use of language where anyone who is positioning himself/herself in a conversation will, at the same time, also position the others. By entering a position in an interactional process, and at the same time offering other participants a position, a moral claim within the relevant discourse is created. The one who gets positioned can choose to accept the moral claim and adapt in terms of entering the given positon, or be critical of the claim, reject it, and modify or change it by a repositioning act (van Langenhove & Harré 1999). The positioning may as such take on a dynamic character, with changing interactional forms in ongoing co-production processes. This points to talk-in-interaction as an in-principle open phenomenon with regard to how the actual reality and meaning are produced. However, the openness is influenced by the institutional context and the participants' positional power. The power to achieve desired positions and action opportunities may differ, implying that participants in power positions can force others to take unwanted positions (Harré & van Lange-hove 1999). The principle of openness in co-production processes is then continuously at risk of being limited. Positioning theory poses a challenge to 'role' as an analytical concept capable of grasping interactional dynamics, and argues for a move to the concept of 'position' in studying people in their everyday world (Harré & van Langenhove 1999). The concept of positioning refers to the assignment of fluid 'parts' or fluid 'roles' to the speaking actors (Harré & van Langenhove 1999), which implies focusing on the way of acting that the actors find appropriate in the current situation. As such, positioning may be seen as forms of role performance. In this chapter, these concepts are used interchangeably in the analysis of how social workers and parents handle and resolve the interactional activities throughout the first meeting of the investigation process.

Positioning is part of how the participants co-ordinate and take part in the verbal realisation of the interactional activities of the actual process. Such activities in child welfare investigations are linked to the speakers' constructions and reconstructions of family problems or resources where parents might be assigned identities they agree on or refute (Midjo 2010). The process of realising interactional activities may then take different forms, e.g. harmonising collaboration, equal or asymmetric negotiations or entrenched conflicts. The performance may involve identity work with attempts to control the impression of themselves to influence others (Goffman 1959).

Methods

This chapter is based on anonymous transcripts of audio recordings of conversations between social workers and parents in child welfare investigations in Norway. The recordings of 114 conversations made between 2004 and 2006 were part of a study of child welfare investigation as an interactional process between child welfare professionals, parents and children. The data follow 17 families in conversations through all stages of a child welfare investigation. The conversations and the participants have been anonymised in different ways, like referring to all social workers as 'she,' rewriting the problems talked about and changing the children's age and gender. The study was approved by the Norwegian Centre for Research Data (NSD).

The analysis is structured around the different interactional tasks or activities as they are introduced by the social worker and realised in the verbal communication and interaction between the social worker and the parents as the investigation unfolds (Gee 1999; Linell 1998). The specific analysis strategy is based on recurring conversational situations or episodes that highlight how these interactional activities take shape and become realised, i.e. mainly situations where social workers and parents negotiate meaning. The analysis in this chapter includes two cases representing dominant participation practices when parents disagree with the notification of concerns about their children.

Findings and discussion

The analysis of the first meeting, referred to as the notification meeting, identified three interactional activities initiated by the social workers, defined as information work, commentary work and contract work (Midjo 2010).

Information work as an interactional activity is characterised by social workers' monologic information to parents about the relationship between the legal-administrative power and their rights as service users and formal parties in the case. It is a complicated interactional activity where the social workers make the legal-administrative power system relevant as a context for the investigation, while at the same time trying to soften the potential power impact by concentrating on the child welfare service as a supportive institution. As such, they are setting the scene for the investigation process, where downplaying the controlling and power dimension might be seen as a strategy to ensure that parents adhere to the investigation, especially those parents who basically have not sought help or do not want further contact. Parents are here primarily positioned as listeners, which they appear to accept by performing various forms of active listening. When parents occasionally withdraw from the silent and passive position they are assigned, they are asked about their knowledge of the child welfare service. Some of the parents use their answering position to initiate an active role performance, like the mother who includes a specific self-positioning when answering the question whether she has been in contact with the child welfare service before:

> I have not been in any contact with the child welfare service previously, but I understand of course what you are doing here, *that* I understand.

The mother's implication that she has some knowledge about this might simply be a rejection of the question, but it could also represent an attempt to distance herself from the potential identity she may be assigned.

Commentary work as an interactional activity implies that parents are given participatory positions where they, in principle, may elaborate, justify and explain the situation or incident which has triggered the concerns about their children. This implies opportunities to contribute with knowledge, experience and their children's needs in their lifeworld, and thus offer perspectives that might influence the picture of the reality brought forward in the notification. Whether parents are positioned as part of the concern for the child or not will highly influence how this interactional activity is managed and coped with.

Voluntary involvement in establishing contact with the child welfare service and agreement to the notification leads to a shared elaboration of the concerns within the investigation process. In such cases, parents rarely challenge the institutional positions available as their stories correspond with the purpose of the interactional activity. As their role performance does not represent any problems related to the realisation of the interactional activity and the investigation process, parents are given space to expand their stories.

However, disagreement with the content of the notification implies a possible threat to the realisation of the interactional activity, as parents initiate the concern that turns the commentary work into a negotiation process. None of the parents who disagreed were aware that the child welfare service had been contacted before they were called to a meeting with them. Disagreement positioning ranges from total rejection of the content of the notification to minor changes. When parents dismiss every single point of the concern, the whole investigation process is at risk. The analysis of the following two excerpts highlights how parents and social workers get involved in negotiation processes related to the notification and concern for the children, and how parents' participation position is both restricted and realised.

The first case analysed is from a notification meeting with a father who has daily custody of his three daughters aged between six and eleven years. Concern for the children is related to the description of a father who is not allowing the children to play with their peers. The social worker has now read the notification to the father, and concluded with an institutional obligation to investigate. The father reacts immediately, agreeing with this conclusion:

Yes, of course you need to investigate such a notification.

This agreement is, however, related to 'such a notification' and not to the notification as a true description of the everyday life of his children. The concerns about his children are then rejected. Through this adherence to the assessment in the notification, the father makes a role performance as belonging to a 'normal parent world'. He is thus creating a position which enables him to show acceptance of the child welfare obligations and rights to act, and simultaneously dissociate the action as relevant to him (Sacks 1992: 44). By labelling the description of the concerns a lie, the father initiates a truth discourse that implicitly raises questions about the basis for the continuation of the investigation. The father is now given space to bring in an alternative perspective by talking about the everyday life of the family and the children, but he is not given acceptance for his alternative story by the social worker. As the father's focus may divert attention from the essence of the commentary work, the social worker closes the father's story by reverting to the concrete concerns about the children described in the notification. As such, she appears to take control over which discourses are valid as commentary discourses. Excerpt 1 shows the initial part of how the social worker refocuses on the commentary work by giving a detailed review of the reported concerns, and how the father now gets positioned in an answering position. The excerpt begins with the social worker initiating a childhood and childcare discourse by referring to one of the claims in the notification (lines 1–2).[Below heading treated as special heading]

Excerpt 1

S: 1 Yes, the notifier says she is concerned about the three girls, that it's very rare that

2 they are allowed to be with the other children in the local community

F: 3 That's pure falsehood the whole thing, you know

S: 4 Hmm

F: 5 I have never refused to let the girls be out with the other kids in the street
6 except when they are doing their homework

S: 7 Yes, it also says here that (introducing a new concern theme)

The father seems to accept the repositioning to an answering position, implying a possible limitation of his role performance. However, he uses this position to continue the truth discourse by rejecting the notification (line 3) and the categorisation of his children and himself (line 5). At the end of his commentary work on this concern, he introduces an alternative interpretation of why he is refusing to let the children go out (line 6). By linking the refusal to let them play to schoolwork, the father adds knowledge to the reported situation at the same time as he positions himself as a responsible parent. The social worker continues her attention to the commentary work by moving on to the next topic of concern described in the notification, without giving attention to the father's information and role performance.

The commentary work continues in the same way, with the social worker positioning the father to answer her questions, and the father accepting this position at the same time as continuing his concern-reduction strategy by expanding his speech position. In this way, the father produces a participation position from which he adds knowledge about the everyday life of the family, thus uncovering an alternative story. However, the social worker continues to show no interest in the knowledge and perspectives introduced by the father.

The second case which is analysed shows a mother using correction as a concern-reducing strategy which implies both rejection and approval of the notification. Excerpt 2 is from a notification meeting with a mother who has daily custody of her seven-year-old daughter. The mother was informed that a report would be sent to the child welfare service. When the social worker reads the notification, describing a situation involving a mother who is very drunk and taking the bus home together with an anxious daughter late at night, the mother gets upset as she has quite another story to tell about the situation. The excerpt starts as the mother is being assigned a commentary position which she enters by initiating a justification account and telling what 'really' happened (line 1). By giving a description of the planned situation and what happened next, the mother positions herself as a responsible mother who had planned a safe evening for her child.

Excerpt 2

M: 1 What really happened that day was that my friend was going to babysit for
me

S: 2 Hmm

M: 3 Yes, and the agreement was that she should put my daughter to bed, call me and I
4 would come home

S: 5 But was your daughter with you then, at the place where you were?

M: 6 No she was with my friend, so she was *not* with me watching me drinking, no

S: 7 No, so she got there together with your friend?

M: 8 Yes and that was not the plan, that she should come to the place where I was having a glass of wine

S: 9 Yes

M: 10 And that was the most stupid thing that happened, she should not have come there

S: 11 No

The mother's correction strategy represents a contextualisation of the event referred to in the notification, where she positions herself as a responsible mother. Her account of the non-intentional course of action brings her into a reflexive self-positioning where she first appears to admit having acted wrongly, but then more explicitly positions the babysitter as the one who is responsible for the changed and unfavourable situation for the child (line 10). The social worker appears to give the mother space and motivation for telling her alternative story by making short comments that show her listening (lines 2, 9 and 11) and by asking supplementary questions (lines 5 and 7).

In both these cases, parents use their commentary position to introduce alternative stories to the notification. But, while the father's participation position gets restricted by the social worker, the mother appears to be encouraged to tell her alternative story. Alternative stories must be defined as relevant, and the two stories here differ with regard to how they meet the institutional regulation of commentary work as an interactional activity. Although the commentary position in principle includes expressing rejection of relevant discourses, accepting such discourses would imply opening a space for criticism and negotiation of the decision by the child welfare service to initiate an investigation. Commentary work as an interactional activity does not include such negotiations. This implies that parents' alternative perspectives are difficult to acknowledge at this stage of the investigation if the commentary work represents a rejection of the notification.

In realising 'commentary work', parents then are to be offered positions that delimit their role performance to accounting for the concern described in the notification, implying the adding of information by explaining, defending or justifying themselves. Such positioning work represents a central dimension of professional discourse practices within welfare services like child welfare and social work (Hall et al. 2006). Despite this regulation, parents' role performance shows that they, on the one hand, adapt to the given position, while on the other hand expand it in ways which allow them to produce their own version of the situation or events that gave rise to the concerns. In this way, they take an active participation position in the investigation process. The status of the alternative story as part of the knowledge-production process in the investigation is, however, uncertain.

Contract work

At the end of the first meeting, social workers have to agree to a 'contract' with the parents on carrying out the investigation as a collaboration project, including how extensive the investigation should be in obtaining information from other professionals and from the children. Obtaining information outside the family raises questions about stigmatisation of children and parents, thus downgrading the position of parents in contexts where parenthood is important, like at school. At the same time, it might be important for the child welfare service to contact childhood institutions. However, it is also important for the child welfare service to carry out the investigation as a voluntary joint project, thus giving the parents the necessary influence to ensure the continuation of the investigation. Although it is difficult to predict how individual cases develop as the social workers obtain more information, the 'contract work' is an important legitimising activity for the further collaboration process. The analysis of the following excerpts shows how social workers and parents negotiate their future contract.

Excerpt 3 takes up the father who has rejected any concern for his children. From the commentary work with a high degree of questioning or ignoring of the father's alternative story, the social worker now takes quite a different approach by transforming the father's rejection of the reported concerns into a possible truth (line 1). In this way, she reinstates the validity of the father's story and positions him as a possible truth-telling actor. The father confirms this positioning by emphasising honesty and openness, and the bad experience of being reported to the child welfare service (lines 2–3).

Excerpt 3

S: 1 It may well be that what you say is actually true, right?
F: 2 Yes, because we have nothing to hide, but it's worrying to get such notifications
3 It's not something you like to have hanging over you

S: 4 No, so how do we deal with this?
F: 5 In one way or another it must be solved
S: 6 Yes
F: 7 The children are old enough now . . . it is possible to talk to them
S: 8 Yes, that is something we could do

The social worker briefly supports the father before she positions him as jointly responsible for the investigation (line 4). By initiating a 'we' perspective, she appears to seek a partnership with the father, which he follows up by entering into an authoritative position pointing to the need for something to be done (line 5). This positioning may be understood as a continuation of his earlier truth discourse. However, his next statement (line 7) shows that he adopts a role performance in accordance with a collaboration perspective, suggesting that one way of resolving the situation might be to talk to his children (line 8).

Constructing the father's story as potentially true, the social worker makes visible two alternative and contradictory stories with different results. She also acknowledges the father as a collaborator, and as such gives him access to a more active participation position.

Excerpt 4 deals with the 'contract work' with the mother from excerpt 2, who partly denied the notification story of her evening of drinking. Before arriving at this interactional activity, the social worker and the mother had talked about the mother's drinking. The mother, who denied having a problem, had proposed closing the case. The social worker, however, had doubts about the mother's denial and wanted to continue the investigation and obtain more information. Excerpt 4 begins after the social worker informed the mother about the child welfare service's different opportunities to obtain more information. The mother is commenting on this information, and the social worker initiates a more powerful strategy by positioning the mother in a situation where she has to define a strategy for working out if she has an alcohol problem (line 1). The strategy places the mother in a forced position, but at the same time gives her a powerful participation position in choosing a further information strategy.

Excerpt 4

S: 1 What do you think we can do to be assured that such things won't happen
      again?
M: 2 As I've said, I agree that you can
      3 if you want to drop in on me anytime to take a look
S: 4 Yes, I was going to ask you whether that would be possible, in order to be
      assured that this is not
      5 still happening
M: 6 Yes, you are welcome any time
S: 7 This is you know authority control to your drinking problem, both announced
      and unannounced?
M: 8 Yes, yes

The mother accepts the participation position of deciding the future strategy, but is also changing her own future position. Positioning the mother with a possible drinking problem, combined with focusing on control measures, implies making visible a client position for the mother. By first underlining that she has herself proposed a visit earlier in the conversation (line 2), and then constructing the controlling home visits from the social worker as some sort of an informal visit (line 3), she appears to perform a more equal role. The social worker acknowledges the mother's proposal by pointing to the need to visit the mother (lines 4–5). However, the mother appears to continue downplaying the status of these visits and places herself in a host position (line 6). The social worker is not sure whether the mother has understood, and enters into an explanatory position by emphasising that the visits are about control (line 7). The mother shows that she understands this aspect through an explicit adherence to the social worker's information (line 8).

In the last excerpt, the mother tries to take control of the negotiation about her future position. She seems to be quite aware of the client position given to her by the social worker; but by her role performance as a host, she might be seen as doing identity work, making it evident that she is a good mother with no drinking problem. As such, she reconstructs her future position as collaborative in relation to the child welfare service.

Although they are placed in forced decision positions, parents are given some opportunities to influence the further investigation. As such, these two excerpts appear to show that at the end of the first meeting, parents are invited into more active and influencing positions than in the former interactional activity work.

As seen in excerpt 3, some parents may have no problems with involving their children in the investigation. Others might be more sceptical. Excerpt 5 represents an interaction about talking with the child where the mother has expressed some doubts about the necessity for this. The excerpt starts with the social worker entering into a justifying position as the child's spokesperson (line 1), a positioning the mother acknowledges (line 2). Then the social worker continues her accountability work by justifying her wish to include the school (lines 3–4).

Excerpt 5

S: 1 Hmm (.) My job is to ensure that your child is doing well

M: 2 Yes I understand that

S: 3 And perhaps (.) in order to learn a little about how your daughter is doing I would like to talk to her at her school

M: 4 Yes, I do not know how you do it (.) at the school (.) if they do it, I do not know (.) I mean (.)

5 do you need to talk to her about this?

S: 6 Are you talking about your daughter?

M: 7 Yes (.) but in any case not on her own

S: 8 No, we do not need that in the first instance

The mother's role performance in this conversation seems related to a concern about the child. In her question to the social worker, she indicates that she is sceptical of involving her daughter (lines 4–5), and in the next statement she explicitly presents specific requirements for talking to her (line 7). She does not appear to deny the social worker the opportunity to talk to her child, but does not want her to talk to the child alone. The social worker does not continue to argue her case, but aligns with the mother (line 8). It is, however, a temporary decision implying that parents might be asked the same question later on.

As part of carrying out the investigation as a collaboration project with parents, social workers appear to depend on parental approval for obtaining information from external professional actors as well as for talking to the children. Social workers are, however, in a position to decide how far parents' wishes and meanings should apply, and may at any time renegotiate the 'contract' with the parents.

Conclusion

From the passive and silent position within the first interactional activity, to the more open but regulated position in the 'commentary work', parents seem to be offered some choice in their position in the last interactional activity. The analysis appears to show how notification meetings gradually take shape as interaction processes, where parents are getting more active and influencing participation positions. However, the analysis also shows the hidden part of social workers' institutional power as they define and regulate how the interactional activities are managed, which positions are available for parents, and what kind of influence they have. This raises the question of what kind of participation is possible within a context where people hold different knowledge and power legitimacy, and mutual understanding is difficult to reach, as in these child welfare investigations.

The participation discourse in child welfare research has given much attention to the complex nature of child welfare as a context for implementing participation principles (Hall & Slembrouck 2001; Thorpe 2008). Others, like D'Cruz and Stagnitti (2008), point to different approaches to participation as a critical factor for participation outcomes by referring to the differences between a practice of professionals working together with service users to identify problems, and a practice where service users are involved in conversations about already-defined concerns. The participation practices analysed in this chapter appear to match both approaches, while giving attention to how parents' participation positions change throughout the process due to different forms of interactions in the different interactional activities.

The interactional perspective in this study makes it possible to identify how the complex participation processes are situated, not only in relation to the institutional context, but also to the interactional activities that could be identified as what participation is about. As such, the perspective also makes it possible to differentiate between participation and activity, which is discussed as a critical aspect in defining participation within the International Classification of Functioning, Disability and Health (ICF) framework (Piskur et al. 2014).

When the situated interaction and participation processes take different forms throughout the investigation, this might be seen as part of the different functions of the three interactional activities (information work, commentary work, and contract work), functions that influence which positions are available for the parents.

A situated interactional framework has the possibility to make visible the otherwise invisible dimensions of participatory processes, and thus represent an important perspective for further research on participation concepts and practices.

References

Arnstein SR (1969) Ladder of citizen participation. *Journal of the American Institute of Planners*, 35(3), 216–224.

Broadhurst K and Holt KE (2010) Partnerships and the limits of procedure: Prospects for relationships between parents and professionals under the new public law outline. *Child & Family Social Work*, 15, 97–107.

Darlington Y, Healy K and Feeney JA (2010) Challenges in implementing participatory practice in child protection: a contingency approach. *Children and Youth Service Review*, 32, 1020–1027.

D'Cruz H and Stagnitti K (2008) Reconstructing child welfare through participatory and child-centered professional practice: A conceptual approach. *Child and Family Social Work*, 14, 156–165.

Forrester D, Kershaw S, Moss H and Rollnick S (2008) Communication skills in child protection: How do social workers talk to parents? *Child and Family Social Work*, 13, 41–51.

Gee, JP (1999) *An Introduction to Discourse Analysis: Theory and Method*. London: Routledge.

Gilbert N, Parton N and Skivenes M (eds) (2011) *Child Protection Systems*. New York: Oxford University Press.

Goffman E (1959) *The Presentation of Self in Everyday Life*. Garden City, NY: Anchor Books.

Hall C and Slembrouck S (2001) Parent participation in social work meetings: The case of child protection conferences. *European Journal of Social Work*, 4(2), 143–160.

Hall C, Slembrouck S and Sarangi S (2006) *Language Practices in Social Work. Categorisation and accountability in child welfare*. London: Routledge.

Harré R and van Langenhove L (1999) The dynamics of social episodes. In Harré R and van Langenhove L (eds) *Positioning Theory: Moral Contexts of Intentional Action*. Oxford: Blackwell Publishers (pp. 1–13).

Healey K and Darlington Y (2009) Service user participation in diverse child protection contexts: Principle for practice. *Child & Family Social Work*, 14, 420–430.

Khoo E, Hyvonen U and Nygren L (2002) Child welfare or child protection: Uncovering Swedish and Canadian orientations to social intervention in child maltreatment. *Qualitative Social Work*, 1(4), 451–471.

Linell P (1998) *Approaching Dialogue: Talk, Interaction and Contexts in Dialogical Perspectives*. Amsterdam: John Benjamins.

Midjo T (2010) En studie av samhandlingen mellom foreldre og barnevernsarbeidere i barnevernets undersøkelse [A study of the interaction between parents and social workers in child welfare investigations.] Phd Theses. Trondheim: Norwegian University of Science and Technology.

Piskur B, Daniëls R, Jongmans MJ, Ketelaar M, Smeets RJEM, Norton M and Beurskens AJHM (2014) Participation and social participation: are they distinct concepts? *Clinical rehabilitation*, 28(3), 211–220.

Sacks H (1992) Lecture 6. The MIR membership categorization device. In Jefferson G (ed) *Lectures on Conversation*. Vol. 1. Oxford: Blackwell (pp. 40–48).

Sheppard M (2005) Mothers' coping strategies as child and family care service applicants. *British Journal of Social Work*, 35, 743–759.

Slettebø T (2013) Partnership with parents of children in care: A study of collective user participation in child protection services. *British Journal of Social Work*, 43, 579–595.

Thorpe R (2008) Family inclusion in child protection practice: building bridges in working with (not against) families. *Communities, Families and Children Australia*, 3, 4–18.

van Langenhove L and Harré R (1999). Introducing positioning theory. In Harré R and van Langenhove L (eds) *Positioning Theory: Moral Contexts of Intentional Action*. Oxford: Blackwell Publishers Ltd. (pp. 14–31).

11 Shout out who we are!

How might engagement in cultural activities enhance participation in everyday occupations for people in vulnerable life situations?

Sissel Horghagen and Clare Hocking

Introduction

> I fled from the war and thought I would start a new life in Norway. After all these years, I still do not know where my journey will end. I am angry and feel that I could do something cruel. I do nothing but wait. I wait for others to decide about my future. Where and when will my long flight from the war end?
>
> (Mimba, a 21-year-old asylum seeker after two years of living in a refugee center, presenting his story to a live audience)

This chapter explores how engagement in cultural activities such as theatre can enhance the participation of people in vulnerable situations in the social, economic and cultural life of the community. Their participation is important. Being part of the community supports people's health and well-being by increasing their social networks and reducing their risk of physical and sexual assault. Participating in culturally meaningful occupations also gives people opportunities to present who they are and hope to be (Wilcock & Hocking, 2015), and to display their competencies (Goffman, 2012). Being included in civic society enhances opportunities to participate in decisions that affect their lives and ensures access to their fundamental human rights (Gavrielides, 2014). Inclusive societies also benefit from having more engaged citizens.

Evidence supporting the impact of participatory theatre projects on participation in society has been building over the last decade. Working across diverse populations, including people made vulnerable by enduring mental health issues and other life circumstances, researchers have drawn on theories spanning recovery principles, positive and community psychology, health promotion and community development. This chapter is grounded in occupational justice, which is underpinned by two important ideas: that occupation is the foundation for health (Wilcock & Hocking, 2015), and that occupation has the power to improve the lives of vulnerable people (Whiteford & Hocking, 2012). From that perspective, removing the barriers to participation that make people vulnerable are key to improving health and well-being. Achieving that outcome will require health practitioners to shift their practice from healthcare settings to initiatives that cross the employment, housing, education and justice sectors, and the arts (WHO, 1986).

Being in vulnerable life situations, however, minimizes possibilities for social participation and reduces people's repertoire of occupations (Molineux, 2011; Whiteford, 2000). For people who are constantly or periodically in vulnerable life situations, the impact can be both immediate and long term. This might be a homeless man, or a young girl staying at a refugee reception center waiting for a residency permit. Both might experience geographic and social isolation and experience daily breaches of their human rights to liberty, security, work, decent housing, privacy, owning property and participation in the cultural life of the community (United Nations, 1948). They might, in addition, have difficulty being believed because people in mainstream society regard them with suspicion.

In this chapter, we argue that engagement in cultural activities such as participatory theatre, also known as community or applied theatre, can enhance people's capabilities and competencies and transform their sense of "what we are and what we can be" (Diba & d'Oliveira, 2015, 1354). We assert that participation in the arts can be a vehicle for social change, helping people in vulnerable circumstances become more visible and accepted (Sonn, Quayle, Belanji, & Baker, 2015). To illustrate that argument, we draw from two studies that explored whether people living in circumstances that severely curtailed their opportunities and resources could occupy or seize their everyday occupations by writing and producing a theatrical performance. Further, could those performances promote participation in society through opportunities to exchange knowledge and experiences between the participants and others in their social environments? To provide context to the chapter, we begin with an overview of the human rights of people in vulnerable circumstances. We then consider theatre as a vehicle for enhancing participation and empowering people.

The human rights of people in vulnerable life situations

Participation as a human, political, and civil right has been formalized through laws, resolutions and conventions (SHD, 1996/97; UN, 2006; WHO, 2001) and outlined in research (Borell, Asaba, Rosenberg, & Whiteford, 2006; Witsø, Eide, & Vik, 2011). Inclusion is one of the basic principles of full and effective participation in society, as described in the UN Convention on the Rights for Persons with Disabilities (2006; Art.3c). This fore fronting of inclusion is a profound paradigmatic shift (Sinclair, 2006), from viewing people with special needs as objects for care and recipients of services, to international recognition of equal rights and opportunities for all. Despite those advances, the human rights of some people in vulnerable situations are not fully realized. Of relevance to this chapter, the human rights to adequate housing and to seek asylum from persecution in another country are identified in the United Nations' Universal Declaration of Human Rights (UN, 1948). Nonetheless, people who are homeless or waiting to be granted status as an asylum seeker can experience breaches of these and other rights which profoundly limit their opportunities for participation.

Theatre as a vehicle for inclusion

Theatre studies! Can that be science?

Some people might question "Why culture? Why theatre?" when we pay attention to people in vulnerable life situations. They have critical arguments about whether cultural occupations can meet the needs of people who experience denigration and exclusion. Are not their needs more basic, they might ask? Others ask if engagement in cultural occupations is a feasible research topic. Is it possible to generate knowledge based on research designs linked to theatre? In response, we draw from two studies where theatre has been used as an occupation to enhance participation and inclusion for people in vulnerable life situations.

The transformational potential of cultural occupations such as theatre

Throughout history, people in all cultures have engaged in song, dance and design. The need for expression through different creative media seems to be an innate aspect of human nature (Langer, 1966). If that is so, Langer suggested that creativity is part of the cognitive, perceptual and emotional architecture necessary for a human's social life. As well as being an expression of creativity, the transformative potential of occupation has long been recognized and channeled to realize personal and societal change (Watson, Tucker, & Drury, 2014). Seen this way, theatre is not a luxury product of civilization, but a medium to change and empower people's everyday lives. Participation in culturally and socially valued occupations can transform people from being victimized to being empowered. In this chapter, we assert that people who fall outside mainstream society for various reasons are entitled to participate in meaningful occupations, including cultural activities that have transformational possibilities.

The transformational possibilities of theatre are seated in the idea of theatre as a subjunctive reality, where unrealized human potential and hypothetical possibilities can be explored without the constraints of known situations and settled facts (Bruner, 1986). As an occupation, theatre invites people to get involved in creative processes through which their experiences and resources can unfold. In applied theatre, there is an intention to use theatre in a non-traditional way that will bring about such changes through direct participation (Thompson, 2003). For example, it might enable participants to interpret the emerging space between cultures in such a way that the performances represent cultural enactments of potential new identities and integrative social actions (Becker, 2004; Kaptani & Yuval-Davis, 2008). Used in this way, theatre can be a means of inspiring ways of thinking, critical reflections, emotional engagement and personal transformation (Gray et al., 2000; Kwon, 2004).

Research into the arts as transformational media

Broad claims have been made about using people's creative abilities to enhance their quality of participation in everyday occupations (Creek, 2009). Supporting those assertions, there is growing evidence that participation in the arts promotes participation. For example, a critical review of research into arts programmes concluded that social recovery relates to an enhanced sense of belonging and overcoming stigma; and occupational recovery is fostered by taking on an identity as an artist and having a sense of contributing to society (Van Lith, Schofield, & Fenner, 2013). Like arts programmes, participating in theatre provides opportunities for people in vulnerable circumstances to discover what they can do as they work together to put on a performance. Amongst the claims made are that performative theatre is a forum for counter-storytelling, in which people who are invisible or ignored can challenge stereotypes and speak back to the broader community (Sonn et al., 2015). Perhaps more importantly, theatre positions them as citizens with the talent and right to access culture, rather than vulnerable and needing assistance (Diba & d'Oliveira, 2015). Theatre has thus been used extensively as a medium to empower people experiencing oppression.

In bringing actors and audience together, participatory theatre also has the potential to promote social change. For instance, arts projects that involve mental health service users in planning and delivering the performance (Heenan, 2006) can promote a sense of connection (Sagan, 2012) and, by creating a bridge to the community (Howells & Zelnik, 2009), promote social inclusion (Hacking, Secker, Spandler, Kent, & Shenton, 2008). Furthermore, by becoming emotionally involved, the audience can feel a sense of ownership over identifying and reflecting on social situations of concern and ways to bring about change (Sloman, 2011). Contemporary research also suggests that participatory theatre is effective in building community capacity to address issues, and to strengthening, energizing and empowering community members to do so (Sloman, 2011).

Various forms of participatory theatre exist. Augusto Boal, a Brazilian, developed *Forum Theatre*, where the audience can suggest different actions for the character who is oppressed and enter the stage to demonstrate their ideas. Observational reports by the theatre ensemble attest that audience members became empowered by imagining and enacting the idea of change to generate social action (Boal, 1998). Boal also cooperated with Paulo Freire, the author of the *Pedagogy of the Oppressed*, to develop *Legislative Theatre*, which is used in neighbourhoods to identify community problems (Freire, 1998). This form of theatre has been used to develop research designs and democratize dialogic processes where environmental health research, community healthcare and education have been integrated (Sullivan & Lloyd, 2006). Taken together, the evidence suggests that theatre can be used as a medium to promote participation and create more inclusive societies. We now move on to describe specific examples of using theatre production to promote participation.

Case studies of transformation through theatre

The form of theatre employed in the two studies we draw from is applied theatre, which is often used in educational contexts. Its theoretical roots can be traced back to key critical theorists, primarily Augusto Boal (1998), Freire (1998), and Sullivan and Lloyd (2006). This form of theatre is intended to promote change in human activity through direct participation (Becker, 2004; Thompson, 2003). Applied theatre involves taking participants' ideas and artwork into the stage production and performing them live (Rowe, 2004). The script for the theatre productions we describe developed out of six months of working with structured activities and improvisations (Johnstone, 1979), along with Tai Chi, voice exercises, drawing, and dramatization of events in the participants' lives. Giving the participants control over the script and the performance ensured that their own experiences and stories, told in ways they determined, were presented to the audience. In this account, we focus on aspects of participation; first, participation in development of the theatre production, and then participation outcomes.

Participants in the first study were 11 asylum seekers who were living in a reception center in a city in Norway (M = 7, F = 4) (Horghagen & Josephsson, 2010). Participants in the second study were four homeless people in the same city (M = 3, F = 1) (Horghagen, 2012). The case examples we describe have been previously published. One explored theatre at an activity center for asylum seekers (Horghagen & Josephsson, 2010). The second explored theatre as an occupation for homeless people (Horghagen, 2012). The instructors were a performance artist and a teacher with cultural expertise. The analysis, which was derived from systematic document analysis (DePoy & Gitlin, 2015), showed that the transformations that occurred through participation in theatrical activities took place on three levels: personal, social and societal. All names given are pseudonyms.

Personal experiences of participating in theatre

Most of the asylum seekers and homeless people who participated in the theatre projects were victims of problematic life situations. When they first met the instructors, their accounts focused on the circumstances that had caused them to lose control of their lives. Some of the homeless people had been neglected as children and sent to special institutions where they experienced sexual and violent assaults (Befring report, 2004). Some experienced mental illness, and some described themselves as completely incompetent. Rather than being concerned about having enough to eat and a place to sleep, they were most concerned with being treated with respect and dignity, and overcoming the stigma of having been institutionalized. Thus, they mostly talked about the past, and seemed stuck in their experiences of occupational injustice. The asylum seekers mostly talked about the present time, appearing frightened of describing what had happened in the past. No one talked about the future. The asylum seekers in particular described how their future was in the hands of the government or that they had handed the future over to fate.

Participating in the applied theatre projects was an opportunity for the participants to take back some control by informing the audience about the injustices they had experienced and having those experiences validated. Part of that experience, for all of the participants in the two studies, was institutional restrictions that deprived them of occupational choice, resources and freedom:

> For me the reception centre is a prison where I am waiting for my future, living on charity. It is 365 days in the year. I have been there for 8 years with no approval, walking to my mailbox with a little hope every day.
>
> (Iris's performance)

Planning what they wanted to say to the audience and learning how they could convey their message enabled the participants to reflect on and question what had happened to them. For example, Arne, one of the homeless men, told this story:

> After my second year at school, the child welfare authorities and the police came to our home. They placed me in an institution for children. I lived there for 9 years and they pigeonholed me, said I was not as smart as the others. How come? I managed to get a drivers license when I was 19 years old! Now I am 49 and I want to get rid of this stigma that has hindered me a lot in life.
>
> (Arne's performance)

Engaging with the theatre was a starting point for personal enablement, but the changes that occurred did not happen immediately. Rather, after some months of active involvement in theatre, several of the participants began to talk about themselves as people with competencies. Where they had initially presented themselves as victims, engaging in the organized activities required to prepare for the show led to them gradually taking more control over other parts of their lives. They took on new roles, re-established daily routines, and learned strategies to cope with everyday events. Involvement in theatre also created opportunities to be pleased with themselves and their achievements. Christiansen and Townsend (2010) emphasized how people understand themselves and create their experiences through their occupational choices. By choosing to participate in applied theatre, the participants in these studies transformed their self-perception (Blair, 2000). Underpinning this transformation, they grew in their understanding of their own situation and came to identify their position as an asylum seeker or homeless person.

Social experiences when participating in theatre

When the theatre projects began, the participants were predictably wary of each other. The homeless participants had been subjected to multiple degradations, and all of the participants had experienced betrayals of trust. The asylum seekers were from different cultures and countries and did not know each other, and the young women (aged 18–25 years old) felt especially unsafe, both during their escape and at the asylum centers. Noting that the participants did not interact, the instructors encouraged them to take care of each other. After weeks of participation in the varied occupations involved in a theatrical production, they gradually began to respond to and help each other, which fostered a sense of affiliation and connect-edness (Mead, Hilton, & Curtis, 2001). One day, during a break in theatre work, Sara told a tragic story about how her brother was killed and about her mother's response. Hearing of this atrocity silenced everybody. Then Temba reflected:

> We have to lift ourselves up from all these sorrows. You cannot live by your hate. We do not move forward by thinking of our dreadful memories. Instead, we must find peace with ourselves, and find our competencies and strengths and use them.

Sharing traumatic incidents from one's past takes courage. In the context of this study, the participants' recounting and responding to past traumas reveals that they felt safe with each other. From this position of safety, they could gradually experience greater peace of mind and stand together to take more power in their lives.

The asylum seekers in particular argued and discussed things, but also worked closely together. They started to share meals after rehearsals, developing ways to be generous with each other and presenting themselves as persons they were proud to be. Over time, their growing relationships impacted their everyday lives beyond the theatre. They became people who had the capability to support others, taking small steps to assist each other to participate, such as making arrangements about which bus to take to the theatre project. In contrast to the isolated lives they had previously lived, they also went to other places together and, with this peer support, became more visible to other members of the community. These shifts align with Townsend (1997), who highlighted the potential of occupation to transform aspects of people's social life.

Societal transformation from participating in theatre

Before the performances, the actors and audience had different views of "the other". For the audience, seeing the asylum seekers or homeless people's competencies, and hearing stories of why they live as they do, challenged existing prejudices and stereotypes. At the time when the homeless participants presented their performance, the authorities apologized for the disrespectful treatment they and other children had received at schools and homes for children with learning problems. In their new characters, the participants themselves dared to say what had happened to them, to place blame with those who were guilty, and to stop blaming themselves. Similarly, at the opening night of the asylum seekers' performance, the mayor of the city arose:

> Thank you for inviting me to this performance. I will honor your performance, through which you have given us new insights by giving your experiences and knowledge-based artistic expression.

This was a special moment: a coming together of those waiting for asylum and the mayor, who represented the authorities. Their roles were reversed; the asylum seekers were the hosts who had invited the citizens to their presentation.

In promoting the active participation of both the performers and the audience, applied theatre breaks down the traditional roles of transmitter and receiver (Becker, 2004). It activates reflection and dialogue between the performers and the audience through their shared experience, so that a social expression of art and an inter-human relationship occurs.

There is a tendency among people from education, art, science, health and social work to instigate projects that integrate art and culture with social challenges (Kwon, 2004). The studies presented in this chapter demonstrate that applied theatre creates possibilities to consider people in vulnerable situations in the light of their historical, social and political context. For example, one way in which that possibility was accentuated was that the asylum-seekers' performance was staged in a fort where members of the resistance were executed by the Nazis during World War II. This venue was chosen to make transparent the similarities between the last war in Norway and the challenges faced by asylum seekers. This brings the little stories along with the great stories of history, enabling transformation at a societal level.

Discussion

Today's health and social challenges often relate to loneliness, poverty and alienation. People in vulnerable life situations risk becoming isolated and passive, rejected and forgotten by society (Mead, Hilton, & Curtis 2001). This was true of participants in the applied theatre productions we report, who were dependent on others and social benefits. They felt victimized and, as Polkinghorne (1996) predicted, some had lost dignity and self-respect, and given up the power to direct their lives. Their opportunities were limited and, as Wilcock (2006) proposed, that meant they were unable to demonstrate who they were and hoped to be.

The term "occupation" means to seize or take possession (Yerxa et al., 1990), and the participants did indeed come to possess the theatre occupations in which they were involved. The practical wisdom gained from doing theatre showed them to be people who had unique knowledge and experiences that others wanted them to share. Slowly, through engagement in theatre occupations, the participants increased their activity levels and developed greater structure to their days, which led to the development of skills and problem-solving abilities. As they began to plan and organize their days, they experienced meaningfulness, responsibility and purposefulness. They came to believe in their abilities and potential; to see themselves as people who could be agents of their own lives, set goals, strive to achieve those goals, overcome obstacles and actualize their ideals (Polkinghorne, 1996). They were enabled to do that by contributing to the achievement of their collective goal: to give a theatre performance. There is no evidence that their transformation had a lasting effect, but they had gained experience of being in a more empowered position.

The personal level: bringing new characters into existence

The vulnerable life situation of the participants excluded them from active citizenship, which was compounded by having acquired roles they were ashamed of or having lost roles. There are substantial identity costs to no longer being recognized as a brother, son, friend, worker, and so on (Briar, 1980), because people think of and experience themselves according to the roles they inhabit and the occupations they do (Kielhofner, 2008). Therefore, it can be a healing process to bring new roles or characters into existence, not necessarily as employed, but within meaningful roles in creative occupations. The participants in study were instructed in theatre methods (Boal, 1998; Freire, 1998; Saldana, 2005; Thompson, 2003) through which they could control their own story and their hopes for the future. They started to imagine and talk about things that could happen, which they had not previously dared to do. Using the subjunctive form of "what if", they started to open their minds, to be proud of themselves, and to see future perspectives of how to handle everyday occupations.

The social level: becoming visible

The invisibility of the participants in both studies was abstract and concrete. Some experienced an inner sense of invisibility, having lost the sense of who they were, and all had low levels of participation in everyday occupations. Through theatre methods (Boal, 1998; Freire, 1998; Saldana, 2005), the participants shifted from being alienated from one another to being well known to each other. They learned how to communicate within the group, discussing things and negotiating, solving disagreements and developing respect for different cultural values. They also began to trust others which, as Smith (2005) found in her research with refugees, develops people's sense of safety. The findings seemed to suggest a strong link between the process of being empowered and becoming visible to others. Such processes can be viewed as part of political processes, which are fundamental to gaining active citizenship (Pollard & Kronenberg, 2008; Whiteford & Pereira, 2012) and reducing stigmatization and invisibility. In addition, engaging in the theatre projects gave the participants opportunities to express their frustration and break down inner and outward oppressions. This was an important transition, given Boal (1998) and Freire's (1998) assertion that people who perceive themselves to be locked into disempowered situations might become destructive.

While we have described the participants as invisible within the broader society, another possibility is that those who were homeless were, in fact, visible but negatively stereotyped. Social stereotypes contain power that builds oppression, particularly when other members of society perceive a group as posing a threat to safety or economic and social stability (Pollard & Kronenberg, 2008). The performances of the asylum seekers and homeless participants eliminated some of those stereotypes and their resultant oppression. The participants were perceived to be individuals rather than a homogeneous group through the public self-representation which evidenced their abilities (Pollard & Kronenberg, 2008).

The societal level: building connections

Theatre can be considered a form of entertainment (similar to poetry, song and dance) (Scott, 2009), but also has a more political form, as it has been used to empower people (Boal, 1998; Johnstone, 1979). The findings reveal how creative activities can support people living in vulnerable situations to handle challenges encountered in everyday life. Perhaps more important, theatre created bonds between the participants and their local community. This outcome showcases the complex structures of everyday occupations and how they are influenced by ecology, power, geography, politics and historical context. Through participation in theatre, the participants learned skills related to the associated activities as well as strategies to handle everyday occupations. These activities were performed in groups, and provided possibilities to learn from other participants. It was these activities that gave the participants and their audience the possibility of taking the step from alienation to social connection.

Conclusion

This chapter presented knowledge about the transformative potential of participation in theatre activities; how it activated changes of personal, social and societal aspects of everyday life occupations. Further, it presented how people's experiences of occupational injustice can be communicated through theatre, and how this can lead to tolerance and respect for "the others". The chapter contributes to understanding how people in vulnerable circumstances can be empowered to participate in their community through the act of doing. However, that can only happen when members of the community acknowledge their vulnerability, come to know them, and because of that, support their participation in the social, economic and cultural life of the community.

References

Becker, K 2004, 'Perspectives for the study of visual culture', *Nordisk Pedagogic*, vol. 24, pp. 242–249.

Befring-rapporten, NOU, 2004:23. *Barnehjem og sentralskoler under lupen. Nasjonal kartlegging av omsorgssvikt og overgrep i barnevernsinstitusjoner 1945–1980*, Statens forvaltningstjeneste, Informasjonsforvaltning, Oslo, Norway.

Blair, SE 2000, 'The centrality of occupation during life transitions', *British Journal of Occupational Therapy*, vol. 63, no. 5, pp. 231–237.

Boal, A 1998, *Legislative theatre: Using performance to make politics*, Routledge, London.

Borell, L, Asaba, E, Rosenberg, L, Schult, M & Townsend, E 2006, 'Exploring experiences of participation among individuals living with chronic pain', *Scandinavian Journal of Occupational Therapy*, vol. 13, no. 2, pp. 76–85. doi:10.1080/11038120600673023.

Briar, KH 1980, 'Helping the unemployed client', *Journal of Sociology and Social Welfare*, vol. 7, pp. 895–906.

Bruner, J 1986, *Actual minds, possible worlds*, Harvard University Press, Cambridge, MA.

Christiansen, C & Townsend, E 2010, 'The occupational nature of social groups' in *Introduction to occupation: The art and science of living*, 2nd edn, eds C Christiansen & E Townsend, Prentice Hall, Thorofare, NJ, pp. 175–210.

Creek, J 2009, *Occupational therapy and mental health*, Churchill Livingstone Elsevier, Philadelphia, PA.

DePoy, E & Gitlin, LN 2015, *Introduction to research: Understanding and applying multiple strategies*, 5th edn, Elsevier Health Sciences, St. Louis, Missouri.

Diba, D & d'Oliveira, AF 2015, 'Community theatre as social support for youth: Agents in the promotion of health', *Ciência & Saúde Coletiva*, vol. 20, no. 5, pp. 1353–1362.

Freire, P 1998, *Pedagogy of freedom: Ethics, democracy and civic courage*, Rowman & Littlefield, Lanham, MD.

Gavrielides, T 2014, October, 'Mapping of barriers to social inclusion of young people in vulnerable situations', *Presentation at Erasmus+ Civil Society Cooperation*, Strasbourg. Available from http://iars.org.uk/sites/default/files/Mapping%20of%20Barriers%20 to%20Social%20Inclusion%20of%20Young%20People%20in%20Vulnerable%20Situations%20Presentation_%20T.G_IARS.pdf.

Goffman, E 2012, 'The presentation of self in everyday life', originally published 1959, in *Contemporary Sociological Theory*, 3rd edn, eds C Calhun, J Gertis, J Moody, S Pfaff & I Virk, Wiley-Blackwell, Chichester, UK, pp. 46–61.

Gray, R, Sinding, C, Ivonoffski, V, Fitch, M, Hampson, A & Greenberg, M 2000, 'The use of research-based theatre in a project related to metastatic breast cancer', *Health Expectations*, vol. 3, no. 2, pp. 137–144.

Hacking, S, Secker, J, Spandler, H, Kent, L & Shenton, J 2008, 'Evaluating the impact of participatory art projects for people with mental health needs', *Health and Social Care in the Community*, vol. 16, no. 6, pp. 638–648. doi:10.1111/j.1365–2524.2008.00789.x.

Heenan, D 2006, 'Art as therapy: An effective way of promoting positive mental health? *Disability & Society*, vol. 21, no. 2, pp. 179–191. doi:10.1080/09687590500498143.

Horghagen, S 2012, 'Theatre as meaning making of the self', *Ergoterapeuten*, vol 2, pp. 54–60.

Horghagen, S & Josephsson, S 2010, 'Theatre as liberation, collaboration and relationship for asylum seekers', *Journal of Occupational Science*, vol. 17, no. 3, pp. 168–176.

Howells, V & Zelnik, T 2009, 'Making art: A qualitative study of personal and group transformation in a community arts studio', *Psychiatric Rehabilitation Journal*, vol. 32, no. 3, pp. 215–222. doi:10.2975/32.3.2009.215.222.

Johnstone, K 1979, *IMPR: improvisation and the theatre*, Methuen Publishing, London.

Kaptani, E & Yuval-Davis, N 2008, 'Participatory theatre as a research methodology: Identity, performance and social action among refugees', *Sociological Research*, vol. 13, no. 5(2). doi:10.5153/sro.1789.

Kielhofner, G 2008, *Model of human occupation: Theory and application*, 4th edn, Williams & Wilkins, Philadelphia.

Kwon, M 2004, *One place after another: Site-specific art and locational identity*, MIT Press, Cambridge, MA.

Langer, SK 1966, 'The cultural importance of the arts', *Journal of Aesthetic Education*, vol. 1, no. 1, pp. 5–12.

Mead, S, Hilton, D & Curtis, L 2001, 'Peer support: A theoretical perspective', *Psychiatric Rehabilitation Journal*, vol. 25, no. 2, p. 134.

Molineux, M 2011, 'Standing firm on shifting sands', *New Zealand Journal of Occupational Therapy*, vol. 58, no. 1, p. 21.

Polkinghorne, DE 1996, 'Transformative narratives: From victimic to agentic life plots', *American Journal of Occupational Therapy*, vol. 50, no. 4, pp. 299–305.

Pollard, N & Kronenberg, F 2008, 'Working with people on the margins' in *Occupational therapy and mental health*, 4th edn, eds J Creek & L Lougher, Churchill Livingstone Elsevier, Oxford, pp. 557–577.

Rowe, N 2004, 'The drama of doing: Occupation in the here and now', *Journal of Occupational Science*, vol. 11, pp. 95–104.

Sagan, O 2012, 'Connection and reparation: Narratives of art practice in the lives of mental health service users', *Counselling Psychology Quarterly*, vol. 25, no. 3, pp. 239–249. doi: 10.1080/09515070.2012.703128.

Saldana, J 2005, *An anthology of reality theatre*, AltaMira Press, Walnut Creek, CA.

Scott, S 2009, *Making sense of everyday life*, Polity Press, Cambridge.

SHD: St.meld. nr. 25. 1996/97, *Åpenhet og helhet* (The Norwegian government's White Paper on mental illness and mental health services), Sosial- og Helsedepartementet, Oslo.

Sinclair, K 2006, 'Occupational therapy worldwide: WFOT', *Australian Occupational Therapy Journal*, vol. 53, pp. 149–150.

Sloman, A 2011, 'Using participatory theatre in international community development', *Community Development Journal*, vol. 47, no. 1, pp. 42–57. doi:10.1093/cdj/bsq059.

Smith, HC 2005, 'Feel the fear and do it anyway: Meeting the occupational needs of refugees and people seeking asylum', *British Journal of Occupational Therapy*, vol. 68, no. 10, pp. 474–476.

Sonn, CC, Quayle, AF, Belanji, B & Baker, AM 2015, 'Responding to racialization through arts practice: The case of participatory theatre', *Journal of Community Psychology*, vol. 43, no. 2, pp. 244–259.

Sullivan, J & Lloyd, RS 2006, 'The forum theatre of Augusto Boal: A dramatic model for dialogue and community-based environmental science', *Local Environment*, vol. 11, no. 6, pp. 627–646.

Thompson, J 2003, *Applied theatre: Bewilderment and beyond*, Peter Lang AG, European Academic Publishers, Bern.

Townsend, E 1997, 'Occupation: Potential for personal and social transformation', *Journal of Occupational Science*, vol. 4, no. 1, pp. 18–26.

United Nations 1948, *Universal declaration of human rights*, United Nations, Geneva.

United Nations 2006, *Convention on the rights of persons with disabilities*, The United Nations General Assembly resolution 60/232 of 23 December, United Nations, Geneva.

Van Lith, T, Schofield, MJ & Fenner, P 2013, 'Identifying the evidence-base for art-based practices and their potential benefit for mental health recovery: A critical review', *Disability and Rehabilitation*, vol. 35, no. 16, pp. 1309–1323. doi:10.3109/09638288.2012.732188.

Watson, R, Tucker, L & Drury, S 2014, 'Can we make a difference? examining the transformative potential of sport and active recreation' in *Diversity, equity and inclusion in sport and leisure*, eds K Dashper & T Fletcher, Routledge, New York, NY, pp. 7–21.

Whiteford, GE 2000, 'Occupational deprivation: Global challenge in the new millennium', *British Journal of Occupational Therapy*, vol. 63, no. 5, pp. 200–204.

Whiteford, GE & Hocking, C eds 2012, *Occupational science: Society, inclusion, participation*, Wiley-Blackwell, Oxford, UK.

Whiteford, GE & Pereira, RB 2012, 'Visioning a way forward' in *Occupational science: Society, inclusion, participation*, eds GE Whiteford & C Hocking, Wiley-Blackwell, Oxford, UK, pp. 187–209.

Wilcock, AA 2006, *An occupational perspective of health*, 2nd edn, Slack, Thorofare, New Jersey.

Wilcock, AA & Hocking, C 2015, *An occupational perspective of health*, 3rd edn, Slack, Thorofare, NJ.

Witsø, AE, Eide, AH & Vik, K 2011, 'Professional carers' perspectives on participation for older adults living in place', *Disability and Rehabilitation*, vol. 33, no. 7, pp. 557–568.

World Health Organization 2001, 'Mental health: New understanding, new hope', *World Health Report. 2001*, World Health Organization, Geneva.

World Health Organization, Health and Welfare Canada, Canadian Public Health Association 1986, *Ottawa charter for health promotion*, WHO, Ottawa, Canada.

Yerxa, E, Clark, F, & Frank, G 1990, 'An introduction to occupational science: A foundation for occupational therapy in the 21st century', *Occupational Therapy in Heath Care*, vol. 6, pp. 1–17.

12 Impacts on work participation of people with mental health disability

Klara Jakobsen, Rosemary Lysaght and Terry Krupa

Introduction

Life goals and opportunities, including work and employment, can be impacted by the presence of a mental health disability due to both functional and participation challenges arising from the health condition, and to environmental obstacles associated with unaccommodating and unwelcoming social environments. Yet, evidence suggests that despite these many challenges, given opportunity and supportive conditions, most people with mental health disabilities would choose to work (OECD 2012a). In addition, work is gaining recognition as an important enabler of recovery, with potential to positively impact on confidence, self-worth, social integration and socioeconomic status (Dunn, Wewiorski & Rogers 2008). These are important drivers for ongoing efforts to enhance work participation.

The purpose of this chapter is to examine the human and environmental factors that influence work participation for people with serious mental illness, and by considering the situation from a variety of philosophical perspectives, to both highlight innovative and successful interventions, and envision novel approaches. The complexity and nuances of these interventions will be highlighted by contrasting the situation of persons with and without workforce attachment, who may experience very different environmental conditions and resources as they strive to achieve satisfying work participation.

The imperative for addressing work participation

The UN Convention on the Rights of Persons with Disabilities (2007) asserts *the right of persons with disabilities to work, on an equal basis with others. This includes the right to the opportunity to gain a living by work freely chosen or accepted in a labour market and work environment that is open, inclusive and accessible to persons with disabilities* (Article 27). Yet, many people with mental health disabilities are not realising this right, and this problem is prevalent across developed societies.

Around 20% of the working-age population in an average Organisation for Economic Co-operation and Development (OECD) country (OECD 2012b) lives with a diagnosable mental health disorder. Most of these individuals are affected by common mental illnesses, such as anxiety and depression (OECD 2014), but around 5% have a serious mental illness, determined both by the presence of a diagnosed mental illness and some form of functional impairment which substantially impacts one or more major life activities. Those with reported mental health disorders are less likely to be employed, and much more likely to be unemployed than persons without mental health disorders. The lack of workforce participation is even more pronounced among individuals who experience serious mental illness, with statistics indicating that in Europe, only 10–20% of that population is employed (Catty et al. 2008). An exit from working life due to a mental health disability can have life-changing implications for the individual, but it also represents a critical social and economic challenge for developed economies. Evidence suggests that people with mental illnesses represent approximately one-third of the people supported financially by government disability benefits (Danziger, Frank & Meara 2009). Work-related disabilities, based on mental health-related conditions, have been on the rise in recent years, and have been reported to constitute the greatest source of disability claims in a number of jurisdictions (OECD 2012a; WHO 2004). Further, the underemployment of people with mental illnesses means that societies, both developed and developing, are not benefiting from the socioeconomic contributions of a significant number of citizens, and ultimately calls into question the extent to which societies are meeting their human rights obligations (Krupa et al. 2009).

Efforts to ensure that people with mental health disabilities gain access to work that meets or exceeds fair and equitable standards for employment have generally lagged behind those directed towards people with disabilities that are primarily physical in nature (Bruyere, Erickson & VanLooy 2004; Hoefsmit, Houkes & Nijhuis 2012; MacDonald-Wilson et al. 2002). There are several reasons for this. Studies of the stigma of mental illness in employment indicate that assumptions about the competence, predictability and legitimacy of people with mental illness can lead to exclusionary attitudes and behaviours from employers and workmates. This can lead to affected individuals being ignored, shunned or directly rejected, and denied progression and advancement on the job (Krupa et al. 2009). Social exclusion is often the hardest barrier to overcome and can be associated with feelings of shame, fear and rejection (Corrigan & Wassel 2008). Beyond stigma, the relatively recent growth of a knowledge-based economy also contributes to exclusion. The knowledge concerning how to best accommodate physical capabilities of workers is well known, but is lacking for workers with mental health disabilities (Bruyere, Erickson & BanLooy 2004).

Labour market participation by people with mental illness – a complex picture

The relationship that individuals have with the labour market can be markedly different depending on the nature of the mental health disability, the age of onset and the opportunities an individual has relative to career development. The following section defines two broad categories to describe the labour market attachment of people with mental illness.

Persons lacking workforce attachment

People with weak or absent workforce attachment have few of the connections and resources that facilitate access to sustained employment. Their employment profile may be characterised by *personal challenges* such as reduced self-esteem, self-efficacy and coping resources that enable work participation; and *occupational issues* such as limited work experiences that provide a solid preparation for working. *Environmental factors* such as limited networks that connect them to work might also have a negative effect if family and other social connections are not supportive of employment. In addition, lack of instrumental resources like clothing, grooming supplies and transportation might have an influence. These factors combined suggest that people with mental health disabilities who have weak or absent workforce attachment have a competitive disadvantage when it comes to securing and maintaining work.

People with serious mental illnesses acquired early in life are perhaps the most significantly barriered group with respect to workforce participation. For individuals living with major mental disorders such as schizophrenia and major affective disorders, the onset of the health condition is often during late adolescence and the years of career entry. This leads to further negative impact due to disrupted career trajectories early in their working lives. In this way, the process of marginalisation from the workforce can begin early, when the experience of mental health disability negatively affects successful completion of basic education and/or workforce training. This is particularly an issue in contemporary knowledge-based economies where knowledge and educational achievement is a growing expectation as a valued human resource for employment (Baron & Salzer 2002). The transition from school to work can be challenging when mental illness affects the development of cognitive, social and academic skills, and thereby compromises these individuals' opportunities for early work experiences. Measures to prevent early school leaving and reintegration of young people into the labour market and education is therefore a matter of high priority. However, young people with mental health disability today are increasingly moving into the disability benefit system, and many stay on benefits throughout their lifetime without ever entering the workforce (Eurofund 2012; Knapp, McDaid & Mossialos 2006; OECD 2012a).

People with serious mental illness who are marginalised from the workforce often experience difficulties across many life domains. Not only do they experience functional impacts of the mental disorder, they often *live under conditions of poverty* that negatively affect health and well-being. They can be subject to victimisation in their communities, compromising their freedom of movement and safety. They may further experience poor housing conditions and insufficient housing stability, factors that provide a foundation for work participation. They typically receive some form of government financial support based on their disability that may socially define them as 'not employable', and that comes with regulations related to allowable earnings. These regulations can place individuals in an untenable situation, because they may actually perceive their financial situation as threatened by employment and subsequently be exceptionally cautious about pursuing employment. This situation is often referred to as *the disability trap* (Stapleton et al. 2006).

Persons with mental illness who have workforce attachment

Compared to people without workforce attachment, persons with mental illness who are attached have only recently been the subject of much discussion in scholarly, practice and policy circles. Many people who experience mental illness are employed, and in fact may hold high-level jobs and are well established in good career paths. With the rise in work-related mental health disability claims and disability leave, there has been growing attention to workplace factors that may be contributing to these work absences. Workplace disability related to mental health has, for example, been associated with high levels of workplace demand and overwork (Waghorn & Chant 2011), and stressful aspects of the work itself (Crompton 2011; OECD 2012a).

While some workers experiencing mental health disabilities will take related long-term leave, many will sustain their employment even while dealing with symptoms or other experiences associated with their mental health condition. In this case, the individual may be present at work but experience 'presenteeism', meaning they are present but not fully engaged in work tasks or situations. Evidence suggests that mental illness, and in particular depression, is one of the leading causes of high costs associated with presenteeism in employment (Goetzel et al. 2004).

For individuals with mental illness who sustain their workforce attachment, work-related decisions will be influenced by many factors. For example, in situations where a worker and his/her family depend on the income from employment, there will be considerable pressure to maintain paid employment. In cases where promotions or career advancement are important to the individual, this can impact decisions related to disclosure of the mental illness, help-seeking and applying for medical leave. When co-workers are also friends outside the workplace, this can influence decisions related to any change in job status. All these situations can be influenced by the extent to which the employee holds self-stigma, a situation where the individual internalises negative stereotypes about mental illness and acts in a self-discriminatory manner characterised by shame (Corrigan & Rao 2012).

Individuals with mental illness can be considered 'attached' to the workforce whether they sustain their ongoing employment activities or leave the workplace on sickness benefits. However, those who are on disability leave from employment are at high risk of long-term marginalisation if the absence from the workforce is protracted and efforts to return to work are not successful.

Situating contemporary responses to mental health disability and work

Disability has been conceptualised in a number of ways, and those philosophical paradigms suggest particular strategies or approaches to the employment conundrum. A summary of the prevalent models of disability, and how they shape thinking towards disability and work, is presented in Table 12.1.

Table 12.1 A summary of prevalent models of disability

Conceptual Model	Underlying Beliefs	Interpretation Relative to Workers with Mental Health Disabilities	Employment Approach Based on Model
Biomedical	Disability is a biomedical issue residing in the individual and resulting in functional impairment. Pathology can be managed or eliminated through the use of medical or rehabilitative therapies.	• Interventions should be directed towards improving function. • Medical determination of work incapacity is a valid response in chronic conditions. • Work tasks should be matched to worker capacity.	• Ongoing pharmaceutical or psychotherapeutic treatment for worker. • Disability compensation for workers whose impairments preclude regular employment. • Individual placement and support in work settings for those seen as competitively employable.
Socio-Political	Social participation is limited by lack of opportunity and oppressive social forces.	• Stigma is a predominant barrier to achieving optimal employment. • Workplace structures should be managed to accommodate worker differences and create opportunity. • People with mental health disabilities can create their own conditions for working.	• Workplace anti-stigma interventions. • Anti-discrimination laws. • Human resources strategies including supportive counselling and accommodated work. • Advent of individual and collective models of empowerment, including worker cooperatives, social enterprises and micro-enterprise.
Economic	People with disabilities are seen as a financial liability due to their support needs and their inability to contribute to the economy.	• Cost burden of disability can be reduced by engaging people with mental health disabilities in work to the extent their disability will allow.	• Disability support payment schemes. • Encouragement of work participation to the point of (societal) cost-benefit.

(*Continued*)

Table 12.1 (Continued)

Conceptual Model	Underlying Beliefs	Interpretation Relative to Workers with Mental Health Disabilities	Employment Approach Based on Model
Philanthropic/ Charity	People with disabilities are seen as passive victims of their impairments who should be cared for by society. May depend on the degree to which the individual is seen as the agent of his or her own destiny (i.e. perceived legitimacy of illness).	• Perpetuates views of people with disabilities as lacking agency and power. • Removes expectations of self-sufficiency and the need to work.	• Disability support payment. • Support of commercial ventures involving people with mental health disability as recognition of effort and admiration.

Biomedical models of disability situate the work challenge in the individual and assume that a medical response is the means to overcome functional impairment (Depoy & Gilson, 2004; McColl & Bickenbach 1998; Smart 2009). While paradoxically this approach is validating and can be reaffirming for people with mental health disabilities who have been subjected to a sense of personal responsibility for their illness, it is particularly disempowering in another sense, in that medicalising the condition shifts responsibility for disability management and recovery to healthcare providers. In addition, the medical provider holds the key to eligibility for disability benefits (Smart 2009).

From this perspective, people with mental health disabilities who are employed are typically removed from the workplace and provided with sickness benefits until treatment of their condition allows them to return to work, and/or accommodations may be provided, to reduce the demands of work that may contribute to symptom exacerbation. For persons lacking workplace attachment, vocational rehabilitation aims at improving their employability if they are seen as ultimately being a candidate for work in a competitive employment market. Those seen as having persistent and severe illness are deemed unable to work and are provided ongoing disability financial support.

Socio-political models of disability, which situate the disability in the social response to impairment and functional differences, are aligned with the consumer movement, and the view that individuals can be the agents of their own destiny. From this vantage point, disability is part of the human diversity and not something to be 'normalised' (Depoy & Gilson 2004; McColl & Bickenbach 1998;

Smart 2009). Adherents to this model will direct their interest towards stigma, pre-conceptions of employment potential, and employer willingness to provide accommodation and supportive workplace structures (Smart 2009). This perspective also supports the notion that people with mental health disabilities may wish to embrace their differences, both their assets and challenges, and create their own work opportunities through small business development and worker co-operatives.

The economic model of disability considers disability as a burden that requires either costly treatment and accommodation, or ongoing individual financial support. From an employment perspective, the debate becomes a cost-benefit analysis weighing the costs of accommodation against the reduced burden in terms of disability payments. For an employer, there are a number of economic advantages and disadvantages to consider relative to hiring or retaining workers with mental health disabilities. If an employee is established within an organisation, human capital such as workplace-specific skills, knowledge and loyalties are resources that will be of importance in decisions on whether to retain an employee or not. It may be advantageous to keep an employee if work capacity remains at a reasonable level such that the worker contributes more than the costs of accommodation, and the employer may see less financial advantage in hiring a new employee who requires accommodation unless that employee holds potential for long-term retention and high productivity. The reputational advantages that may be associated with employing workers with disabilities are less clear in the instance of mental health disability, where the impairment is often less visible or definable.

Finally, *the philanthropic or charity model* merits mention here, as this view underlies social policy concerning disability support payments. This type of support is seen as compensation for intractable incapacity and a means of correcting social inequity. Social support for this model is weaker for disabilities that are perceived as self-inflicted, or when the disability lacks credibility.

How employment challenges are currently addressed

Efforts in the area of *service provision* are rapidly advancing. Interventions have been developed for those with mental health disabilities who have experienced employment marginalisation and are unattached to an employer, and for those who are sustaining employment or intending to return to work. In order to establish positive workplace connections and employment experiences for persons who lack workforce attachment and are employment-marginalised, explicit principles have been developed for service providers to ensure that interventions are targeting fair and equitable employment within the broader community. The approach 'supported employment' includes six underlying principles: (1) maintaining a focus on competitive employment, (2) ensuring that eligibility for services is based on consumer choice, (3) rapid job search and placement, (4) integration of rehabilitation and mental health services, (5) attention to consumer preferences in the selection of jobs and supports, and (6) time-unlimited and individualised support (Bond 2004). These principles have been developed specifically to counter traditional biomedical approaches that have assumed that long-term pre-vocational training and rehabilitation are necessary to prepare people for employment. By directing service interventions, the aim is assertively to integrate people with mental illness into work situations in their communities while providing them with focused support (Burns et al. 2007; Crowther et al. 2001).

In the mental health system, the most widely studied form of supported employment is the Individual Placement and Support (IPS) model (Bond 2004). In the IPS model, a team of employment support staff work collaboratively with individuals with mental illness who have been marginalised from employment. By facilitating their expressed interest in employment, the people with mental illness are assertively integrated into situations in the community while providing them with focused support. IPS services are guided by a set of fidelity criteria to facilitate the faithful implementation of the approach, as well as a range of practice resources to inform service development and provider practices (Bond 2004).

Recently the application of supported employment programs has been extended to young people who experience their first episodes of mental illness, and there are concerns about the potential course of the disorder. There is a strong emphasis on keeping youth connected to work to avoid marginalisation and enable a positive vocational career trajectory. The model of supported employment for this population has also been modified to include supported education, with a view to providing an assertive approach to sustaining their engagement in education and training as a foundation for future careers. These models of supported education and employment for youth, based in the socio-political ideology, have demonstrated positive outcomes compared to those receiving the usual mental health services (Bond, Drake & Luciano 2015).

Other approaches to addressing employment marginalisation among people with serious mental illness have been directed to actually *creating employment opportunities* within the broader community. Social firms or work integration social enterprises (WISEs) are like conventional businesses in that they produce and exchange goods and services in a marketplace. In addition to their economic goals, they are intended to create employment and entrepreneurial opportunities for marginalised groups, and have been widely deployed among people with mental health disabilities (Lysaght, Jakobsen & Granhaug 2012; Warner & Mandiberg 2006). To the extent that they are developed as legitimate business ventures, WISEs can be viewed as real work experiences with the potential to develop work-related knowledge and skills that are valued by the workforce (Krupa et al. 2016). Newer approaches to employment generation are promoted in various ways. They may be proactive means of reducing economic demand on the social system, as charitable, socially beneficial services drawing on the benevolent support of the general public. Moreover, in the case of consumer-run businesses, they may act as entities that create a socio-political advantage and empowerment for the persons with mental illnesses.

Similarly, microcredit approaches are based on the idea that through the creation of small, low-interest loans, many individuals with mental health disabilities can build their own entrepreneurial skills by developing ideas for products or services into self-directed businesses (Yunus 2011). These microcredit approaches largely originated in international anti-poverty initiatives, particularly in developing countries where they are considered potentially powerful means of development by building the capacities of those who are poor and disenfranchised. However, they have since been applied in developed countries to address the social-economic needs of groups of people who experience poverty and social exclusion, including those with mental health disabilities (Kreimer-Eis & Conforti 2009). Finally, the development of specialist peer positions within the mental health system has led to a new job classification which defines lived experience of mental illness as a resource and strength to be used to enable health and well-being of others in the system. Not only are these new positions viewed as a means to add significant value to the mental health service system, they also provide affirmative employment positions embedded within integrated employment structures.

Overall, this movement to assertive approaches to enable rapid and supported entry to employment positions for persons with mental health disabilities who are marginalised is being extended throughout the mental health systems of many countries. These approaches challenge the biomedical approach, identifying participation as a right, and demanding environmental change. For example, evidence-based community services, such as Assertive Community Treatment, Strengths-Based Case Management and Peer-Support Initiatives, are being used to help engage people with serious mental illness who experience long-term unemployment in considering work participation and to ensure that they receive the interventions that are likely to sustain work participation (Gold et al. 2006).

Interventions are expanding rapidly, but they are still in the early stages of development and implementation for employees with mental health disabilities who are employed or on disability leave from their positions. These approaches are similar to those applied to people who are employment-marginalised and/or unattached to the workforce, in that they are oriented to promoting worker choice and involvement, keeping people at work and/or reducing the amount of time on work-related disability leave. This responds to the evidence that lengthy separation from work reduces the chances that workers will return from sick leave, and that work separation can influence self-confidence and relationships with co-workers and supervisors. To increase chances of a successful return to work, the interventions must be consistent with contemporary disability management practices. Proactive supportive processes and accommodations will encourage a workplace-based orientation dependent on assertive communication between health and rehabilitation service providers, the employee, the employer and workplace management structures (American College of Occupational and Environmental Medicine 2006; Franche et al. 2005; Jakobsen & Lillefjell 2014).

A range of *person-focused intervention approaches* to enable a return to work in the context of mental illness has emerged. As workers with depression continue to experience functional impairments even after the lifting of depressive symptoms, a cognitive work hardening program providing an opportunity for participants to engage in individualised work-related tasks and dealing with common functional issues is developed (Lagerveld et al. 2012; Wisenthal & Krupa 2014).

Other services have delivered work-focused cognitive behavioural therapy in conjunction with workplace interventions, including time management and priority setting (Lystad et al. 2016; Rose & Perz 2005). Still others have combined clinical treatment interventions, such as medications and psychotherapy, with rehabilitation interventions (such as occupational therapy) and with work-focused interventions (Hees, de Vries & Koeter 2013).

A growing interest has been seen in developing and evaluating specific individual-level interventions that can complement strategies concentrating on worker empowerment. Individual training and counselling may be useful in ensuring that people are fully aware of the rules and their rights with regards to disability benefits, with a view to supporting work participation (Tremblay et al. 2006). Furthermore, supporting workers to manage disclosure of their mental health disability is receiving increasing attention. This concerns both helping workers understand and reflect on the options that are open to them, and advancing an understanding of how employment-related supports and services can be offered regardless of the disclosure decision (Allott et al. 2013; Toth & Dewa 2014).

At the *policy level*, the World Health Organisation (2000) has recognised the importance of making mental health and work a top priority internationally, and highlighted the need for countries to strengthen relevant policies and legislation. Governments are increasingly committed to reducing the burden associated with mental health problems and to enabling the development and implementation of best practices in employment services and support. The rights of people with mental health disabilities are explicitly identified in policies, rules and regulations in many countries. For example, policies protecting the rights of workers with disabilities to reasonable work accommodations are widespread. Ultimately, familiarity with not just the law related to reasonable accommodations, but also to the broad range of potential accommodations, will influence the extent to which people with mental health disabilities experience work equity (Schultz et al. 2011).

The link between work and mental health has attracted substantial *research interest*. Practical applications of this research-based knowledge include the development of standards for psychological safety in the workplace (Shain, Arnold & GermAnn 2012), interventions to reduce the stigma of mental illness in the workplace, promotion of help-seeking among employees in distress, and ensuring supportive and equitable workplace policies and practices. Szeto and Dobson (2010) systematically reviewed stigma interventions and identified a broad range of approaches being implemented internationally. While these anti-stigma interventions use a wide range of learning strategies, like teaching about mental illness, increasing awareness of the presence of mental health issues, and building coping and communication strategies, one approach in particular, namely contact-based education, has demonstrated effectiveness. This involves developing opportunities for employees to have direct contact with someone who speaks openly about their experience of mental illness in a manner that personalises the issue to encourage empathy, and demonstrates hope and recovery (Shepherd, Boardman & Slade 2008).

Shifting the response – rethinking work and mental illness

Work is a complex social construct, and the International Classification of Status in Employment (ICSE) identifies five different classifications for work participation: (1) paid work in an employer-employee relationship, (2) self-employment, (3) serving as a member of a workers' co-operative, (4) working in family-owned businesses, and (5) other types of work, for instance workers in educational and training situations and in the voluntary sector (ILO 1993).

In addition to these socially recognised forms of employment, there are parallel economies that are socially prevalent but not formally recognised. For people who are marginalised from recognised forms of work, including those with mental health disabilities, these less-recognised forms of work may be an integral part of their daily lives and an important means of subsistence. In some cases, these work activities may be socially acceptable forms of trade, such as collecting recyclable products for profit, but they may include socially illegitimate forms of activity, such as begging or the sale of drugs, including prescribed medications.

Individuals involved in the parallel economy are vulnerable to crime, personal injury and poor health, but they may persist in the work due to its financial/economic benefits. They are not typically considered in our understanding of individual productivity despite the work often requiring considerable skills and energy (Kindle & Caplan 2015). To the extent that the work activities of people with mental health disabilities are ignored, their potential will be underestimated and low expectations for employment are likely to prevail.

A new dialogue and means of framing the approach to work and mental illness is necessary if societies are to move towards inclusion and optimisation of human potential. Overall, the social response to disability is shaped by prevailing beliefs, and has led to the combination of strategies described above. If fair and equitable opportunities for paid work are to be extended to people with mental health disabilities, we need to move further towards adoption of a social model of disability that recognises the strengths and weaknesses of other models, and tackles inconsistencies and system failures. Critical dialogues are required relative to employment and mental illness, in particular including the following points:

- How do we effectively reduce the stigma of mental illness?
- How can workers with mental health disabilities best be empowered to be agents of their own futures?
- How do we define careers in contemporary terms that respond to the multiplicity of work types and employment situations?
- Are there ways to recognise and advance social capital using an asset-based approach to employment and career planning?

Conclusions

Mental health disability presents some of the greatest challenges to workforce participation. Recognition of the magnitude of mental health disability suggests that failure to harness the productive potential of this population represents a sizable loss to our economies and social structures. A broad range of factors are associated with the reduced productive engagement of people with mental health issues, and these may be understood by considering the ways in which individual and environmental factors intersect to create or remove participation barriers. Those participation challenges may present quite differently for those who are workforce-attached and have certain individual and environmental advantages to draw upon, and those who lack current or past employment attachment and are severely employment-marginalized.

Society's response to this issue reflects the different philosophical attitudes to disability that have emerged historically, and most of these are still active today. A number of strategies and best practices have thus evolved, and these have effectively moved people with mental health disabilities from being sheltered in community-based employment, and instigated the accommodation of disability in the workplace as a legal and moral requirement. Much remains to be done, however, if we are to achieve the work participation goals of fairness and equity as outlined by the UN's Convention on the Rights of Persons with Disabilities.

A broad-based approach is needed that is based on personal, social, political and economic factors, allowing flexible work options and acknowledging the need for a strategic shift. Given the diversity of the sizable population with mental health disabilities, one approach cannot fit all, yet many options are possible. We need to exploit these various options and work towards empowering people to believe in the possibility of participation in whatever form is supportive of optimal mental health.

References

Allott, KA, Turner, LR, Chinnery, GL, Killackey, EJ, & Nuechterlein, KH 2013, 'Managing disclosure following recent-onset psychosis: Utilizing the individual placement and support model', *Early Intervention in Psychiatry*, vol. 7, no. 3, pp. 338–344.

American College of Occupational and Environmental Medicine 2006, 'Preventing needless work disability by helping people stay employed', *Journal of Occupational & Environmental Medicine*, vol. 48, no. 9, pp. 972–987.

Baron, RC & Salzer, MS 2002, 'Behavioral sciences and the law', *Behavioral Science & Law*, vol. 20, pp. 585–599.

Bond, GR 2004, 'Supported employment: Evidence for an evidence based practice', *Psychiatric Rehabilitation Journal*, vol. 27, pp. 345–359.

Bond, GR, Drake, RE, & Luciano, A 2015, 'Employment and educational outcomes in early intervention programmes for early psychosis: A systematic review', *Epidemiology and Psychiatric Sciences*, vol. 24, no. 5, pp. 446–457.

Bruyere, SM, Erickson, W, & VanLooy, S 2004, 'Comparative study of workplace policy and practices contributing to disability nondiscrimination', *Rehabilitation Psychology*, vol. 49, no. 1, pp. 28–38.

Burns T, Catty J, Becker T, Drake RE, Fioritti A, Knapp M, Lauber C, Rössler W, Tomov T, van Busschbach J, White S, & Wiersma D. 2007, 'The effectiveness of supported employment for people with severe mental illness: A randomised controlled trial', *Lancet*, vol. 370, pp. 1146–1152.

Catty, J, Lissouba P, White S, Becker T, Drake RE, Fioritti A, Knapp M, Lauber C, Rössler W, Tomov T, van Busschbach J, Wiersma D & Burns T 2008, 'Predictors of employment for people with severe mental illness: Results of an international six-centre randomised controlled trial', *The British Journal of Psychiatry*, vol. 192, no. 3, pp. 224–231.

Corrigan, PW & Rao, D 2012, 'On the self-stigma of mental illness: stages, disclosure, and strategies for change', *Canadian Journal of Psychiatry. Revue anadienne de psychiatrie*, vol. 57, no. 8, pp. 464–469.

Corrigan, PW & Wassel, A 2008, 'Understanding and influencing the stigma of mental illness', *Journal of Psychosocial Nursing*, vol. 48, no. 1, pp. 42–48.

Crompton, S 2011, *What's stressing the stressed? Main sources of stress among workers*. Ottawa: Statistics Canada. Available at: http://www.statcan.gc.ca/pub/11–008-x/2011002/article/11562-eng.htm [Accessed 10 May 2016].

Crowther, RE, Marshall, M, Bond, GR, & Huxley, P 2001, 'Helping people with severe mental illness to obtain work: Systematic review', *British Medical Journal*, vol. 322, pp. 204–208.

Danziger S, Frank RG, & Meara E 2009, 'Mental illness, work, and income support programs', *American Journal of Psychiatry*, vol. 166, no. 4, pp. 398–404.

Depoy, E & Gilson, SF 2004, *Rethinking disability: principles for professional and social change*. Belmont, CA: Thomson/Brooks/Cole.

Dunn, E, Wewiorski, NJ, & Rogers, ES 2008, 'The meaning and importance of employment to people in recovery from serious mental illness: Results of a qualitative study', *Psychiatric Rehabilitation Journal*, vol. 32, pp. 59–62.

Eurofund 2012, *NEETs – Young people not in employment, education or training: Characteristics, costs and policy responses in Europe*. Luxemburg: Publications Office of the European Union. Available at: http://www.eurofound.europa.eu/sites/default/files/ef_files/pubdocs/2011/72/en/2/EF1172EN.pdf [Accessed 20 January 2016]

Franche, RL, Cullen, K, Clarke, J, Irvin, E, Sinclair, S, Frank, J, & Institute for Work & Health (IWH) Workplace-Based RTW Intervention Literature Review Research Team 2005, 'Workplace-based return-to-work interventions: A systematic review of the quantitative literature', *Journal of Occupational Rehabilitation*, vol. 15, no. 4, pp. 607–631.

Goetzel, RZ, Long, SR, Ozminkowski, RJ, Hawkins, K, Wang, S, & Lynch, W 2004, 'Health, absence, disability, and presenteeism cost estimates of certain physical and mental health conditions affecting US employers', *Journal of Occupational and Environmental Medicine*, vol. 46, no. 4, pp. 398–412.

Gold, PB, Meisler, N, Santos, AB, Carnemolla, MA, Williams, OH, & Keleher, J 2006, 'Randomized trial of supported employment integrated with assertive community treatment for rural adults with severe mental illness', *Schizophrenia Bulletin*, vol. 32, no. 2, pp. 378–395.

Hees, H, de Vries, G, & Koeter, M 2013, 'Adjuvant occupational therapy improves long-term depression recovery and return-to-work in good health in sick-listed employees with major depression: results of a randomized controlled trial', *Occupational and Environmental Medicine*, vol. 70, no. 4, pp. 252–260.

Hoefsmit, N, Houkes, I, & Nijhuis, FJN 2012, 'Intervention characteristics that facilitate return to work after sickness absence: a systematic literature review', *Journal of Occupational Rehabilitaton*, vol. 22, no. 4, pp. 462–477.

International Labour Organization (ILO) 1993, *Fifteenth International Conference of Labour Statisticians, Report of the Conference*. ICLS/15/D.6 (Rev. 1). International Labour Office, Geneva 1993. [Accessed 20 January 2016]

Jakobsen, K & Lillefjell, M 2014, 'Factors promoting a successful return to work; from an employer and employee perspective', *Scandinavian Journal of Occupational Therapy*, vol. 21, pp. 48–57.

Kindle, PA & Caplan, MA 2015, 'Understanding fringe economic behavior: A Bourdieu-sian-informed meta-ethnography', *Journal of Sociology and Social Welfare*, vol. 42, no. 1, pp. 49–71.

Knapp, M, McDaid, D, & Mossialos, E 2006, *Mental health policy and practice across Europe*. Berkshire, UK: McGraw-Hill Education.

Kreimer-Eis, H & Conforti, A 2009, *Microfinance in Europe: a market overview*. Available at: http://www.eif.org/news_centre/publications/EIF_WP_2009_001_Microfinance.pdf [Accessed 10 May 2016]

Krupa, T, Howell-Moneta, A, Lysaght, R, & Kirsh, B 2016, 'Employer perceptions of the employability of workers in a social business', *Psychiatric Rehabilitation Journal*, vol. 39, no. 2, pp. 120–128.

Krupa, T, Kirsh, B, Cockburn, L, & Gewurtz, R 2009, 'Understanding the stigma of employment in mental illness', *Work*, vol. 33, pp. 413–425.

Lagerveld, SE, Blonk, RW, Brenninkmeijer, V, Wijngaards-de Meij, L, & Schaufeli, WB 2012, 'Work-focused treatment of common mental disorders and return to work: A comparative outcome study', *Journal of Occupational Health Psychology*, vol. 17, no. 2, pp. 220–234.

Lysaght, R, Jakobsen, K, & Granhaug, B 2012, 'Social firms: A means for building employment skills and community integration', *Work*, vol. 41, no. 4, pp. 455–463.

Lystad, JU, Falkum, E, Haaland, VØ, & Bull, H 2016, 'Neurocognition and occupational functioning in schizophrenia spectrum disorders: The MATRICS Consensus Cognitive Battery (MCCB) and workplace assessments', *Schizophrenia Research*, vol. 177, no. 1, pp. 143–149.

MacDonald-Wilson, KL, Rogers, ES, Massaro, JM, Lyass, A, & Crean, T 2002, 'An investigation of reasonable workplace accommodations for people with psychiatric disabilities: quantitative findings from a multi-site study', *Community Mental Health Journal*, vol. 38, no. 1, pp. 35–50.

McColl, MA & Bickenbach JE 1998, *Introduction to disability*. London: WB Saunders Company.

OECD 2012a, *Sick on the job? Myths and realities about mental health and work. Mental Health and Work*. Paris: OECD Publishing. Available at: http://dx.doi.org/10.1787/9789264124523-en [Accessed 20 January 2016]

OECD 2012b, *Sickness, disability and work: breaking the barriers. A synthesis of findings across OECD countries*. Paris: OECD Publishing. Available at: http://dx.doi.org/10.1787/9789264088856-en [Accessed 20 January 2016]

OECD 2014, Health policy studies. Making mental health count. The social and economic costs of neglecting mental health care. Paris: OECD Publishing. Available at: https://www.oecd.org/els/health-systems/Focus-on-Health-Making-Mental-Health-Count.pdf [Accessed 20 January 2016]

Rose, V & Perz, J 2005, 'Is CBT useful in vocational rehabilitation for people with a psychiatric disability?' *Psychiatric Rehabilitation Journal*, vol. 29, no. 1, pp. 56–58.

Schultz, IZ, Milner, RA, Hanson, DB, & Winter, A 2011, 'Employer attitudes towards accommodations in mental health disability', Chapter 17, pp. 325–340, in Schultz Z, Milner RA, Hanson DB & Winter A (Eds), *Work accommodation and retention in mental health*, New York: Springer.

Shain, M, Arnold, I, & GermAnn, K 2012, 'The road to psychological safety legal, scientific, and social foundations for a Canadian national standard on psychological safety in the workplace', *Bulletin of Science, Technology & Society*, vol. 32, no. 2, pp. 142–162.

Shepherd, G, Boardman, J, & Slade, M 2008, *Making recovery a reality*, Policy Paper, Sainsbury Centre for Mental Health, London.

Smart, J 2009, 'The power of models of disability', *Journal of Rehabilitation*, vol. 75, no. 2, pp. 3–11.

Stapleton, DC, O'Day, BL, Livermore, GA, & Imparato, AJ 2006, 'Dismantling the poverty trap: disability policy for the twenty-first century', *Milbank Quarterly*, vol. 84, no. 4, pp. 701–732.

Szeto, AC & Dobson, KS 2010, 'Reducing the stigma of mental disorders at work: A review of current workplace anti-stigma intervention programs', *Applied and Preventive Psychology*, vol. 14, no. 1, pp. 41–56.

Toth, KE & Dewa, CS 2014, 'Employee decision-making about disclosure of a mental disorder at work', *Journal of Occupational Rehabilitation*, vol. 24, no. 4, pp. 732–746.

Tremblay, T, Smith, J, Xie, H, & Drake, RE 2006, 'Effect of benefits counseling services on employment outcomes for people with psychiatric disabilities', *Psychiatric Services, Am Psychiatric Association*, vol. 57, no. 6, pp. 816–821.

UN General Assembly 2007, *Convention on the rights of persons with disabilities (CRPD): Resolution/adopted by the General Assembly*, 24 January 2007, A/RES/61/106. Available at: http://www.refworld.org/docid/45f973632.html [Accessed 20 January 2016]

Waghorn, G & Chant, D 2011, 'Overworking among people with psychiatric disorders: Results from a large community survey', *Journal of Occupational Rehabilitation*, vol. 22, no. 2, pp. 252–261.

Warner, R & Mandiberg, J 2006, 'An update on affirmative businesses or social firms for people with mental illness', *Psychiatric Services, Am Psychiatric Association*, vol. 57, no. 10, pp. 1488–1492.

WHO 2000, Mental health and work: impact, issues and good practises. Available at: http://www.who.int/mental_health/media/en/712.pdf [Accessed 20 January 2016]

WHO 2004, *The global burden of disease; 2004 update*. Geneva: World Health Organization. Available at: http://www.who.int/healthinfo/global_burden_disease/2004_report_update/en/ [Accessed 20 January 2016]

Wisenthal, A & Krupa, T 2014, 'Using intervention mapping to deconstruct cognitive work hardening: a return-to-work intervention for people with depression', *BMC Health Services Research*, vol. 14, no. 530, pp. 1–11. DOI: 10.1186/s12913–014–0530–4.

Yunus, M 2011, Sacrificing microcredit for megaprofits. *The New York Times*. Available at: http://www.nytimes.com/2011/01/15/opinion/15yunus.html?_r=0 [Accessed 20 January 2016]

13 Mental health, participation and social identity

Toril Anne Elstad and Gundi Schrötter Johannsen

This chapter aims to contribute to an understanding of the social dimension of the concept of participation and the meaning participation can have for mental health and identity. In order to increase participation, it is important to support the personal recovery process of each individual. However, since participation can function as a link between individuals and society, health and welfare services should also provide opportunities for social inclusion and reciprocal relationships. According to the theories of Goffman (1967) and Mead (1934/1967), face-to-face interaction is of central importance for identity formation. Breakwell (1986) studied how people act when they feel that their identity is threatened. If you have a mental disorder, it is very likely that both the disorder itself and the reaction from the outside world will increase this feeling of threat. This is in line with Goffman (1963), who pointed out how people with mental illness protect their identities through concealment in order to avoid stigmatisation. Changes in the organisation of mental health services, from a mainly hospital-based psychiatry towards mental health work in local communities, have highlighted issues of participation, social inclusion and integration for people who live with mental health problems. Aiming to support people in daily life, community mental health services that facilitate active participation are encouraged internationally (WHO 2001b, 2005, 2013). From these perspectives, we will present our studies from a Danish and a Norwegian community mental health service, and relate our findings and the discussion of them to the overall themes of participation, social identity and mental health.

Introduction

The International Classification of Functioning, Disability and Health (ICF) (WHO 2001a) definition of participation as *involvement in a life situation* is a broad description that can also be seen as vague. A need for a broader theoretical understanding of the concept of participation has been identified (Cornwall 2008, Eide et al. 2007, Hammel et al. 2008). Dijkers (2010) links participation to the social model of disability rather than a medical model, but also states that the field is still in need of a consensus definition of the concept. According to

Hammel *et al.* (2008), the ICF definition ignores people's complex interactive processes and subjective experiences of participation, and the meaning of their involvement is therefore lacking. Another, similar criticism is that the ICF definition does not include peoples' social relationships and involvement in society, and that it therefore should be redesigned in the direction of social roles (Piskur *et al.* 2014). Although the concept of 'social participation' does not exist in the ICF, it is increasingly used in the research literature (Piskur et al. 2014). In a study of the meaning of participation for people with disabilities, participation was conceptualised as meaningful engagement, social connections, and choice, control, access and opportunity (Hammel *et al.* 2008). Other main themes in this study were related to personal and societal responsibilities and opportunities to support others. To be appreciated and be able to contribute to and mean something for others has been identified as important for experiencing participation among people with a diagnosis of schizophrenia (Yilmaz *et al.* 2009). The importance of reciprocal relationships and belonging to a social fellowship have also been reported in research from community mental health services called 'recovery centers' in the USA (Whitley & Campbell 2014, Whitley & Siantz 2012a, Whitley *et al.* 2012), and from 'low threshold' services in Norway (Elstad 2014, Elstad & Eide 2009, Elstad & Kristiansen 2009).

Mental health problems, social inclusion and participation

Across different perspectives and fields, there is general agreement that mental health and illness have important social dimensions and consequences. A main finding from research over several decades is that a life situation with few social ties and a lack of supportive social relationships has negative effects on mental health in populations (Cobb 1976, Dohrenwend & Dohrenwend 1969, Faris & Dunham 1939, Fisher 1982, Leighton 1959, Srole et al. 1962). Both stigmatising responses from others and fear of being stigmatised can lead to social exclusion and difficulties in establishing social relationships (Allman 2013, Corrigan *et al.* 2009, Lingsom 2008, Norvoll 2013, Scambler 2009). Such processes can lead to various degrees of social isolation and a lack of hope and meaning, as well as low self-esteem, lack of motivation and reduced opportunities to develop and sustain social skills (Boyd 2008, Rogers & Pilgrim 2005, Sayce 2000). Long periods of social isolation can threaten people's experience of being a whole person with a positive social identity (Allman 2013, Elstad & Norvoll 2013).

When addressing social integration, inclusion and participation in the field of mental health work, emphasis has often been put on enhancing the personal recovery processes of individuals and their rights to have control in their daily life situations (Anthony 1993, Borg 2007, Borg & Kristiansen 2004). However, whether living in the community leads to social contact and relationships also depends on how inclusive local communities are (Bricout & Gray 2006, Granerud & Severinsson 2006). A vision of full participation in society is increasingly recognised as central in rehabilitation (Allman 2013, Bjørk-Åkesson & Granlund 2004, Molin

2004). A Danish definition of the rehabilitation process has a strong focus on collaboration between the disabled person, his or her social relationships, and the service providers involved:

> Rehabilitation is a goal-directed and time-limited collaborative process between the disabled person, the person's relatives and the professionals involved. The aim is that people with disabilities, who have, or are at risk of acquiring, severe limitations in their physical, psychological and/or social levels of functioning, can live independent and meaningful lives. Rehabilitation is based on the disabled person's total life situation and decisions, and consists of a coordinated, coherent, and knowledge-based support system.
>
> (Hjortbak *et al.* 2011: 11)

This definition points to independence and meaningfulness as key issues in the rehabilitation process. The term 'relatives' is used in a broad sense, where relatives can be family members or persons who are meaningful others for the service user (Hjortbak *et al.* 2011). The important issue is that only the service user can define who the important others are. According to Hjortbak *et al.* (2011), this triangulation between service providers, service users and relatives implies a new and challenging position for each of the participants. In addition to supporting individuals, an important question on a larger scale is how to also develop inclusive societies (Gustavsson 2004, Madsen 2005, Oliver 1990). The ICF does relate to the impacts that a lack of participation, in addition to individual impairments, can have on people's life situations. This perspective can, however, be seen as too superficially treated in the ICF.

Participation and social participation

The ICF manual does not define 'social participation', and a commonly accepted definition is lacking. The concept is, however, increasingly used in publications from research (Piskur et al. 2014). The concepts of participation and social participation are often used interchangeably, and both are often linked to 'involvement in society and concepts of social integration, social inclusion or social activity' (Piskur et al. 2014: 213). Levasseur et al. (2010: 10) have proposed the following definition: 'Social participation can be defined as a person's involvement in activities that provide interaction with others in society or the community.' This way, mental health work and rehabilitation that support processes of social participation can also be seen as means to enable social inclusion for people who live with mental health problems. Participation in social activity is often described in similar ways to social inclusion, but participation is more often used in a rights-based perspective, such as rights to be involved in decision-making about treatment, individuals' rights to self-determination, and society's responsibility to provide conditions that enable this (Piskur et al. 2014).

According to Mead (1934/1967), self-consciousness and identity develop during processes of social experiences and common activity, as a result of individuals' relations to the processes themselves and to other individuals who take part.

Developing a 'self' depends on an awareness of other people's attitudes towards us and the common social activity we engage in. Goffman (1961, 1963) also describes identity as a subjective experience of one's own personality, which develops through social interaction, and how our 'unique selves' are produced through 'common, ceremonial acts'. In Goffman's theory, mutual trust is established through face-to-face interaction in concrete social situations. Through rituals of politeness and respect, such as greetings, people recognise one another and confirm one another's dignity (Goffman 1967), while being ignored threatens our experiences of being valuable individuals. Both face-to-face interaction and the social frameworks surrounding people's daily life can have an influence on people's identity. Theories about social interaction can shed light on such processes and add to an understanding of what meaning participation may have for social identity and mental health.

Social identity theories

According to Jenkins (2008: 59), 'Both mind and selfhood must be understood as embodied within the routine interaction of the human world, neither strictly individual nor strictly collective', and in this way our sense of who we are is subject to how other people treat us. This is in line with Mead (1934/67), who understands processes of mind and selfhood as an internal-external dialectic. Goffman (1963) and Jenkins (2008) both understand identity as processes of identification: that is, trajectories of being and becoming, which place interaction between people as 'the *a priori* of consciousness, rather than *vice versa*' (Jenkins 2008: 143). According to Breakwell (1986), groups that people belong to are important sources of pride and self-esteem through a sense of belonging to the social world and a sense of social identity. As group membership is a central part of identity, competition between groups can also be about competing identities. If we see social identity as the part of individuals' self-concept that stems from perceived membership in a social group, their group should compare favourably with other groups in order to maintain the self-esteem of its members (Tajfel & Turner 1979).Within social psychology, Stryker and Burke (2000) describe how identity theory can add to our understanding of how social structures affect our 'selves' and how the self affects social behaviours. Lynch (2011) refers to individuals' sense of selfhood both as their inner, personal experience of themselves, and as their sense of self related to the surrounding world. The 'self' is a core issue involved in emotional distress, and recovery of one's sense of selfhood is central for mental health and recovery from mental illness. According to Lynch (2011), if this is overlooked, people's life history and experiences, and their ways of dealing with the world around them, are also overlooked. To create relationships is a key human need, and a sense of selfhood is essential for our ability to enter and maintain social relationships (Lynch 2011). Social processes of identity formation, as described above, mean that our 'social identity' is connected to how other people see us and respond to us, which can be based on the groups we belong to as well as on institutions, organisations, power and self-identification.

Identity and experiences of threat

According to Breakwell (1986), our identity is simultaneously based on self-concept vs. self-evaluation, self-as-object vs. self-as-subject, social-self vs. spiritual-self, and real-self vs. ideal-self. Our identity is therefore constituted as a dialectical interaction between a personal and a social identity, and our current personal identity is a product of the interaction of past personal identities with present social identities (Breakwell 1986). Our identity is guided by three prime principles which we constantly try to maintain and develop. These principles are related to a feeling of uniqueness, as well as feelings of continuity across time and situation, and to personal worth and social value. These three principles will act and be visible on three levels: an intra-psychic, an interpersonal and an inter-group level. Seen in relation to the main issue of participation, Breakwell's key point is that our identity is visible as active actions in our relationship with other people, and that the proposals of identity we bring into different relationships can either be recognised or not be recognised by others.

In an interpersonal relationship, the feeling of uniqueness can be seen as a feeling of personal sovereignty. Just as nations invoke sovereignty, a personal boundary depends on acceptance from others. A feeling of continuity is related to continuity in a life span. At the same time as I recognise myself in my personal history, I also believe that this feeling of continuity will reach into the future. In an interpersonal relationship, this means: which possible opportunities and positions could potentially and legitimately be mine? Again, this has to be accepted by others. The last principle has to do with a feeling of self-esteem. What a person experiences as the essential 'me' and his/her personal contributions to a social context have to be recognised and not seen as only a kind of pseudo-contribution (Breakwell 1986; Johannsen & Pedersen 2014). If these three principles cannot be maintained, the person will experience it as a threat to identity. Breakwell (1986: 46–47) defines a threat to identity this way:

> A threat to identity occurs when the processes of identity, assimilation-accommodation are, for some reason, unable to comply with the principles of continuity, distinctiveness and self-esteem, which habitually guide their operation.

These kinds of threats can be described as a second handicap for people with mental illness. If participation becomes a new language in social and health services, it will be necessary for service providers to include an experience of threat to identity as a possible obstacle to active participation. When people experience a threat to identity, they will activate different coping strategies. Isolation can be one such strategy, a way of action, so that no one will recognise the threat and the marginal position. Another, which is described by Goffman (1963), is a passing strategy. But also negativism, or outright conflicts with anyone who would challenge the identity structure, have been described as strategies used by users of mental health services (Breakwell 1986, Johannsen 2002). Related to the concept of participation, these strategies must be identified and understood as helping strategies by service providers.

Participation and empowerment: related terms in mental health services?

When talking about participation in mental health services, one should also consider empowerment processes. User participation in mental health services can be a challenge for professionals and service users. Many who live with mental health problems have experienced marginalisation processes and often describe themselves as persons placed in an unprivileged position, which can lead to difficulties in being active participants (Andersen, Brok & Mathiasen 2000). Empowerment has a focus on power relations, which highlights a potential to enhance experiences of participation and power in one's own life situation. In the mental health field, it can therefore be fruitful to locate the concepts of participation and rehabilitation within an empowerment perspective. Supporting processes of participation and social inclusion is central to a psychosocial approach in mental health work (Borg & Karlsson 2013, Corrigan et al. 2009, Elstad & Norvoll 2013, Ramon & Williams 2005). According to Craig (2006: 15), the cornerstone of all mental health care should be 'goal-directed therapy managed in partnership and provided in real situations in a culture of empowerment and optimism'.

Inspired by Paulo Freire (1970), we use the concept of empowerment about processes whereby people who are in a weak position can acquire the strength and power to take control over their own lives through handling material, structural, social and cultural factors which keep them in a powerless and oppressed position. The aim is that this will lead to processes of increased awareness as well as active changes towards more egalitarian roles and increased participation. Empowerment consists of three levels (Andersen, Brok & Mathiasen 2000). An individual level based on individual strength can be seen as identity empowerment. A fellowship or community level is based on experiences of power related to sharing common experiences; Elias and Scotson (1994) highlight how collective identities are necessary in order to change processes of marginalisation. A third level is a societal perspective, where groups of people who are in a marginalised position acquire increased influence on political decisions. This level is based on real power and can be seen as political empowerment, which is a particular responsibility of service-user organisations. This makes it necessary for professionals in mental health services to treat user organisations as equal partners.

A central point is that one cannot empower others, but one can organise the professional contribution in ways that enhance the empowerment of individuals and groups. Empowerment is, however, also an ambiguous concept. An empowerment perspective provides opportunities for individuals to influence the services they receive, but it also imposes upon the individual a responsibility to participate and seek influence. This responsibility could end up as a case of 'blaming the victim'. Findings from a Danish study showed that working with rehabilitation is not an easy task, and that the education of service providers is an important issue if participation, inclusion and empowerment are to become general perspectives in social and health services (Mogensen, Bylov & Johannsen 2010). This is also in line with Hjortbak et al. (2011). Supporting processes of participation and social inclusion is central to a psychosocial and relational approach to mental health work (Borg & Karlsson 2013,

Corrigan et al. 2009, Elstad & Norvoll 2013, Ramon & Williams 2005). However, as peoples' experience of, and wishes for, participation varies, what participation in their life situations means must be judged by each individual (Bjørk-Åkesson & Granlund 2004, Sayce 2000). The social dimensions of participation should therefore be further explored and supplemented by other perspectives, such as the meaning different forms of participation have for individuals (Gustavsson 2004).

Mental health, participation and the need for recognition

In Honneth's (1995) theory, 'recognition' has the following three main dimensions: *love* relates to early development and *rights* relates to citizenship, while *solidarity* is about being recognised as capable human beings through participation and mutuality in situated fellowships. His concept of solidarity makes the theory relevant to the above discussions of participation and social inclusion, meaning and mental health. Experiences of not being recognised equals being met with 'disrespect' (Honneth 2007), which means that one is visually observed, but not 'really seen' as a person who deserves respect and recognition for one's uniqueness and capabilities. Such responses can lead to social withdrawal and isolation, while relationships of recognition can enhance people's opportunities for 'self-realisation'. According to Oliver *et al.* (2006), valued and meaningful participation can support experiences of connectedness and belonging, and may foster resilience, positive mental health and well-being. To be met as capable human beings has been identified as important for people's processes of recovery from mental health problems (Anthony 1993, Borg 2007, Deegan 1996, Jacobsen & Willig 2008). Being able to contribute to others and receive recognition for this contribution leads to experiences of self-worth, which are central to identity formation and positive mental health (Antonovsky 1996).

Linking social support to the concept of participation and theories of recognition allows for a broader understanding of participation. Community mental health services that support active participation have been encouraged internationally. Some such recent developments have been 'low threshold', flexible services with an open and accessible organisation, often based on a mix of professional and peer support (Conradson 2003, Kristiansen 2000, Parr 2000, Whitley & Campbell 2014, Whitley & Siantz 2012a, Whitley *et al.* 2012). These changes suggest new roles for people with mental health problems: from being viewed mainly as patients towards active participation as service users and increased agency and control in their own life situations (Corrigan et al. 2009, Craig 2006, Johannsen 2002, Sayce 2000). This also highlights the need for an everyday life perspective and to meet individuals' need for support in their daily life situations (Borg & Karlsson 2013, Elstad & Norvoll 2013).

Participation in community mental health services: examples from Norway and Denmark

Participation, social inclusion, mental health and identity have been central themes in this chapter. How mental health work can support such processes for people who live with mental health problems is an important issue. To illustrate mental health work aiming to support participation, we will present two brief examples from our studies in a Danish and a Norwegian service.

In a Norwegian city, an ethnographic field study was conducted within a community mental health service with an open and flexible, low-threshold approach (Elstad 2014, Elstad & Eide 2009, Elstad & Kristiansen 2009). Mutual sharing of practical advice relating to daily life in the service users' homes and the local community was a central part of the social conversations at the centres. The need for support or challenges varied between people and fluctuated over time for individuals, which meant that an open and flexible approach to mental health work was important. To attend the service according to their own choice and perceived needs was of central value for the service users, as this made it possible to receive support without being subjected to control and surveillance. The low-threshold approach of the service provided opportunities for receiving help and support when needed, as well as opportunities to take on more active roles. For some, managing to attend the service was described as 'mastery' in itself, seen in the light of their mental health problems. Some attended the centres due to their felt needs for social support and company, others were leading and planning activities, and a few took on roles as user representatives. Some service users were, however, worried in case efforts to increase user participation might lead to reduced professional help and too much responsibility.

What attending the service meant for their experiences of participation in daily life was a central theme in both field conversations and individual interviews with key informants. A central finding across observations and interviews was a strong emphasis on the importance of the social milieu. This was about feeling supported and safe in a psychological sense. For many, active participation in the service and participation in the wider community depended on available social support and help from mental health professionals. For some, this ongoing support had prevented admission to psychiatric hospitals. A central theme in field conversations and interviews was the importance of having a place where one could spend time with others who shared experiences of living with mental health problems. For some, to be able to contribute to, as well as be supported by, others who 'knew what it was like' was important. This was related to sharing positive experiences and advice as well as illness experiences, and also to developing mutual relationships and sometimes friendships. In field conversations, some service users who were working and only 'dropped in' occasionally said this was important in order to 'relax from strain', which further supported this finding. Other examples from more regular service users were about not having to feel ashamed of, for example, being young and receiving a disability pension. As one young man put it: '[H]here there are no losers.' For many, attending events in the wider community together also enhanced participation outside the centres. This gave them something to talk about with others, also outside the centre.

A Danish study supports the above study's findings about the importance of participation in everyday life for people with mental health problems (Mogensen, Bylov & Johannsen 2010). A project called 'Relational competence and inclusive fellowships' combined education and service development in group homes that were part of a community mental health service. The aims of the project were to implement changes from an institutional culture based on mainly healthcare towards a culture with a focus on personal development and participation. The project was organised as action research and designed to create transformative learning processes for the staff. A framework for the study was Brookfield's 2005 theoretical orientation within a critical scientific tradition, where individuals problematize their own and others' assumptions as well as the context surrounding their actions: 'those taken-for-granted ideas, common sense beliefs and self-evident rules of thumb that inform our thought and action' (Brookfield 1990: 177). According to Brookfield (1987: 7), critical thinking has four components: (1) identifying and challenging assumptions, (2) challenging the importance of context, (3) imagining and exploring alternatives, and (4) imagining/exploring alternatives leading to reflective scepticism.

Combining the lecturers' theoretical knowledge, the staff's practical knowledge and the residents' experience created opportunities for processes of imagining and exploring alternatives. In addition to teaching, the project included minor innovations at the institution, where staff and residents together created changes based on the residents' active participation in and influence on a daily life that would be more based on their own wishes. These small projects were all different: one was about having a concrete influence on changes to the building; another project was about 'social gatherings'; a third was about power relations. These innovative projects challenged the staff to think differently about their practice and discover the residents' own resources in a new way. The teachers also functioned as consultants in the development projects. This meant that transfers could be created between theory and practice, and that staff members could imagine alternatives which could be tried out in co-operation with the residents. These reflections resulted in a practice which was based on participation and created a space with opportunities for supporting the residents' empowerment processes.

This change in practice also led to the residents' explicit wish to receive the same theoretical lectures as the staff. Participation from residents in the lectures was a challenge for all parties. Lecturers who were used to teaching *about* people in marginalised positions, now had to theorise *with* them. For the residents, the challenge was often whether their contributions and personal experiences were going to be valued on equal terms with the contributions from the staff. Challenges for the staff were generally about changes in the positions of staff and resident. All of a sudden, they found themselves in an equal position as students. An important result from the project was the development of more egalitarian relations between staff and residents, illustrated by the following quote from one of the residents: 'It has been exciting to meet the staff in a new and different way, as equals. This gives a different kind of relationship, which functions well both ways.' Participation in the project strengthened the residents' self-awareness and identities as being more than patients with a diagnosis. This opened up new ways of positioning themselves: as individuals and as a group, in relation to the staff. Related to the aspect of identity, a young female resident said:

> I get a lot out of taking part in the lectures together with the staff. When one is mentally ill, there are many things one cannot do. But I have discovered t that I can still learn. I am not only a diagnosis, I am also someone with an intellect. Since the lectures are not about my illness, but about ordinary human things – about you and me – I no longer see myself as primarily mentally ill, but as a human being who definitely has some difficulties – but who also has just as many opportunities. This actually makes me feel better.

This quote shows that being able to leave behind a negative self-concept as primarily mentally ill can be related to Breakwell's (1986) three principles of identity: a strengthened continuity in seeing oneself as getting better; a feeling of being unique and not just a diagnosis; and, as a result, also acquiring a more general feeling of increased self-worth.

We have presented the two studies above as examples of how social identity, empowerment and opportunities to receive recognition should be considered central principles for developing mental health services that are based on participation. The study from Norway shows the importance of mutual recognition through participation in a setting where one's contributions are valued. Another important finding was how attending a service based on one's own choice and felt needs can enhance experiences of participation in one's own life situation in general. Developing friendships that reach across from the mental health service into everyday life in the community also contributes to participation outside service settings. Both these studies illustrate how opportunities for contributing positively to a fellowship is meaningful for social identity. The quote from the Norwegian study, 'here there are no losers', can be seen as an illustration of a movement away from experiences of a life lived in a marginalised position. In the Danish study, participating as equals in theory lectures together with mental health professionals contributed to positive changes in self-concept among residents in a mental health service, and also to being perceived more positively by others. Processes of empowerment become especially clear in the study from Denmark, as participation in the lectures was the result of an explicit idea and wish from the residents themselves, and not a therapeutic intervention by the staff. Participation in an empowerment perspective can potentially function as a link between individuals and society. The development of mental health services which provide opportunities for social participation and reciprocal relationships are therefore encouraged.

Conclusion

Perspectives from the mental health field, based on experiences and views from both service users and professionals, could potentially broaden the theoretical understanding of the meaning of participation. Mental health work and community mental health services should be flexible, available and responsive to the needs of service users. Different types of 'low-threshold' services offering ongoing support in daily life can be valuable resources in daily life for many. Support from community mental health services, combined with opportunities for active participation in an empowerment perspective, should be available to those who experience this as important in order to cope with challenges in their everyday life situation. It is also important to acknowledge peoples' varying experience of illness and wellness. Further knowledge about practice and social interaction within such services is needed, as well as how such support can enhance social inclusion for people with mental health problems in local communities and society at large.

References

Allman, D. (2013). *The Sociology of Social Inclusion.* DOI: 10.1177/2158244012471957. Downloaded February 19th 2013 from: http://sgo.sagepub.com/content/3/1/2158244012 471957.

Andersen, M. L., Nørlund Brok, P. & Mathiasen, H. (2000). *Empowerment på dansk (Empowerment in Danish).* Frederikshavn, DK: Dafola Forlag.

Anthony, W. A. (1993). Recovery from mental illness: The guiding vision of the mental health service system in the 1990s. *Psychosocial Rehabilitation Journal,* 16(4), 11–23.

Antonovsky, A. (1996). The salutogenic model as a theory to guide health promotion. *Health Promotion International,* 11(1), 11–18.

Bjørk-Åkesson, E. & Granlund, M. (2004). Delaktighet – ett centralt begrepp i WHOs klassifikation av funktionstillstånd, funktionshinder och helsa (ICF) (Participation – a central concept in WHO's International Classification of Functioning, Disability and Health (ICF)). In: Gustavsson, A. (Ed.): *Delaktighetens språk.* Lund, SE: Studentlitteratur, pp. 29–48.

Borg, M. (2007). The Nature of Recovery as Lived in Everyday Life: Perspectives of Individuals Recovering from Severe Mental Health Problems. Doctoral thesis, Trondheim: NTNU Norwegian University of Science and Technology.

Borg, M. & Karlsson, B. (2013). *Psykisk helsearbeid. Humane og sosiale perspektiver og praksiser (Mental health work. Humane and social perspectives and practices).* Oslo: Gyldendal Akademisk.

Borg, M. & Kristiansen, K. (2004). Recovery-oriented professionals: Helping relationships in mental health services. *Journal of Mental Health,* 13(5), 493–505.

Boyd, M. A. (2008 4th ed.). *Psychiatric Nursing. Contemporary Practice.* Philadelphia, Baltimore, New York, London, Buenos Aires, Hong Kong, Sydney, Tokyo: Wolters Kluwer. Lippicott, Williams & Wilkins.

Breakwell G. M. (1986). *Coping with Threatened Identities.* London: Methuen & Co. Ltd.

Bricout, J. C. & Gray, D. B. (2006). Community receptivity: The ecology of disabled persons' participation in the physical, political and social environments. *Scandinavian Journal of Disability Research,* 8(1), 1–21.

Brookfield, S. D. (1987). *Developing Critical Thinkers – Challenging Adults to Explore Alternative Ways of Thinking and Acting.* Milton Keynes: Open University Press.

Brookfield, S. D. (1990). Using Critical Incidents to Explore Learners' Assumptions. In: Mezirow, J. (Ed.): *Fostering Critical Reflection in Adulthood.* San Fransisco: Jossey-Bass, pp. 177–193.

Cobb, S. (1976). Social support as a moderator of life stress. *Psychosomatic Medicine,* 38(5), 300–314.

Conradson, D. (2003). Spaces of care in the city: The place of a community drop-in centre. *Social and Cultural Geography*, 4(4), 507–524.

Cornwall, A. (2008). Unpacking 'participation': Models, meanings and practices. *Community Development Journal*, 43(3), 269–283.

Corrigan, P. W., Larson, J. E. & Rusch, N. (2009). Self-stigma and the "why try" effect: Impact on life goals and evidence-based practices. *World Psychiatry*, 8, 75–81.

Craig, T. (2006). What Is Psychiatric Rehabilitation? In: Roberts, G., Davenport, S., Holloway, F., Tattan, T. (Eds.): *Enabling Recovery: The Principles and Practice of Rehabilitation Psychiatry*. London: Gaskell (Royal College of Psychiatrists), pp. 3–15.

Deegan, P. (1996). Recovery as a Journey of the Heart. *Psychiatric Rehabilitation Journal*, 19(3): 91–97.

Dijkers, M. P. (2010). Issues in the conceptualization and measurement of participation: An overview. *Archives of Physical Medicine and Rehabilitation*, 91(9), 5–16.

Dohrenwend, P. B. & Dohrenwend, B. P. (1969). *Social Status and Psychological Disorder: A Causal Inquiry*. New York, London, Sydney & Toronto: John Wiley & Sons.

Eide, A. H., Jelsma, J., Loeb. M. E., Maart, S. & Ka' Toni, M. (2007). Exploring ICF components in a survey among Xhosa speakers in Eastern & Western Cape, South Africa. *Disability and Rehabilitation*, 30(11), 819–829.

Elias, N. & Scotson, J. L. (1994). *The Established and the Outsiders*. London: Sage Publications.

Elstad, T. A. (2014). Participation in a 'Low Threshold' Community Mental Health Service: An Ethnographic Study of Social Interaction, Activities and Meaning. PhD thesis, NTNU Trondheim: Norwegian University of Science and Technology.

Elstad, T. A. & Eide, A. H. (2009). User participation in community mental health services: Exploring the experiences of users and professionals. *Scandinavian Journal of Caring Sciences*, 23, 674–681.

Elstad, T. A. & Kristiansen, K. (2009). Mental health centres as 'meeting-places' in the community: Exploring experiences of being service users and participants. *Scandinavian Journal of Disability Research*, 11(3), 195–208.

Elstad, T. A. & Norvoll, R. (2013). Sosial inklusjon og eksklusjon (Social Inclusion and Exclusion). In: Norvoll, R. (Ed.): *Samfunn og psykisk helse. Samfunnsvitenskapelige perspektiver (Society and Mental Health. Social Scientific Perspectives)*. Oslo: Gyldendal Akademisk, pp. 118–147.

Faris, R. E. & Dunham, H. W. (1939). *Mental Disorders in Urban Areas: An Ecological Study of Schizophrenia and Other Psychoses*. Chicago: University of Chicago Press.

Fisher, C. S. (1982). *To Dwell among Friends – Personal Networks in Town and City*. Chicago: University of Chicago Press.

Freire, P. (1970). *Pedagogy of the Oppressed*. New York: Herder and Herder.

Goffman, E. (1961). *Asylums. Essays on the Social Situations of Mental Patients and Other Inmates*. Harmondsworth: Penguin Pelican Books.

Goffman, E. (1963). *Stigma. Notes on the Management of Spoiled Identity*. New York: Penguin Books.

Goffman, E. (1967). *Interaction Ritual. Essays on Face-to-Face Behaviour*. New York: Pantheon Books.

Granerud, A. & Severinsson, E. (2006). The struggle for social integration in the community – The experiences of people with mental health problems. *Journal of Psychiatric and Mental Health Nursing*, 13, 288–293.

Gustavsson, A. (Ed.) (2004). *Delaktighetens språk (The Language of Participation)*. Lund: Studentlitteratur.

Hammel, J., Magasi, S., Heinemann, A., Whiteneck, G., Bogner, J. & Rodriguez, E. (2008). What does participation mean? An insider perspective from people with disabilities. *Disability and Rehabilitation*, 30(19), 1445–1460.

Hjortbak, B. R., Bangshaab, J., Johansen, J. S. & Lund, H. (2011). *Udfordringer til rehabilitering (Challenges in Rehabilitation)*. Copenhagen: Rehabiliteringsforum Danmark.

Honneth, A. (1995). *The Struggle for Recognition: The Moral Grammar of Social Conflicts*. Cambridge, UK: Polity Press.

Honneth, A. (2007) *Disrespect: The Normative Foundations of Critical Theory*. Cambridge, UK & Malden USA: Polity Press.

Jacobsen, M. H. & R. Willig (Eds.) (2008). *Anerkendelsespolitik (Politics of Recognition)*. Odense: University Press of Southern Denmark.

Jenkins R. (2008, 3rd ed.). *Social Identity*. London and New York: Routledge.

Johannsen, G. (2002). Kulturel marginalisering og social deltagelse – eksemplificeret ved mennesker med en sindslidelse (Cultural Marginalisation and Social Participation – Examples from People with Mental Health Problems). Unpublished thesis in pedagogy, Copenhagen, DK: Denmarks University of Pedagogy.

Johannsen, G. & Pedersen, M. (Eds.) (2014). *Unges livsvilkår (Young Persons' Life Situations)*. Copenhagen: Akademisk Forlag.

Kristiansen, S. (2000). Interaction patterns among users of a Danish community care centre. *International Social Work*, 43(3), 325–336.

Leighton, A. H. (1959). *My Name Is Legion: The Stirling County Study of Psychiatric Disorder and Sociocultural Environment*. New York: Basic Books.

Levasseur, M., Richard, L., Gauvin, L. & Raymond, E. (2010). Inventory and analysis of definitions of social participation found in the ageing literature: Proposed taxonomy of social activities. *Social Science & Medicine*, 71, 2141–2149.

Lingsom, S. (2008). Invisible impairments: Dilemmas of concealment and disclosure. *Scandinavian Journal of Disability Research*, 10(1), 2–16.

Lynch T. (2011). *Selfhood: A Key to the Recovery of Emotional Wellbeing, Mental Health and the Prevention of Mental Health Problems*. Limerick, Ireland: Mental health Publishing.

Madsen, B. (2005). *Socialpedagogik – Integration og inklusion i det moderne samfund (Social Pedagogy – Integration and Inclusion in Modern Society)*. Copenhagen: Hans Reitzel.

Mead G. H. (1934/1967). *Mind, Self and Society from the Standpoint of a Social Behaviorist*. Chicago: University of Chicago Press.

Mogensen, F., Bylov, F. & Johannsen, G. (2010). *Uddannelse og udvikling på professionshøjskoler (Education and Developments in University Colleges)*. Esbjerg, DK: UC Vest Press.

Molin, M. (2004). Delaktighet inom handikappområdet – en begreppsanalys (Participation in the Area of Disability – A Concept Analysis). In: Gustavsson, A. (Ed.): *Delaktighetes språk (The Language of Participation)*. Lund S: Studentlitteratur, pp. 61–81.

Norvoll, R. (2013). Samfunnsvitenskapelige perspektiver på psykisk helse og psykiske helsetjenester (Social Scientific Perspectives on Mental Health and Mental Health Services). In: Norvoll, R. (Ed.): *Samfunn og psykisk helse. Samfunnsvitenskapelige perspektiver (Society and Mental Health. Social Scientific Perspectives)*. Oslo: Gyldendal Akademisk, pp. 38–72.

Oliver, M. (1990). *The Politics of Disablement*. Basingstoke, UK: Macmillan.

Oliver, K. G., Collin, P., Burns, J. & Nicholas, J. (2006). Building resilience in young people through meaningful participation. *Australian e-Journal for the Advancement of Mental Health*, 5(1), 5–7. ISSN: 1446–7984.

Parr, H. (2000). Interpreting the 'hidden social geographies' of mental health: Ethnographies of inclusion and exclusion in semi-institutional places. *Health & Place*, 6, 225–237.

Piskur, B., Daniels, R., Jongmans, M. J., Ketelaar, M., Smeets, R. JEM, Norton, M. & Beurskens, A. JHM (2014). Participation and social participation: Are they distinct concepts? *Clinical Rehabilitation*, 28(3), 211–220.

Ramon, S. & Williams, J. E. (Eds.) (2005). *Mental Health at the Crossroads: The Promise of the Psychosocial Approach*. Aldershot: Ashgate Publishers Limited.

Rogers, A. & Pilgrim, D. (2005, 3rd ed.). *A Sociology of Mental Health and Illness*. Berkshire & New York: Open University Press.

Sayce, L. (2000). *From Psychiatric Patient to Citizen. Overcoming Discrimination and Social Exclusion*. Houndmills, Basingstoke: Palgrave MacMillan.

Scambler, G. (2009). Health-related stigma. *Sociology of Health & Illness*, 31(3), 441–455.

Srole, L., Langer, T. S., Michael, S. T., Kirkpatrick, P., Opler, M. K. & Rennie, T. A. C. (1962). *Mental Health in the Metropolis: The Midtown Manhattan Study*. New York: McGraw-Hill.

Stryker S. & Burke P. J. (2000). The past, present and future of an identity theory. *Social Psychology Quarterly*, 63(4), 284–297.

Tajfel, H. & Turner, J. C. (1979). An Integrative Theory of Intergroup Conflict. In: W. G. Austin & S. Worshel (Eds.): *The Social Psychology of Intergroup Relations*. Monterey, CA: Brooks/Cole, pp. 33–47.

Whitley, R. & Campbell, R. D. (2014). Stigma, agency and recovery amongst people with severe mental illness. *Social Science and Medicine*, 107, 1–8. DOI: 10.1016/j.socscimed.2014.02.010.

Whitley, R. & Siantz, E. (2012). Recovery centers for people with a mental illness: An emerging best practice? *Psychiatric Services*, 63(1), 10–12.

Whitley, R., Strickler, D. & Drake, R. E. (2012). Recovery centers for people with severe mental illness: A survey of programs. *Community Mental Health Journal*, 48, 547–556.

WHO (2001a). *International Classification of Functioning, Disability and Health (ICF)*. Geneva: World Health Organization.

WHO (2001b). *Mental Health: New Understanding, New Hope. World Health Report*. Geneva: World Health Organization.

WHO (2005). *Promoting Mental Health. Concepts – Emerging Evidence – Practice*. Geneva: World Health Organization.

WHO (2013). *Mental Health Action Plan 2013–2020*. Geneva: World Health Organization.

Yilmaz, M., Josephsson, S., Danermark, B. & og Ivarsson, A. B. (2009). Social processes of participation in everyday life among persons with schizophrenia. *International Journal of Qualitative Studies on Health and Well-Being*, 4, 267–279.

14 Digitalised communication and social interaction

New opportunities for young disabled people's participation

Sylvia Söderström and Helena Hemmingsson

During the last decades, methods of communication and interaction have developed and changed contemporaneously with technological progress. Information and Communication Technology (ICT) has become a vitally important aspect of people's lives, and its usage has evolved to confirm and underline identities and values, making technology and society mutually constitutive (MacKenzie & Wajcman 2005; Räsänen 2008). Post-modern social life is characterised by the domestication of technology. This refers to the process of users adapting new technologies to their own requirements, and making technology a natural and taken-for-granted part of their everyday life (Sørensen 2004). Additionally, post-modern life is also characterised by individual choices, multiple identities and mobility (Hughes, Russell & Paterson 2005). The liquidity and mobility that seem to mark the lives of most people in Western societies are not so apparent in the lives of disabled people. However, while Hughes, Russell and Paterson (2005) conclude that young disabled people have little or no option but to consume segregated leisure in segregated places, we find that young people's domestication of technology has provided young disabled people with multiple options and new opportunities for participation and social interaction.

In this chapter, we investigate participation in the everyday life of young disabled people in relation to ICTs through an interactional perspective. We perceive participation as involvement in life situations, which means taking part, being accepted, belonging, being included, being engaged in an area of life, or having access to needed resources (ICF-CY 2007). Thus, participation is a dynamic process that takes place as an interaction between individuals and contextual factors (Noreau & Fougeyrollas 2000). We also recognise that there are different types of participation, such as for example participation in activities (opportunities to perform the same activities as peers) and social participation (opportunities for interaction with and a feeling of belonging to a peer group), and that young people often prioritise social participation (Asbjörnslett & Hemmingsson 2008).

Furthermore, we concur with Bossaert et al. (2013) and other scholars who emphasise that social interaction is a vital aspect of participation. Taking this perspective on participation as our point of departure, we investigate how young people's domestication of ICTs influences the opportunities for young disabled persons to participate in their everyday life.

The aim of this chapter is to provide new insights into the field of participation research by investigating the impact of ICTs on the opportunities available to young disabled people for social participation. Our perspective on participation in this chapter highlights participation as an individual experience of being a part of a social environment and being actively involved in valued life situations (Hemmingsson & Jonsson 2005). Thus, the relation between disability, ICTs and society is under scrutiny, and our investigation takes place at the crossroads between the fields of Disability Studies and of Science, Technology and Society (STS) studies (Ravneberg & Söderström in press). Further, our investigation draws on empirical examples from several studies in Sweden and Norway, both quantitative and qualitative, on the significance of ICTs on young disabled people's social interaction and participation in everyday school life and leisure activities.

Our perception of disability is in accordance with the Nordic relational model of disability as a mismatch between a person's capabilities and the functional demands of the environment; or in terms of a gap between an individual and societal, environmental and contextual demands. The important point in this perspective is that disability emerges in interpersonal relationships, in encounters between individuals and the environment, and in encounters between individuals and society (Gustavsson, Tøssebro & Traustadòttir 2005). Thus, people are not disabled all the time, but they are made and unmade able and disabled in particular situations, under particular conditions, and in particular practices and relations (Moser 2006). When considering disability as something relational that displays itself differently in different encounters and relationships, the empirical context in which this takes place becomes of great analytical importance. Thus, we will give a short insight into available knowledge in the field of young disabled people and the significance of ICTs in their social interactions and participation, and then provide some empirical images of how young disabled people experience and perceive their ICTs. In conclusion, we will discuss the significance of ICTs as markers of identity and distinction, and the concept of social interaction in a digitalised society.

Young people and digitalised social interaction

Young disabled people are primarily ordinary young people with the same desires, aspirations and needs as any other young people. The significance of ICTs for young disabled people is thus quite similar to that of other young people. This means that ICTs are above all valued for their social, interactive and communicative potential in social interaction and participation in the peer group (McMillan & Morrison 2006; Söderström & Ytterhus 2010). Furthermore, it is very likely that ICTs as social media are of even greater importance for disabled young people than for their non-disabled peers. This is especially the case for those who have mobility limitations and may have difficulties with participating in leisure activities outside the home. When comparing engagement in Internet activities among young people with disabilities and a reference group in the same age, it was found that a higher proportion of young people with motor impairments was engaged in

ICT activities than young people in general (Lidström, Ahlsten & Hemmingsson 2010). In particular, social Internet activities were more common among young people with impairments. For example, a higher proportion of boys and girls with disabilities visited online communities such as social networking sites compared with non-disabled peers (Lidström, Ahlsten & Hemmingsson 2010). Moreover, research also demonstrates that the use of the Internet is a predictor for meeting friends face to face, and the probability of meeting friends increases if children and youth participate in social Internet activities such as visiting online communities and e-mailing (Lidström, Ahlsten & Hemmingsson 2010; Söderström 2009). For young people with attention-deficit hyperactivity disorder (ADHD), participating in Internet activities also provides opportunities for establishing communication with friends which may be complementary to traditional means of meeting face to face (Bolic-Baric, Kjellberg, Hellberg & Hemmingsson online).

This potential of ICTs does, however, lead to a permeability of the virtual and the material world. The material world and the virtual world are no longer separate entities, but are permeable, mutually constituted and embedded in the everyday life of young people (Buckingham 2006; Peter & Valkenburg 2006; Söderström 2013). This permeability is an expression of how new digital technologies are being domesticated. However, the domestication of ICTs and permeability of the material and virtual present some challenges to the social interaction and participation of young disabled people. One of these challenges is usability of the ICTs. While accessible ICTs are those that a person can operate, usable ICTs are those that this person can use for the purposes he or she wishes (Söderström 2009). Thus, accessible ICTs are not necessarily usable. This is especially the case for young blind people (Söderström & Ytterhus 2010) or young people with severe physical impairments (Borgestig et al. in press). Another challenge is the continuous dependency on usable ICTs which the permeability of the virtual and the material leads to (McMillan & Morrison 2006). This dependency is a double-edged sword inasmuch as it embraces more and more of young people's everyday lives. Consequently, while the social, interactive and communicative use of ICTs are vital for young people's social interaction and participation in the peer group, a withdrawal from the use of ICTs or an inability to engage in digital forms of communication represent dangers of exclusion for young people (Livingstone & Helsper 2007; McMillan & Morrison 2006).

Assistive ICT devices

Many young disabled people are dependent on various kinds of assistive technologies (ATs) to make ICTs accessible and usable. In fact, a survey study by Lidström and colleagues (2012) found that 44% of young disabled people used a computer-based AT device, making it more common than mobility devices for this group. ATs are defined as any item, piece of equipment, or product that is applied to secure, increase, maintain or improve functional capabilities (Wielandt et al. 2006). ATs are technologies used to improve, expand or extend people's performances, actions and interactions, and might thus be experienced as an extension of the body (Moser 2006; Winance 2006). Assistive ICTs may be hardware devices such as enlarged keyboards or braille keyboards, or software programs such as screen magnifiers or eye-tracking communication programs. In the Nordic countries, authorities allocate ATs to disabled people free of charge for use at home, school, work or leisure, and for disabled people of all ages. However, using ATs involves more than overcoming environmental barriers; it also involves symbolic, historical and cultural contexts. ATs are loaded with collective cultural traditions, symbols and values, and subjective feelings and meanings assigned to the technology (Wielandt et al. 2006). This symbolic connotation turns out to be the case also for assistive ICT software programs which are not immediately conspicuous, such as screen magnifiers, which are perceived to symbolise old age (Söderström & Ytterhus 2010). From the perspective of young people with disabilities, the utility of an assistive device is related to whether or not it facilitates participation in real-life situations where psychosocial aspects, such as how the device influences self-images and peer reactions to the device, are of outmost importance. Thus, from the young person's perspective, a usable AT enables functioning in everyday activities without threatening or complicating social participation with peers (Hemmingsson, Lidström & Nygård 2009).

Theoretical point of departure

Investigating how young people's domestication of ICT influences the opportunities available to young disabled persons for participation in their everyday life, we employ two different, but closely related, theoretical perspectives. The chosen perspectives correspond with our relational understanding of disability and our interactional understanding of participation, and we therefore find them suitable for our investigation.

The first theoretical perspective represents an interactionist approach (Blumer 1998). An interactionist approach enhances our insight into how meaning is constituted, confirmed, maintained and spread, as well as into the significance of shared values and symbols. The most significant dimension of symbols is that they have meaning only to the extent that individuals share the belief that the symbol possesses that particular value. It is through young people's everyday acceptance or rejection of symbols that their identity in a peer group is determined (Dennis & Martin 2005), and thus their opportunities for social participation, which is the central phenomenon in symbolic interactionism (Blumer 1998).

The second theoretical perspective employed in this chapter is an actor-network theory (ANT) perspective (Latour 2008). According to ANT, any object, artefact or person who generates an effect by making a difference is an actor. Actors may indicate, encourage, permit, influence, make possible, determine or obstruct actions. Therefore, who and what enter into an action, or a social practice, need to be carefully scrutinised. While human actions, communication and symbols only constitute one part of social practices, things, objects and technologies constitute the other part. In social practices, the connections and joining of actions create network effects that constitute social structure. The challenge is to follow the actors, reveal their actions, and show how the social is created (Latour 2008). Such socio-material practices may be how young disabled people use their assistive ICT, how the assistive ICT influences their possibilities for actions, interactions and participation, and how these possibilities affect them.

The significance of ICTs in young disabled people's social interactions and participation

The empirical data elaborated and discussed in this section are derived from several disability studies carried out in Sweden and in Norway. All descriptions are real, the excerpts are rendered as literally as possible, and the data illustrate common features of the studies. The names, however, are fictional. We will now look more closely into how young disabled people in Sweden and in Norway experience the use of ICTs and assistive ICTs, and what they think of their experiences.

Opportunities in leisure activities

The ability to interact with peers is of utmost concern for most young people, disabled or not. Moreover, young people's peer communities are characterised by extensive permeability between the virtual and material worlds, and the use of ICTs is central in both areas (Buckingham 2006; Söderström 2013). In different ways, young disabled people seize every opportunity to present themselves as ordinary, competent and independent. They do this above all by using ICTs in the same way and for the same purposes as any other young person, i.e. communicatively, socially and interactively. Eivind is a 17-year-old partially sighted boy. Eivind presented himself as a passionate computer games player, and he explained:

> I play World of Warcraft. Sometimes I can play for six hours. Sometimes I play with local friends and sometimes with people from England and the Netherlands. We play and talk at the same time. It's fun to get to know other people. You get to know them quite well when you play and talk with them almost every day.
>
> (Söderström 2009, p. 135)

Eivind made arrangements, sometimes with his friends in the neighbourhood and sometimes with his online friends, about when to play and who to play with. Sometimes he and his friends played World of Warcraft in face-to-face settings as a team, and other times he played the game alone with online partners. Another boy is Jacob, who is 16 years old. Jacob has comprehensive mobility difficulties and uses a powered wheelchair. His biggest interest is computers. He explained:

> My friends and I gather at my place. I have three mates. We have common interests; it's all about computers. We get together at my place about every

other weekend. Everybody brings along at least one computer each. Then it's all about computers all through the weekend. It is like a social happening.

(Söderström 2009, p. 135)

Young disabled people are like other young people. Most of them attend the local school and grow up in neighbourhoods where non-disabled young people surround them. Thus, the identity references of young disabled people are similar to those of young non-disabled people. This means that it is very important for young disabled people to blend in with their peers, and especially to avoid standing out in a negative manner (Hemmingsson, Lidström & Nygård 2009). However, the digitalisation of society places young people in different discourses: the same young person is 'ordinary' in some settings and 'disabled' in others (Wielandt et al. 2006).

Jacob took charge and initiated activities of his own choices. In this way, Jacob created alternative opportunities for participation and interaction with other boys, alternatives that were made possible due to the boys' common interest in technological devices. On these occasions, Jacob was not disabled and excluded; rather, he was in full control and was able to participate in valued activities with friends and like-minded peers. Thus, the socio-material practices made possible by ICTs have provided young disabled people with opportunities to demonstrate competence, abilities and independence – properties that contradict common stereotypes of disabled people as restricted, dependent and in need of care (Söderström & Ytterhus 2010).

Opportunities in everyday school life

Lisa is a girl with severe mobility difficulties, attending fifth grade in a mainstream school. Lisa uses a powered wheelchair and a lot of assistive ICTs at school. One assistive ICT is a software mathematics program on her computer, and another is a joystick replacing the keyboard. In maths classes, the tasks appear on the screen one by one, proposing several possible answers. Lisa uses the joystick to click on the answer she thinks is correct. Clicking on the right answer, she is given points, more points for more difficult maths tasks. Lisa navigates a marker quite quickly around the screen using the joystick. Because she has some involuntary movements in her upper limbs, it is sometimes a little hard for her to stop the marker exactly at the correct answer. However, most of the time she manages to do this, and at the end of the maths class, she has a lot of points. Lisa proudly shows her points total to some of her classmates, who stop at her desk and compliment her.

In this maths class, the assistive ICT Lisa uses functions as an actor enabling her to participate in an ordinary class activity, and to show a positively valued identity as a competent student. In this way, the assistive software mathematics program and the assistive joystick function as an actor empowering Lisa to participate in an everyday school activity. When assistive ICTs work as expected, disabled students find them very intriguing. When asked what they think of assistive ICTs, expressions such as '*I think ICT is an ingenious invention*', '*I would be lost without it'*, and *'It would be a boring life without it'* illuminate the central role played by technologies in the everyday school lives of disabled students (Söderström 2012, p. 33).

Participation is, however, not an activity done by one actor alone. Participation involves many actors, human and non-human, in a network of connections (Latour 2008). In that respect, the opportunities for participation which are provided to disabled students by useful and compatible assistive ICTs are made possible by a set of actors in a network of connections. Lisa's participation in her maths classes is thus not solely due to the properties of the technologies used. It is also due to the combined interaction between, and properties of, Lisa, of the assistive ICTs, and of the total classroom setting. Thus, Lisa's participation is made possible through three interrelating circumstances: (1) her mastering of the useful and compatible assistive ICTs, (2) her presence and participation in the classroom, and (3) her classmates' acknowledgement of her competence.

However, assistive ICTs in school also pose special challenges for the students who receive an AT device to be used in school. Schools are an arena for intensive social interaction and identity negotiation among young people of about the same age. The young people are organised in groups, and there are rules and regulations that all students have to accept. Unlike home, school is an environment where young people have very few personal possessions. Being the only one in class to receive something special like a computer might present a challenge. Jenny, an 11-year-old girl who had been given a computer in order to be able to write in class, told us what happened when she received it as an assistive device:

> In the beginning all the boys in the class were jealous because I'd been given a computer, but then I told them why they'd given it to me and they said OK, but it's unfair anyhow.
>
> (Hemmingsson, Lidström & Nygård 2009, p. 468)

As this example shows, arrangements aiming to increase participation in learning activities might receive a negative reaction from peers. Students with a disability might be teased because they are carrying out a school task, such as writing, differently from their peers, or peers might be jealous and think it is unfair that someone should receive something they themselves do not have access to in school, as in the example above. When this happens, it counteracts the effort of the student with disability to enter into identity negotiations with classmates, and he/she is ascribed an identity as disabled. This in turn might result in the student with disability being reluctant to use the device, although fully appreciating the advantages for learning. From the student's perspective, a good relationship with peers often takes priority, and therefore becomes more important than, for example, optimal opportunities for reading and writing. Such circumstances are sometimes the reason for young people's refusal to use assistive devices in school, despite the benefits teachers and parents expect the devices to bring (Hemmingsson et al. 2009). Another example is a 15-year-old girl, Alice, who was very much aware of the fact that being able to write fluently was extremely important for her future opportunities. She said:

> It is important, because in today's society you cannot manage without being able to write. Do you really think that you can get a job if you come with your CV and it says: weaknesses: cannot write! Then I don't think you'd get a job.
> (Breivik & Hemmingsson 2013, p. 353)

Alice wrote faster with the ICT device than by hand, and the spelling program really helped her. Nevertheless, after a while she felt that the device made her stand out in class. She was the only one not writing by hand, and she felt different and deviant and chose to manage without it, although it impacted on her results in school. As students with disabilities, Jenny and Alice experienced that assistive devices, or other arrangements aiming to increase their opportunities in school, are not always fully accepted by peers. Adolescents view peer relations as one of the most significant factors affecting their quality of life (Helseth & Misvær 2010). For that reason, they weight the utility of the learning device against the possible negative social consequences (Hemmingsson et al. 2009; Söderström & Ytterhus 2010).

Opportunities to pass as ordinary

Many disabled young people make use of the opportunities provided to them by assistive ICTs to display digital skills and competencies, and to participate in meaningful settings with peers. By doing this, they display similarities to peers. Furthermore, by doing ordinary things, young disabled people neutralise disability and pass as ordinary young people (Goffman 1967). It is, however, vital to recognise that usability is not solely an attribute of the AT itself, but that the human-device-environment interaction is equally important. Iselin is a 17-year-old blind girl who told this story:

> I got a mobile phone for Christmas some years ago. I had wanted one for some time because everybody else had one. However, I do not really understand why I got it, because I couldn't read anything on it. My brother got very annoyed with me because he had to read all the text messages aloud for me. Then I got Talks, and that really rescued me. Then I felt like oooh . . . how nice, now I can finally be like an ordinary young person.
> (Söderström & Ytterhus 2010, p. 309)

Young people constantly use mobile texting to express their sense of self, and to build and maintain peer relationships, co-ordinate social gatherings and define who belongs to important social communities (Lonkila & Gladarev 2008; Söderström 2011). It is therefore vital to young people to be able to read and write text messages, and through this, young disabled people perform their symbolic work by doing ordinary things, displaying their belonging and thus pass as ordinary. The AT Talks gave Iselin the opportunity to overcome a technological barrier to social interaction and inclusion in her peer group.

While the symbolic value of technologies may be perceived as 'to have is to be' (Hocking 2000), it appears that the nature of the link between having and being lies in the way the technologies are used, i.e. in the actual and continual symbolic work of negotiating and maintaining identity (Dennis & Martin 2005). The mobile phone did not provide Iselin with the opportunity to perform this symbolic work, given its inaccessible visual interface. However, Talks enabled Iselin to hear text messages by herself and to keep in touch with and be available to her friends while maintaining her privacy. Now she could use her mobile phone in the same way as her friends, and simultaneously perform her symbolic identity work by passing as ordinary (Goffman 1967). Thus, Talks enabled Iselin to participate in text messaging. This participation made Iselin feel rescued, and ultimately like an ordinary young person. She could pass as normal. Later on, Iselin elaborated on the significance of assistive ICTs:

> Both the mobile phone and the computer have helped a lot of people, and me too, to be more accepted. These technologies have helped us to get in touch with people, and to show them that we are interested in interaction, and that we are interesting people to interact with. It would have been a very boring life without them.
>
> (Söderström & Ytterhus 2010, p. 310)

Through her interactive use of assistive ICTs, Iselin engages in symbolic work as a member of the youth community and displays herself as an interesting and ordinary person to other members of this community. The domestication of ICT – and corresponding assistive ICTs – has provided many young disabled people with opportunities they did not previously have to pass as normal. Both Buckingham (2006) and Hocking (2000) point out that because technology and its objects are also cultural objects, it is important to use the 'right' technology in the 'right' way. This is especially true for young people, who are at a stage of their lives during which most of them consider passing as 'normal' and being included in the peer group most important. ICT is technology inscribed with the qualities of competence, independence and youth, and the 'right' use of ICT is a key element in young people's negotiation of identity and belonging (Buckingham 2006; Söderström & Ytterhus 2010).

Discussion

The primary focus by far among young people with disabilities is the social benefits which the use of assistive ICTs provides them. More than anything, they want to pass as ordinary young people, participating in ordinary peer relationships. However, in doing so in the digital arena, they are at continuous risk, especially those with visual impairments, of falling short. ICTs might, on the one hand, facilitate social participation by providing new opportunities for some young disabled persons; but on the other hand, they may represent new challenges and new barriers that were previously not an issue. For example, young visually impaired persons face challenges with graphic interfaces, inaccessible websites and the speed of digital communication. Another group that may experience increased barriers with the move of social participation to the web is young people with intellectual disabilities. Social participation that relies on written messages and ability to navigate in a changeable digital landscape may be a hindrance for young people with intellectual disabilities, as they may have lower digital competences, such as word-processing skills, than their peers.

Nevertheless, for most young disabled persons, the potential to pass as ordinary by participating in the digital arena overshadows the risks of falling short (Söderström & Ytterhus 2010). Moreover, participating in the digital arena also involves a dependency on accessible and usable assistive ICTs. From the young person's perspective, this means that while accessible ICT is ICT you can operate, usable ICT is ICT you can use for whatever purpose you want. Thus, accessible ICT refers to the design of a product and is ICT you can operate. Usable ICT, on the other hand, refers to a product's 'seaworthiness' in terms of the extent to which the ICT, and related AT, meet the user's own priorities. These two characteristics of ICT might turn out to be two quite different characteristics (Söderström 2009). Consequently, one may sometimes be fooled into believing that *accessible* ICT serves as a facilitator to participation when it actually is *unusable* ICT, which serves as an inhibitor to participation.

The domestication of ICT by young people in general has provided young disabled people with increased opportunities for participation in leisure activities. This might be participation in the digital arena, such as in the case of Eivind, who engaged in online computer games. It might also be participation in face-to-face settings, such as in the case of Jacob, who organised computer gatherings with friends at home. Employing an ANT perspective, ICT turns out to be a vital actor in providing young disabled people enhanced opportunities for social participation with peers. Very often, young people's social participation takes place with or *about* digital technologies. This strong connection between technology and participation has, however, altered the context, style and frequency of participation. According to the Swedish Media Council, which has followed young people's media habits since 2005 and publishes a report every other year, the frequency of meeting friends (face to face) after school has decreased substantially. In the Swedish Media Council's first report from 2006, meeting friends was the most common activity after school among young people, but in 2010 it was only number three. In 2006, 74% stated that they usually met friends after school, compared to 64% in 2008. In 2010, the wording of the question was modified to clarify that it referred to face-to-face meetings, and the number for that year was 58% (Hemmingsson 2015). During the same period, social websites expanded tremendously, and it is likely that some social interaction has moved to the web. In 2012–2013, a comparison of media habits of young persons in Sweden and Norway was conducted, and there were considerable similarities between the two countries. In both countries, young people aged 13–16 years spent about three hours every day on social media. Moreover, children start to use the Internet at an early age, at approximately 2–3 years (Swedish Media Council 2014). This makes it plausible to assume that disabled children also become familiar with digital technologies at an early stage, and that this development has increased their opportunities for social participation.

Social participation on the web may give more freedom. As you can have multiple remote friends, you are in a position to choose which parts of your personality you make visible, and in that way influence the responses of your interaction partner. The Internet could also provide an opportunity for communication without time pressure, and this might be an advantage for some young people with disabilities. During adolescence, the need to conform to one's peers is particularly important, and standing out from the majority has a significant negative impact (Grue 2001; Söderström & Ytterhus 2010). In this respect, the use of assistive technologies, that is technologies designed especially for disabled people, might be a risky business. The cases of Jenny and Alice, who use assistive technologies at school, illustrate how this might take place. These cases illuminate how we are identified, categorised and valued through our use of technologies, and how this influences our opportunities for participation. Several studies have found that young disabled people value social participation and acknowledgement over the academic achievement and/or functional convenience that assistive technologies may provide them with (Söderström & Ytterhus 2010; Wielandt et al. 2006). This does not necessarily mean that it is the assistive technologies as such that define the values, categories and identities connected to them. Rather, it is our associations, beliefs and prejudices that make these connections between the technologies and the persons using them. This may indicate that in cases where assistive technologies resemble ordinary technologies, assistive technologies may promote the social participation of young disabled people. It might, however, also indicate that when non-disabled people perceive assistive technologies as just alternative versions of ordinary technologies, the same outcome is achieved. We find that in order to facilitate social participation for young disabled people, there is a need for increased involvement and awareness of the importance of both the technological and the attitudinal aspects of participation.

Concluding remarks

One case alone, whether human or non-human, does not constitute participation; neither is participation a stable or fixed state. Participation is dynamic, flexible and relational, involving persons, objects, technologies, places and contexts, all in a network of connections. For most people, participation is a natural everyday experience which includes the domestication of technology. In this chapter, we have investigated young disabled people's social participation in their peer group in light of young people's domestication of ICT.

The implementation of new, and increasingly advanced and complex, technologies and assistive technologies might be perceived as experiments with established categories, such as the category of disability. Sometimes such an implementation leads to increased participation and social interaction for disabled people, and at other times it is a barrier to the same. Nevertheless, technological development, implementation and domestication provide us with opportunities to gain enhanced insight into the process of constructing and re-constructing dichotomies such as us–them and able–disabled, and the significance this has on people's opportunities for participation.

One of the challenges we face is that if technology is to promote social inter-action and participation for disabled people, we must recognise that disability and ability are not a dichotomy. People are made able or disabled in many different ways in different situations. The question is not how ICTs and advanced technological solutions may normalise human functions and actions. Rather, the question is how technology may create effects that help change the way we think about – and distinguish between – able and disabled, and thus facilitate new opportunities and new forms of social participation.

References

Asbjörnslett, M., & Hemmingsson, H. 2008, Participation at school – experienced by teen-agers with physical disabilities. *Scandinavian Journal of Occupational Therapy*, 15(3), 153–161.

Blumer, H. 1998, *Symbolic interactionism: Perspective and method.* Englewood Cliffs: Prentice Hall.

Bolic-Baric, V., Hellberg, K., Kjellberg, A., & Hemmingsson, H. online, "Internet activities during leisure: A comparison between adolescents with ADHD and adolescents from the general population", *Journal of Attention Disorder.*

Borgestig, M., Sandqvist, J. Ahlsten, G. Falkmer, T., & Hemmingsson, H. online, "Gaze-based assistive technology in daily activities in children with severe physical impair-ments – an intervention study", *Developmental Neurorehabilitation.*

Bossaert, B., Colpin, H., Pijl, S.J., & Petry, K. 2013, "Truly included? A literature study focusing on the social dimensions of inclusion in education", *International Journal of Inclusive Education*, 17(1), 60–79. doi:10.1080/13603116.2011.580464.

Breivik, I., & Hemmingsson, H. 2013, "Experiences of handwriting and using a comput-erised ATD in school: Adolescents with Asperger syndrome", *Scandinavian Journal of Occupational Therapy*, 20(5), 349–356.

Buckingham, D. 2006, "Children and new media", in L.A. Lievrouw & S. Livingstone (eds.) *The handbook of new media updated student edition*, pp. 75–91. London, UK: Sage.

Dennis, A., & Martin, P.J. 2005, "Symbolic interactionism and the concept of power", *The British Journal of Sociology*, 65(2), 191–213.

Goffman, E. 1967, *Interaction ritual – essays on face-to-face behaviour.* New York: Pan-theon Books.

Grue, L. 2001, *Motstand og mestring Om funksjonshemming og livsvilkår* (Resistance and coping. On disability and life conditions, not available in English). Oslo, NO: Abstrakt Forlag AS.

Gustavsson, A., Tøssebro, J., & Traustadòttir, R. 2005, "Introduction: Approaches and per-spectives in Nordic disability research", in A. Gustavsson, J. Sandvin, R. Traustadòttir &

J. Tøssebro (eds.) *Resistance, reflection and change: Nordic disability research*, pp. 23–44. Lund: Studentlitteratur.

Helseth S., & Misvær, N. 2010, "Adolescents' perception of quality of life: What it is and what matters", *Journal of Clinical Nursing*, 19, 1454–1456.

Hemmingsson, H. 2015, "Trendsetters and followers: Disabled young people computer use during leisure time", in R. Traustadottir, B. Ytterhus, S. Egilson & B. Berg (eds.) *Childhood and disability in the Nordic countries: Being, becoming, belonging*, pp. 167–178. Sheffield: Palgrave Macmillan.

Hemmingsson, H., & Jonsson, H. 2005, "An occupational perspective on the concept of participation in the international classification of functioning, disability and health – Some critical remarks", *American Journal of Occupational Therapy*, 59(5), 569–576.

Hemmingsson, H., Lidström, H., & Nygård, L. 2009, "Use of assistive technology devices in mainstream schools: Students' perspective", *The American Journal of Occupational Therapy*, 63(4), 461–470.

Hocking, C. 2000, "Having and using objects in the Western world", *Journal of Occupational Science*, 7(3), 148–157.

Hughes, B., Russell, R., & Paterson, K. 2005, "Nothing to be had 'off the peg': Consumption, identity and the immobilization of young disabled people", *Disability & Society*, 20(1), 3–17.

ICF-CY 2007, *International classification of functioning, disability and health. Children & youth version ICF-CY*. Geneva: WHO ISBN 978 92 4 1547321.

Latour, B. 2008, *En ny sociologi for et nyt samfund Introduktion til Aktør-Netværk-teori* (a new sociology for a new society: Introduction to Actor-Network theory). København: Akademisk Forlag.

Lidström, H., Ahlsten, G., & Hemmingsson, H. 2010, "The influence of ICT on the activity patterns of children with physical disabilities outside school", *Child: Care, Health & Development*, 37(3), 313–321.

Lidström, H., Almqvist, L., & Hemmingsson, H. 2012, "Computer-based assistive technology device for use by children with physical disabilities: A cross-sectional study", *Disability and Rehabilitation: Assistive Technology*, 7(4), 287–293.

Livingstone, S., & Helsper, E. 2007, "Gradations in digital inclusion: Children, young people and the digital divide", *New Media & Society*, 9(4), 671–696.

Lonkila, M., & Gladarev, B. 2008, "Social networks and cell phone use in Russia: Local consequences of global communication technology", *New Media & Society*, 10(2), 273–293.

MacKenzie, D., & Wajcman, J. 2005, "Introductory essay: The social shaping of technology", in D. Mackenzie & J. Wajcman (eds.) *The social shaping of technology*, second edition, pp. 3–27. Berkshire: Open University Press.

McMillan, S.J., & Morrison, M. 2006, "Coming of age with the Internet: A qualitative exploration of how the Internet has become an integral part of young people's lives", *New Media & Society*, 8(1), 73–95.

Moser, I. 2006, "Sociotechnical practices and difference on the interference between disability, gender and class", *Science, Technology & Human Values*, 31(5), 1–28.

Noreau, L., & Fougeyrollas, P. 2000, "Long-term consequences of spinal cord injury on social participation: The occurrence of handicap situations", *Disability & Rehabilitation*, 2, 170–180.

Peter, J., & Valkenburg, P.M. 2006, "Research note: Individual differences in perceptions of Internet communication", *European Journal of Communication*, 21(2), 213–226.

Räsänen, P. 2008, "The aftermath of the ICT revolution? Media and communication technology preferences in Finland in 1999 and 2004", *New Media & Society*, 10(2), 225–245.

Ravneberg, B., & Söderström, S. in press, *Disability, society & assistive technology*. Surrey, UK: Ashgate Publishing Group.

Söderström, S. 2009, "The significance of ICT in disabled youth's identity negotiations", *Scandinavian Journal of Disability Research*, 11(2), 131–144.

Söderström, S. 2011, "Staying safe while on the move: Exploring differences in disabled and non-disabled young people's perceptions of the mobile phone's significance in daily life", *YOUNG Nordic Journal of Youth Research*, 19(1), 91–109.

Söderström, S. 2012, "Disabled pupils' use of assistive ICT in Norwegian schools", in F.A. Auat Cheein (ed.) *Assistive technologies*, pp. 25–48. Kroatia: InTech. ISBN 978–953-51–0348–6.

Söderström, S. 2013, "Digital differentiation in young people's Internet use – Eliminating or reproducing disability stereotypes? *Future Internet*, 5, 190–204. doi:10.3390/fi5020190.

Söderström, S., & Ytterhus, B. 2010, "The use and non-use of assistive technologies from the world of information and communication technology by visually impaired young people: A walk on the tightrope of peer-inclusion", *Disability & Society*, 25(3), 303–315.

Sørensen, K.H. 2004, "Tingenes samfunn. Kunnskap og materialitet som sosiologiske korrektiver" (in English: The Society of Things. Knowledge and Materiality as Sociological Corrections), *Sociologi i dag (Sociology Today)*, 34(2), 5–25.

Swedish Media Council and Medietillsynet 2014, *Barn och medier i Sverige vs Norge: Informationsblad* (Children and media in Norway versus Sweden: Information sheet). Stockholm: Statens Medieråd.

Wielandt, T., McKenna, K., Tooth, L., & Strong, J. 2006, "Factors that predict the post-charge use of recommended assistive technology (AT)", *Disability & Rehabilitation: Assistive Technology*, 1(1–2), 29–40.

Winance, M. 2006, "Trying out the wheelchair: The mutual shaping of people and devices through adjustment", *Science, Technology & Human Values*, 31(1), 52–72.

15 Participation in everyday life as lived negotiations

Challenges and opportunities within a situated understanding of participation

Sissel Alsaker, Staffan Josephsson and Virginia Dickie

> I'm very good at managing my illness, but not the other things in my everyday life; it requires too much energy . . . and nobody asks me about that.
>
> (Alsaker, 1998)

> Wallander set out to change his habits and had a small evening meal: He was concentrating so hard on making sure that only the right things found their way onto his plate that he forgot he had signed up for the laundry, and by the time he remembered it was too late.
>
> (Mankell and translator, 1997/2003, p. 35)

The above vignettes are from different sources showing involvement in life situations. Liv was a participant in an ethnographic study on how meaning is established in the everyday lives of women living with chronic rheumatic disease, and Kurt Wallander is the protagonist of popular Swedish crime series.

We draw from these two sources with a specific mission to unpack *the practice of participation* in the everyday lives of individuals. Participation was developed as a professional concept with the aim of broadening the understanding of health to encompass the everyday lives of people (Cornwall, 2008; Hammel et al., 2008; Yilmas et al., 2009). But how is participation established, and how does it function at the most ordinary, mundane level of people's lives? Knowledge about this is limited, and there are many questions to be answered. What does it mean for individuals to be involved in life situations? Who are the actors in the participation? Is participation in the everyday clearly defined and easy to read, or is it rather opaque and mundane? What characterises the practice of participation in the everyday? How does individual participation meet with challenges regarding the intersections of everyday living, health conditions and service provision? Is it that 'involvement in life situations' is something that must be negotiated through the ever-changing situations of everyday life? As seen from this short list of queries, there are many issues that need to be addressed regarding participation in everyday life which seems to be characterised by complexity. This chapter sets out to explore some aspects of this complexity. We will do this by drawing from existing literature on participation and everyday life, and use these resources to present and analyse material from the two stories in the introductory vignettes. The stories are presented more extensively below, and originate from two different textual genres: literature and empirical data. Wallander was created by the Swedish writer Henning Mankell (1997/2002) in a series of popular Swedish crime novels, and Liv is a woman living with chronic rheumatic disease who participated in an observational study focusing on her everyday living (Alsaker, 1998). The purpose of this chapter is to unpack the practice of participation, specifically aiming to describe how participation works in the everyday lives of individuals. We use the example from Mankell's book in order to show how everyday participation is portrayed in contemporary culture. The example from the ethnographic study will add scientifically grounded material to deepen our reasoning and understanding of everyday participation.

From both these resources, our path into elaborating on participation goes through the everyday, exemplified by the complexities, contradictions and challenges that Wallander and Liv meet in their everyday involvements. By the word 'everyday', we mean the situations and actions that make up the daily lives of individuals. In the literature on participation which grounds this book, there is a growing interest in broadening the concept of participation; and by linking the term to the everyday, we hope to contribute to this by exploring participation as a set of resources available to individuals in their everyday lives. To illustrate the first of the resources, we return to Mankell's novel. In order to paint a nuanced picture of how participation is simultaneously situated and ongoing within the lives of people, we will show you some glimpses of Wallander's everyday life.

> On Wednesday, 7 August, 1996, Kurt Wallander came close to being killed in a traffic accident just east of Ystad. . .. As he calmed down he realised what had happened. He had fallen asleep at the wheel.
>
> (p. 9)

> At midnight he went to bed. He had a meeting . . . the next day and he had to go to the doctor. He lay awake in the darkness for a long time. Two years ago he had thought about moving from the flat. . .. He had dreamed of getting a dog, of living with Baiba. But nothing had come of it. No Baiba, no house, no dog.
>
> (p. 21)

The following day, Wallander capably handles various work responsibilities, and the stage is set for the discovery of horrible crimes as the book progresses. He goes to the doctor, where he learns that he has diabetes. He goes to the library and reads up on the disease.

> He realised he had only himself to blame. The food he ate, his lack of exercise, and his on-and-off dieting had all contributed to the disease. He put the

book back on the shelf. A sense of failure and disgust came over him. He knew there was no way out. He had to do something about his lifestyle.

(p. 34)

Then he returns to work.

This excerpt from the novel *One Step Behind* shows how Henning Mankell uses everyday ordinary activities such as eating, doing chores and spending time with family as a means of embedding his character, Kurt Wallander, in the everyday world in which he lives and works. When Wallander is not actively solving a crime, Mankell devotes considerable writing to the humdrum daily concerns that occupy his time – selling his father's house, finding public restrooms or a private place to pee (a hint of the diabetes diagnosis to come), cleaning his flat, not finding a TV programme that interests him as he flips through channels, and so on. But in his writing about Wallander's everyday activities, Mankell has also set Wallander apart from the everyday world of 'others' (just as Liv expresses her sense of difference later in this chapter). Wallander is often portrayed as not very good at participating in the everyday, even if he is a brilliant policeman who tunes into the everyday activity patterns of crime victims and perpetrators. In many of the Wallander mysteries, we read about Wallander either forgetting to sign up for laundry time, or forgetting to use the time he signed up for – lapses that are meaningful to Swedish apartment dwellers. Wallander, who is divorced, spends much of his leisure time alone, and often ruminates about his health and the need to watch what he eats. Nonetheless, he forgets to buy food, and often settles for convenience food that he knows is not good for him. When he learns that he has diabetes, he tries to take on this new identity and the responsibilities it entails. These glimpses of Wallander's everyday life show him struggling, and often lonely. He is different from others and less capable of managing his life than they seem to be. And yet he is a considerate supervisor of those who work with him, and he demonstrates a keen understanding of how others think, feel and act.

As shown in the above example, Mankell has given us a brilliant description of how a person is deeply participating in his life through everyday occurrences. These everyday actions and happenings provide the reader with material to interpret and understand who Wallander is, the choices he makes and how he prioritises and involves himself in everyday living. Most of us will read several moral issues into our interpretation of the texts; perhaps he has few friends, he does not exercise, he is lonely, he does not take care of his health. As professionals, we will probably see a future patient or a person in great need of health prevention strategies on many levels, both medically and socially. Wallander's example sets the stage for exploring the varied and often complex and contradictory situations that occur in everyday participation. To broaden our understanding of everyday participation, we need to delve into theory as well as the ethnographic study of Liv's everyday life.

How do we understand that something is simultaneously situated and ongoing? Situated understanding has its origins in feminist theory (Haraway, 1991). The argument that all knowledge is situated implies that every interpretation that is made, be it from lay people or researchers, is by necessity an interpretation from a particular point of view. However, one aspect that distinguishes scientific knowledge from lay knowledge is that researchers need to clarify their interpretative framework. This means that interpretative work from social and material life must be grounded and located in an embodied framework of experiences, concepts, beliefs and standards. Explanation of that framework may add to or support our interpretation and make it more transparent.

This chapter will also bring forward resources clarifying what we mean by the everyday as situated and ongoing. This implies showing everyday participation through empirical examples of a complicated and intricate practice that is situated, emergent and negotiated. We hereby hope to contribute to the knowledge base on which this book is founded, and to an expansion of the current understanding of participation as a concept that shows involvement in life situations as something that occurs and is constantly negotiated in local contexts – merging and emerging among persons, spaces, narratives and actions within what we call the everyday.

Living and acting in the realm of the everyday involves both being engaged in and able to make use of whatever resources are available in time and localities. Such resources may be natural as well as man-made objects, and of course persons and animals, together with moral and cultural issues. Traditionally, involvement in life situations is mostly measured or assessed historically in the form of individuals' overall experiences, or regarding specific issues in society (Hart & Heatwole Shank, 2016), or individuals' perception of the possibility of participation in certain activities or societal circumstances (Yilmaz et al., 2008).

However, here we will address participation as emerging and ongoing, implying that the everyday resources are made available to individuals through their experiences, actions and/or intentions. Consequently, we run into issues regarding what is pre-planned or not necessarily predictable. This lack of predictability is a complicating issue when talking about participation in everyday circumstances. With regard to involvement in life situations, the current conceptualisation of participation in the International Classification of Functioning, Disability and Heal (ICF) framework points towards the everyday as an important matter for both individuals and health service providers (Cornwall, 2008; Hammel et al., 2008), but does little to explain and develop the concept of the everyday. We will identify some gaps and dilemmas in the knowledge on participation in the everyday, and suggest some paths for future studies in this matter.

The everyday

The everyday is the ordinary, mundane things and activities that people do throughout their waking hours. In the frame of the everyday, human life emerges through what people do, how they do it, and with whom, where and when, in a seemingly endless stream marked by habitual as well as unknown situations. There is movement from one thing to another, among people, indoors and outside, in natural or man-made surroundings, shifting seasons and weather; at home, at work, in recreational time spent with family, friends and colleagues, locally and further afield. Thus, the everyday implies predictable as well as unpredictable situations. The situatedness of this everyday perspective is commonly understood through the concept of culture, local as well as global. Culture and its content of everyday social acts is thus viewed as ongoing and continuously changing, in contrast to a view of culture as something set or clearly framed (Gullestad, 1996). Consequently, the everyday comprises what people do throughout their ordinary days, individuals who at any time may be considered to belong to a particular population in a particular culture.

The concepts of everyday life and everyday activities are rarely defined in the literature, but the terms are often used interchangeably, and we will here compress these two terms into 'the everyday'. Traditionally the term 'everyday activities' means what individuals do as time is passing (Hasselkus, 2006, 2011). Also included in this use of the term is the manner in which individuals perform, where they perform, and the assumption that such activities are embedded with meaning. Scientific approaches to the area of everyday activities are connected to a notion of everyday life. They are relatively few and did not appear in the social science literature until recently, even if some philosophers had previously talked about everyday practice or pragmatism (Lawlor, 2006; Polkinghorne, 2004; Pollio et al., 1997). Based on Schüts's ideas of the social interaction in everyday life (Borg et al., 2007), Berger and Luckman's (Berger & Luckman, 1967) theories of the dialectic between the individual and society came to have considerable influence. Concepts of everyday life were further developed in Goffman's *The Presentation of Self in Everyday Life* (Goffman, 1992), which is widely used in health and social sciences. Here, Goffman introduced theatre metaphors such as 'back stage' and 'front stage' to develop the ever-changing and ongoing situatedness that characterise the everyday as well as the individual's opportunities to take part in and influence changing circumstances and content. Goffman's ideas recognised everyday life as a scientifically interesting subject of study, produced results showing how structure and content characterised everyday life, and described what kind of meaning and values people ascribed to it. Gullestad (1996) understood everyday life as social acts (Gullestad, 1996; Gullestad, 1989) happening in a culture. She posited that culture in itself is not a set phenomenon but is created, adjusted and negotiated by acting people in what she called local circumstances. Inspired by Gullestad, we use the concept of local culture to characterise the experience of everyday life in specific, identifiable localities. This is in contrast to global cultures, in which the phenomenon of everyday life is identifiable globally in many geographic localities (Frerer & Vu, 2007), and is of a more generic character. Local culture comprises ordinary people's interpretation of what to do and how to act in the circumstances of their everyday living, their moral values and interests, and their feelings of appropriateness and comfort, close to the above presentation of situatedness. Another aspect to consider is routines and habits, which in the literature is often linked to the everyday (Clark, 2000; Clark et al., 2007). The concept of habit in the everyday might be said to describe routine, repetitive and unintended aspects of people's everyday life. However, habits are the foundation of what people do and render it possible for people to act and participate in activities that are not pre-planned or that need to be acted upon on the spur of the moment. The knowledge and actions of many activities such as shopping, dressing appropriately for the weather, driving or riding a bike are learned consciously and then become relatively automatic habits requiring little thought and effort. Habits play a central part in participation because they occur as responses to familiar situations. The complicated and often contradictory content of the everyday that we have presented here shows that everyday participation can be challenging for the actors who may easily stumble and get off track. Recently, the everyday has received a great deal of attention in general publications in Scandinavian culture, arguably due to our welfare states, where almost everyone belongs to a class of 'ordinary people' with opportunities to live good everyday lives. The linking of the everyday with the idea and quality of ordinariness represents a normative or general understanding of the everyday in a culture and its population. Inherent in it are the activities and the practical and moral aspects temporally ascribed to ordinariness (Kralik, 2002). Gullestad (1996) notes that everyday life is people's ways of establishing integration in their immediate world by setting up and maintaining a meaningful connection between social roles, activities and circumstances, an understanding which this chapter draws upon. From Gullestad's reasoning, it follows that the mundane or ordinary aspects of everyday life might be different for people not belonging to what is thought of as the general population, clearly of relevance for individuals living with health issues. The individual, the health service and the policymakers aiming for everyday participation might all find challenges here.

There are also reasons to question our understanding of the content of the everyday/everyday life in the light of the way the public sphere nowadays tends to link varied entities to the concept of 'everyday', for example everyday-people, everyday-safety, everyday-reality, everyday-opportunities, everyday-habits, everyday-'whatever'. This might mean that the concept in itself is open to interpretation, and that 'everyday' captures important values, norms and content in the public sphere. On the other hand, when used to characterise many aspects in the human realm of daily life, it may also weaken its scientific value as a concept. Recent literature tends to understand everyday life as grounded in social constraints that may create a longing for something 'outside' these constraints (Baklien et al., 2015). This means that what seems to be mundane and ordinary for most people might be strange and extraordinary for others, and 'everyday' might therefore be difficult to pin down (Scott, 2009). To address this challenge, we will try to situate our theoretical argument through an empirical example of the situatedness that is necessary to understand a practice of participation in local contexts.

The practice of participation

'Participation as a praxis is, after all, rarely a seamless process; rather, it constitutes a terrain of contestation, in which relations of power between different actors, each with their own "projects", shape and reshape the boundaries of action' (Cornwall, 2008, p. 276). Cornwall states that a praxis of participation is ongoing, complicated and contested, not just between the actors, but also in relation to morals, meaning and values as well as objects and circumstances. This is an important argument, which points towards a practice of participation that is situated in individual, social, societal and material contexts. In the everyday, individual participation requires a constant making and unmaking in terms of the many issues that emerge. This way of negotiating everyday participation challenges the somewhat simplistic understanding of the everyday as something uncomplicated and effortless, and raises questions about how to unpack and understand individuals' participation in the everyday.

How can we examine participation in relation to everyday? We have stated that 'involvement in a life situation' is the way participation is defined in the ICF. Consequently, we argue that a 'life situation' may take place in the 'everyday,' meaning that the everyday consists of situations where people occupy a space and relate to and interact in a context, namely a local culture. By studying people who experience issues around participation in their everyday lives, as shown in the case of Liv later in this chapter, we will attempt to illustrate how the practice of participation actually happens.

Above we have outlined theoretical resources that we find useful in unpacking an understanding of participation in the everyday. From this, it appears that the practice of everyday participation involves different processes. Some of these are easily detectable because they are pre-planned. An example of this would be, e.g. deciding to go and see a film the following day. This would probably involve checking out what was on at the local cinema, how the scheduled times fitted in with other activities, and working out who else might want to come. In this example, the participation praxis is structured and pre-planned. Another example shows a more in-the-moment scenario, for example bumping into a friend in the street and ending up listening to a story of something that has happened in his life lately, and quite unexpectedly finding oneself involved in the friend's situation. One difference between these types of everyday praxis is that individual control is greater in the first, whereas the second requires action on the spot, due to the emergence of the situation. On the other hand, the kind of interaction/participation that is emerging may seem to have a different quality regarding involvement, and exemplifies how involvement in a life situation may have a wide range of qualities.

To further address participation from within, we need to look into an understanding of participation as social connection, meaning and values. Yerxa eloquently developed the issue of 'the infinite distance between the I and the It' (Yerxa, 2009, p. 490), pointing towards the vastness of the space between how people experience the everyday and how the surrounding world perceives it, with regard to bodily functions, morality or objects. How such I-phenomena meet with the everyday may be seen as something that constantly needs attention regarding a practice of participation.

Understanding how participation happens means studying particular situations where it is enacted, and where participation is at stake through negotiating between the I and the It, between the experiencing person and the everyday. Here everyday context is situated in this particular moment of time and place, where it is possible for the acting human to engage with, express and create meaning in a particular participatory practice.

We will now turn to the stories from Liv's everyday life. They are examples of how participation is situated, and we intend to describe and discuss how Liv negotiates participation in her everyday context. The stories describe living everyday life with a rheumatic condition and the struggle between the need for both structure and spontaneity, and demonstrate how Liv is situated in relation to her local culture.

Liv's story

A good day for me is when I do something I enjoy at my own pace and have time at my disposal. Over the years it has been very difficult for me to stick to my preferred rhythm in my everyday life . . . but now I have organised everything the way I like and that gives me the necessary variation between rest and work. I sometimes wonder if I am too organised, and if I occasionally need to practise a bit of disorder in my everyday life, it is probably smart to be a bit more flexible . . .

My partner also has a chronic disease, but he is in paid employment. That is why I do most of the housework. . .. However, he has made several adjustments to the house and garage to make life easier for me, and it gives me a lot of freedom to come and go as I want. Just imagine, I can now decide to drive into town to do the shopping or go and see a film if and when I want!

This may sound as if I just do what I like and make other people do the rest, but I can assure you that I always consider my relationships with my partner and friend when I prioritise activities. Family and friends are important for me, but we do not need to meet every day. We don't live that near each other, but I keep in regular touch by phone.

I also need to tell you about my crossword friends. You see, we are a group of friends who love to do the newspaper crosswords, and then we call each other and discuss the solutions . . . It is very nice to share an activity like that, and as there is a new crossword every week, it gives us a lot of opportunities for socialising . . .

I spend a lot of time and do a lot of preparation for my everyday life, something you healthy people do not need to worry about. Even if our society is now fairly well adjusted to disabled people, there are still a large number of tasks that I still cannot just decide to do on the spur of the moment, I cannot, for example, refuel my car without help because I am unable to manage the self-service pumps.

You know, first we have to learn to live with the disease, then we must learn how to move our bodies, and then we need to learn how to move around in our local community (Alsaker, 1998, unpublished field notes).

In the account of her challenges with her illness, Liv gives us examples of how she negotiates everyday participation. In addition, she contrasts her situation with 'you healthy people', situating herself as different, belonging to certain 'others'. However, the complex everyday that Liv faces may also be experienced by 'others' without obvious illness or disability, if we look at the number of everyday issues that are prominent in local Scandinavian culture.

Discussion

Considering Liv's story, we can identify some overall negotiations around her particularity (Alsaker & Josephsson, 2003, 2011). She considers herself to have challenges in her everyday living which differ from those of ordinary people, her neighbours, colleagues, et cetera (the population in her context). This means that she places herself apart from the general population when it comes to everyday participation. This is interesting in view of the way participation is defined as 'involvement in life situations', and how her story is all about involvement. She is involved in the content, pace, habits and structure of her everyday life, her relationship with her partner and the practical arrangements she needs to make and which her partner prepares and fulfils for her. However, she says that she has considered the impact this has on her relationships with both her partner and her friends. In our interpretation, she has actually given considerable thought to the issue of her contribution versus her dependence on the contributions of others. We see this as her way of negotiating participation in her everyday life, but always relating to her health issues. This shows that participation for Liv situates her in the 'unhealthy' category. We find it opportune to ask if this is a challenge to the idea of participation as a global concept. Liv shows how situated participation appears in her everyday life, and how her most important negotiations are very closely related to the consequences her medical condition has for her ability to become involved in the everyday chores and activities that we know make up individuals' experiences of participation.

If we accept the dichotomy healthy-unhealthy as part of Liv's everyday life, we can say that Liv's negotiations are grounded in her everyday doing. She situates her participation by way of being 'not healthy' as opposed to 'those who are healthy', and her expression points out that she thinks there is a difference in the quality or experience of participation between herself and the 'others'. She also reasons around the pace of the everyday, and seems to position herself as opposite to something. Liv embraces her options for user involvement; she considers herself an 'expert by experience' regarding her everyday participation. She demonstrates an ability to manage and negotiate her participation situated in what we think is a rather ordinary local context. On the other hand, she shows how challenging everyday participation is when it comes to practical issues, doing ordinary things in ordinary ways. She also struggles with identity issues; she wants to be and act like everyone else (Alsaker & Josephsson, 2003).

We further identify two challenging and in many ways contradictory negotiations: first, participation as intent; and second, participation in ongoing, everyday practice, activities, which include her planning for participation, both socially and in practical matters. In the following paragraphs, we will address these two kinds of negotiation.

First, Liv shows us her reasoning around her everyday life. Here she demonstrates how she enables herself to participate. Even if she situates herself as 'unhealthy' and is not able to do paid work, she manages to live a fairly ordinary everyday life. For her, this means living on a disability pension in a suburban family home with her partner, just like her neighbours and friends. She talks about herself as a person who puts great effort into enabling herself to live and participate; she considers herself as an actor. The following statement is typical: *I spend a lot of time and do plenty of preparation for my everyday life, something you healthy people do not need to worry about.* She goes on to give examples of how she needs to plan her participation to a greater extent by relating that she needs help to refuel her car, as she cannot manage the weight of the service-pump. In order for her to take the car and go to visit a friend, go shopping, or undertake other similar outings, she needs to put in quite a bit of effort to plan ahead to be sure that the car has enough petrol. That may mean that she needs to involve her partner, or she needs to find out whether there is a staffed petrol station nearby, something that she cannot expect in today's society.

On the other hand, Liv values the enormous freedom the car gives her. She can leave home on an impulse; she has a choice in her everyday participation which confirms her agency. In most people's everyday lives, this is part of their habitual repertoire and taken for granted. If the car is there, you can just drive to the shops to pick up your groceries when you need to. By doing this, Liv is experiencing everyday participation, however tailored to her situation, as it requires planning and time use far beyond that of the 'healthy' people.

At a glance, such negotiations may not seem particularly problematic and time-consuming. However, living with a chronic condition as Liv does means they are always there, all through her everyday life, and they are bound to affect her opportunities to be involved. It might be difficult for the 'healthy' population to understand the issues she is having to deal with. However, for Liv, negotiating her everyday participation means addressing very particular and mundane issues. Given the social and material context in which she is situated, she needs to plan her everyday very carefully. Liv manages to participate by enabling herself to be involved, but she must also prioritise and discuss how much time she has available, and adjust her everyday participation accordingly. On the other hand, it could be said that her considered choices add more meaning and quality to her everyday participation. Unpacking participation in the everyday from Liv's story shows that the value of freedom that is present in everyday participation may be lost or limited, and is not negotiable for many individuals. Challenges and contradictions are inherent in everyday participation for everyone; however, for those who do not belong to the 'healthy' population, the phenomenon takes on a greater complexity which needs to be addressed in research, service delivery and policy.

Epilogue – participation in the everyday as contradictory and incomplete

By including the case of Wallander, we add an example from contemporary fiction. We cannot know Mankell's intentions when he wrote so much about Wallander's participation in the mundane activities of the everyday, and how this participation failed to meet cultural expectations. But as readers, we interpret, and it is our perspective that makes this meaningful. From a transactional perspective, Wallander lives in a world which expects things to be done in a certain way, and he does not always manage to fully meet those expectations. That makes him both 'different', but also a lot like us, the readers. Without directly saying so, the novel plays on the norm that people are expected to do certain things: eat well, get enough sleep, sign up for laundry. It also places his extraordinary life of solving horrible crimes in a more ordinary place, where the fridge is empty and the laundry basket is full. Readers can relate to that, even if it doesn't make for the most exciting prose. The familiarity of it pulls us into the story, even if the rest of it is mostly beyond our experience. By not being terribly successful with participation in the everyday, Wallander is fallible and real. Maybe there is a lesson to be learnt here about participation in the everyday.

References

Alsaker S. (1998) *Aktivitet, roller og identititetshåndtering i hverdagslivet til mennesker med kroniske revmatiske lidelser. Psykologisk Institutt, Helsevitenskap.* Trondheim: NTNU, 104.

Alsaker S and Josephsson S. (2003) Negotiating occupational identities while living with chronic rheumatic disease. *Scandinavian Journal of Occupational Therapy* 10: 167–176.

Alsaker S and Josephsson S. (2011) Stories stirring the quest of the 'good': Narratives of women living with chronic rheumatic conditions. *Scandinavian Journal of Disability Research* 13: 53–70.

Baklien B, Ytterhus B and Bongaardt R. (2015) When everyday life becomes a storm on the horizon: Families' experiences of good mental health while hiking in nature. *Anthroplogy & Medicine* 23(1): 42–53.

Berger P and Luckman T. (1967) *The social construction of reality.* London: Penguin Group.

Borg T, Runge U, Tjørnov J, Brandt Å and Madsen AJ. (2007) *Basisbok i ergoterapi* [*Basisbook in occupational therapy*]. København: Munksgaard Danmark.

Clark F. (2000) The concepts of habits and routine: A preliminary theoretical synthesis. *OTJR – Occupational Therapy Journal of Research* 20: 123–135.

Clark F, Sanders K, Carlson M, Blanche E and Jackson J. (2007) Synthesis of habit theory. *OTJR – Occupation, Participation and Health* 27: 7S–23S.

Cornwall A. (2008) Unpacking 'participation': Models, meanings and practices. *Community Development Journal* 43: 269–283.

Frerer K and Vu CM. (2007) An anthropological view of powerty. *Journal of HUman Behavior in the Social Environment* 16: 73–86.

Goffman E. (1992) *Vårt rollespill til daglig* [*The presentation of self in everyday life*]. Norway: Pax Forlag a/s.

Gullestad M. (1989) *Kultur og hverdagsliv* [*Culture and everyday life*]. Oslo: Scandinavian University Press.

Gullestad M. (1996) *Everyday life philosophers*. Oslo: Scandinavian University Press.

Hammel J, Magasi S, Heinemann A, Whiteneck G, Bogner J and Rodriguez E. (2008) What does participation mean? An insider perspective from people with disabilities. *Disability & Rehabilitation* 30: 1445–1460.

Haraway DJ. (1991) *Simians, cyborgs and women: The reinvention of nature*. New York: Routledge.

Hart EC and Heatwole Shank K. (2016) Participating at the mall: Possibilities and tensions that shape older adults' occupations. *Journal of Occupational science* 23: 67–81.

Hasselkus BR. (2006) The world of everyday occupation: Real people, real lives. *The American Journal of Occupational Therapy* 60: 627–640.

Hasselkus BR. (2011) *The meaning of everyday occupation*. Thorofare, NJ: Slack Inc.

Kralik D. (2002) The quest for ordinariness: Transition experienced by midlife women living with chronic illness. *Journal of Advanced Nursing* 39: 146–154.

Lawlor MS. (2006) William James's psychological pragmatism: Habit, belief and purposive human behaviour. *Cambridge Journal of Economics* 30: 321–345.

Mankell H and (Translator) STM. (1997/2003) Faceless killers. *http://www.goodreads.com/book/show/935308.Faceless_Killers*.

Polkinghorne D. (2004) *Practice and the human sciences: The case for a judgement-based practice of care*. New York: State University of New York Press.

Pollio HR, Henley TB and Thompson CJ. (1997) *The phenomenology of everyday life*. Cambridge: Cambridge University Press.

Scott S. (2009) *Making sense of everyday life*. Cambridge: Polity Press.

Yerxa EJ. (2009) Infinite distance between the I and the It. *American Journal of Occupational Therapy* 63: 490–497.

Yilmaz M, Josephsson S, Danermark B and Ivarsson AB. (2008) Participation by doing: Social interaction in everyday activities among persons with schizofrenia. *Scandinavian Journal of Occupational Therapy* 15(3): 162–172.

Yilmas M, Josephsson S, Danermark B and Ivarsson AB. (2009) Social processes of participation in everyday life among persons with schizophrenia. *International Journal of Qualitative studies on Health and Well-being* 4: 267–279.

16 Barriers to participation

Time, social and physical obstacles for students with disabilities

Eva Magnus, Ulla Kroksmark and Kersti Nordell

Introduction

Time, as a universal dimension, guides and structures the human experience of activities. The patterns of activities in which people engage have a temporal rhythm as they occur in and through time. Meaningful and purposeful activities may promote health and well-being (Meyer, 1922/1977; Wilcock, 2010; Wilcock & Hocking, 2015). Patterns of time uses can provide information about cultural values and ecological variables that influence activity constructed by individuals on a day-to-day basis. The intention of this chapter is to illuminate how desirable participation for students with disabilities is influenced both by their time use in everyday life activities and by environmental obstacles.

Participation in activities involves dynamic interaction between people and their cultural, social and physical environment (Frank, Block, & Zemke, 2008; Hammel et al., 2008). Through participation, people gain skills and capability, connect with peers and the community, and find purpose and meaning in life. By structuring time, routines and physical space efficiently, people can decrease daily stress and maintain healthier relationships (Hammel, 2009). Time is of crucial relevance for participation. The availability of time might thus be a key condition for the opportunity to participate in activities people choose, where the activities take place and with whom. Further, in studying participation, a time-geographic approach can be useful through its focus on what people actually do within their various daily contexts, and what kind of restrictions they experience. Such a method provides access to a concrete dimension of participation. This chapter contributes to a discussion on time and participation by presenting the time-geographic method (TGM) as a tool to access concrete everyday participation. The TGM was originally developed by Torsten Hägerstrand, a Swedish professor in human geography (Hägerstrand, 1985). The TGM is a holistic approach which examines people's everyday activities and movements in time and space. The method was further developed by Kajsa Ellegård (Ellegård, 1999) to study individual activity patterns and the subjective dimension (Nordell, 2002), and has been used in various areas of research, for instance studying young people's everyday life (Alsaker et al, 2006; Kroksmark & Nordell, 2001; Magnus, 2009).

Active participation is a main political goal in the politics of disability in Norway and other Western countries. Participation in society involves equal opportunities in education, employment, leisure and social situations. At the same time, it is known that individuals with disabilities meet barriers to desirable participation, either as physical obstacles or through excluding attitudes in human relations (Shakespeare, 2006). It is globally agreed that disability is a complex phenomenon. The UN Convention on the Rights of Persons with Disabilities (CRPD) states: 'that disability is an evolving concept and that disability results from the interaction between persons with impairments and attitudinal and environmental barriers that hinder their full and effective participation in society on an equal basis with others' (UN, 2006, p. 2). Also, the International Classification of Functioning, Disability and Health (ICF) demonstrates how disability is a result of the interaction between the health condition of a person and their environment (WHO, 2001), although attitudes are absent from the classification system.

This chapter will illuminate how time use and environmental barriers can influence participation in higher education for students with disabilities in Norway. We begin with the stories of Heidi and Harald, which will illustrate elements of the everyday life of students with disabilities.

Everyday life of Heidi and Harald

Heidi and Harald were two university students living in Norway. Like most students, their intentions in life were to graduate, and then get a job in order to be economically independent. They both enjoyed being students and living on their own for the first time. Heidi and Harald recorded their daily activities in a diary during one week, in accordance with the TGM. The following are short descriptions of how they spent their time.

Heidi was a female student who lived in a flat not far from the university. Due to movement restrictions, she used an electric wheelchair. Her physical capability influenced her everyday activities, such as caring for herself, leisure activities and studies. Dyslexia also influenced her ability to study. To assist her in activities at home, in studies and in leisure, she had a personal assistant and a student assistant for altogether 65 hours a week, with more hours on weekdays than on Saturdays and Sundays.

On weekdays, Heidi got up between 7 and 8 am. Getting out of bed and doing her morning routines took her one and a half hours. After a quick breakfast, she went by taxi to the university. She spent time in the classroom following the courses. Her personal assistant supported her by putting her books and laptop in the right position, assisting her in the canteen and the library, and with toilet visits. Heidi spent quite a lot of time organising her everyday life on weekdays. She needed to set up time schedules for her personal assistants, visit health professionals, make phone calls to public service agencies, and deal with transport issues. Most afternoons and evenings were spent studying and watching television. Before the assistant left in the afternoon, the assistant helped Heidi put the laptop and audiobook in the right position, making sure that Heidi could reach and use the things she needed during the hours she spent alone. Another routine task was to plan the next day for her personal assistant. Around 11 pm, a home-care assistant came to help her go to bed.

Weekends were different, as Heidi slept longer in the morning. Usually she studied by herself and went out with her assistant, sometimes for a meal. In the evenings, she watched television and studied until the care assistant arrived around 11 pm.

Heidi spent most of her time at home, at the university and at the health service or other official places like the post office or the Norwegian Labour and Welfare Administration (NAV). She used a taxi to get around, spending nearly an hour a day travelling. Even if she had access to a taxi, she often had to wait because it did not arrive at the right time. Heidi spent most of her time either with her personal assistant, with healthcare personnel or by herself.

Harald was a male student. He shared a flat with three other male students. He wrote the following at the end of his diary:

> Summing up, I can say that I have been short of energy the whole week. It's also important for me to state that despite my cerebral palsy I don't feel lonely. I have good friends who I can talk to. The problem is that I often don't have the energy when they want me to come along to different activities. Because of my disability, there are also some extra tasks to be done in connection with my accommodation, and so on.

Harald had no services in his home. He was surprised how much time he had to spend on administration of his studies and the accommodations he needed to make.

Due to the cerebral palsy, Harald needed more time to do his part of the housework than his flatmates. He moved around without any kind of support, but he moved more slowly and unsteadily, and therefore needed more time than other students to get around, both inside the buildings and on campus.

Being a student requires time and perseverance in reading. Harald also had binocular vision, which affected both his reading and writing. He had developed a strategy for efficient reading, with regular 15-minute breaks every hour to prevent headaches. This strategy was important to ensure time for other activities, like being with friends. The first semester, Harald studied nearly full time. The second semester he reduced his study progression to half-time, as he realised that he needed more time to rest than other students. He spent 11 hours each day sleeping and resting, sleeping late in the mornings and often resting an hour during the day. In addition, he needed extra time for many of the ordinary daily activities, both for his studies and for managing his accommodations. Consequently, he did not see his friends and his physiotherapist as often as he would have liked, and needed.

Heidi and Harald are two out of 18 students with disabilities who participated in a Norwegian study of the everyday life of students with disabilities in Norway

(Magnus, 2009). Data collection consisted of time-geographic diaries of one week, individual interviews (Holstein & Gubrium, 1995) and focus groups (Krueger, 2009).

The time-geographic method

Even if participation in political terms is defined as the opportunity to participate on one's own terms in a society that is open to different ways of functioning, it is well known that persons with disabilities meet barriers such as physical obstacles or excluding attitudes. To understand and analyse the particular types of barriers to participation which young adults with disabilities encounter, a time-geographic approach can be useful. In time geography, all activities performed by an individual are integrated into contexts (Ellegård, 1999). The everyday context constitutes the sequence of all activities performed by a person within a certain time period; the social context indicates when a person is together with other people; the geographical context shows where people perform activities and their movement during the day. Finally, the project context shows how different performed activities are connected by their objectives. The all-embracing project for everyone is living one's life; and within that context, people are involved in all kinds of long- and short-term projects, such as preparing food, getting an education, caring for children, gardening, etc. These projects, and the activities in time and space that constitute them, are restricted by circumstances. During most of what an individual does, she or he will sometimes experience restrictions which indicate what is possible and what is not possible for that person to do. Hägerstrand (1985) identifies three kinds of restrictions or constraints that influence our choices and what we actually do:

- Capacity – that is, the individual's biological, economical, material, cognitive and mental resources.
- Coupling – the necessity for individuals, tools and aids assistance to meet at given times and places.
- Authority – rules and laws to be followed, set up by an authority.

With the everyday lives of Heidi and Harald in mind, it is obvious that these three areas of restriction have a greater significance for young students with disability than they do for other students.

Procedure

Using the time-geographic diary method (Ellegård, 1999; Nordell, 2002), the 18 students with disabilities, aged between 18 and 35, recorded *When* (the time of day), *What I do* (activities), *Where I am* (where), *Together with* (with whom) and *Comments* in a notebook. Starting when they woke up in the morning, they noted activities, movements, places visited and interactions with other people throughout the week. Beneath the heading *Comments*, they were free to comment on the situations described. Diaries from one week provided information about the incidence of their main activities over time, of places they had visited and of togetherness. In this way, the time-geographic diary method describes both their activity context and their social and geographical context.

The diaries were individually coded using a code book in accordance with the diary method. The code book shows how the activities (more than 700) are classified in seven activity spheres (care for oneself, care for others, household care, recreation, travel, procurement and preparation of food, and work/school), which altogether constitute the all-embracing project of 'living one's life'.

The codes are adapted through a computer program called 'Everyday Life'. A new tool – Aday System – is an up-to-date version of Everyday Life. The Aday App makes it easy to note down daily activities, and the Aday Evaluation Tool manages the processing of the diary entries that are automatically sent from the app (Kroksmark & Nordell, 2013).

The program enables the study of daily life through a frequency table. The graphs show activities and movements during one weekday. Time is shown on the vertical axis, the codes assigned to activities are on the horizontal axis, and the irregular path illustrates the actual activities. The path is read from bottom to top. The vertical line represents time spent in an activity, whilst the horizontal line shows a change of activity. The graphs of geographical and social context show places the person has spent time in, and time spent alone and together with other people. The frequency table indicates how many times each activity is performed and for how many minutes each time. Studies of the graphs of activities, movements, social and geographical context and frequency tables, raise questions and reflections on the everyday life of the individual.

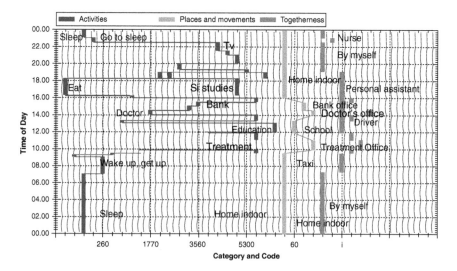

Figure 16.1 Heidi – Thursday

Following completion of the diaries and their analysis, in-depth face-to-face interviews were conducted. The diary method reveals regularities and content of daily life, but not priorities, motives, barriers and the degree to which the individual had to make choices contrary to what was actually desired. The starting point of the interview was subjects from the diary, followed by themes prepared in an interview guide. When the researcher met a person for an interview, information about the coding and studying of the graphs was the first step. In this process, the person most often started talking about or reflecting on situations or conditions described in the diary. In this way, the diary functioned as what McCracken calls 'an auto-driving', a prompting strategy that can bring elements into the interview which otherwise might be difficult or forgotten (McCracken, 1988). In different ways, the participant and researcher had already started the process of constructing an understanding of how elements of single activities influence everyday life. They had some shared descriptions from which they could continue talking about actions and processes shaping the everyday life. Both the diary and the interview guide were prompts during the interview.

The analysis began by looking into time use in activity spheres, places and togetherness, followed by reading the interview transcripts to search for both activity patterns and the main projects of the individuals.

Participants' main project

The diaries illustrate that the everyday life of the participating students are both the same and different from other students These young adults spent more time in rest and sleep, in ordinary daily activities, alone, and in planning their days than was the case with non-disabled occupational and physiotherapy students (Alsaker et al., 2006). However, they spent at least as many hours studying as other students (Aamodt, Hovdhaugen & Opheim, 2006).

The amount of time spent in some activities influences time use in other activities, and what can be understood as projects in a time-geographic vocabulary. In accordance with the understanding of projects (i.e. all the activities a person carries out to reach a goal), analysis also found three main projects to be central elements of the everyday life of these students:

* Qualifying for employment.
* Making everyday life work.
* Caring for my health.

Qualifying for employment

All these 18 participating students loved being students and studying. The motivation was two-sided. They described learning as a pleasure, and the long-term aim was employment and independent living. The other side of their motivation was a desire to show other people that they could manage, despite negative expectations from others. In an interview, Harald said:

> I want to show society that I can contribute despite my problems, and that I am no different from others. So, if people think that they can stereotype me they are wrong.

Harald had to demonstrate that he had the will and the competence to participate, despite disabilities that others thought would stop him. He was happy about his studies and being a student, but on the other hand, he had worked hard to get the accommodations and support he needed. In particular, household tasks were difficult and took time for him to carry out, and he considered hiring someone to do his part of the chores. Harald's goal was to find a balance between studying, daily activities, rest, hanging out with friends, and physiotherapy treatment.

In order to qualify for employment, students in general have to work hard. Even if most of the students were studying part time, they spent as many hours studying during a week as an average full-time Norwegian student, namely 30 hours (Aamodt et al., 2006), and sometimes more. Two universities in Sweden (Nilsson-Lindström, 2003; Stockholms University, 2006) reported similar findings. The majority of students in the current study needed extra time for reading, writing or doing the practical things in-between, like finding a book in the library, getting accessible literature, using the photocopier, taking notes or moving between different buildings and rooms.

Harald was permitted to record his lectures because he needed extra time writing. The tape was transferred to the computer at home; he listened to it again and made additional notes. In an interview, Harald said:

> So, it creates some extra tasks. Quite a few extra things that most people don't understand, but that is how it is!

Kjell, a male student with vision loss, knew that he could manage to read 50 pages a day before the exam. He decided to concentrate on the central part of the syllabus and hoped that this would be enough. Kari, a female student, also with vision loss, used audiobooks. She pointed to the fact that it is more time-consuming using an audiobook than an ordinary book because it is difficult to skim. This means that reading speed is reduced, even with the aid of a dictation machine, an audiobook or audio-described television. Accommodations will not completely remove the restrictions the student experiences, but they may contribute to a reduction in energy and time use, and thus a better learning outcome.

Qualifying for employment most often means that the students move from their parental home and have to cope by themselves. Included in the project of qualifying for employment is therefore also a need to learn how to access services and accommodation. This involves meetings with counselling offices, the administration and the responsible lecturers at the university, and other public authorities, as well as acquiring knowledge about disability rights and opportunities. In the past, parents and the school system had taken responsibility for these matters, which the students now have to deal with themselves.

Making everyday life work

Daily activities are described as activities we can see but do not notice (Hasselkus, 2006, 2011). These are activities that are present in our lives all the time and in all places. Even if these are activities carried out by all of us – e.g. hoovering the living room, preparing supper or putting away the laundry – each individual finds his or her own way of doing them.

For some students, these were time-consuming and demanding activities. Peter used Sundays for washing his clothes. The laundry was in a building a few hundred metres from where he lived. He also used the tumble dryer, which meant he had to walk to and from the building several times. He called himself one-handed, and was able to use the other arm as a support. Because he walked slowly due to cerebral palsy, he needed time to walk between the laundry and his flat, and time for other parts of this activity. In an interview, Peter said:

> Even if the actions do not demand a lot of strength, using fine motor skills is often just as difficult. I can spend a whole hour folding clothes that come out of the tumble drier.

Peter had no skills in doing these activities when he left home. Now he was happy to learn new skills, even if he saw that many activities were more time-consuming for him than for other students. In an interview, Peter said:

> Cleaning the flat, doing the dishes, washing my clothes, cooking – these are all activities I have to leave extra time for. I have discovered what I CAN do and what I CANNOT do. This means that meals are simple, but I try to maintain a variation.

When the lectures started early in the morning, Peter went home afterwards to have breakfast. He did not have difficulty dressing, but making breakfast in addition was too much. In an interview, Peter described the move away from home like this:

> It was both a positive and a negative experience. It is a bit difficult to explain, but there were a lot of surprises. I had to do everything myself. But I can do it simply, and I learn things that I would not have learned if I hadn't moved here. Well, I discovered that I actually had to do it all myself in order to make my everyday life work.

Many of the ordinary daily activities can be experienced as demanding for students with disabilities. Mostly they are not difficult, but they can be tiring because they require extra time and energy. At the same time, these activities are part of an everyday life experience, and it is necessary to be conscious of them when moving from home to live independently. For Heidi, these activities were administered by her and carried out by assistants. By writing the diary, Heidi experienced how much time she spent administering other people in order to make her everyday life work. She said:

> I would like to have a social life and to make myself a network. But organising everyday life takes up all my time and energy.

Heidi prioritised spending her time making it possible for her to study. This meant that she had little time for activities that other students characterise as important, such as making friends and building networks. Other students in the study made the same reflections about how they managed to make their everyday lives work.

Caring for my health

This project involved activities such as physiotherapy and other kinds of treatment, but also activities linked to well-being, pleasure and new energy. One finding was that the students with disability spent more time in rest and sleep than the non-disabled occupational and physiotherapy students (Alsaker et al., 2006) and more than the general Norwegian average, which is 8.5 hours (Rønning & Våge, 2002). Harald slept 11 hours on average, Heidi 9 hours, and Bjørn, who suffered from chronic pain after an accident, slept for 9.5 hours. The need for rest and sleep can be seen as a result of disabilities, which made university and ordinary daily activities more time-consuming than they were for other students. Reasons were also linked to diagnoses that caused pain or fatigue due to the side effects of medicines. The project 'Taking care of my health' also includes activities linked to keeping the body fit, by training with the physiotherapist or visiting the hospital regularly to keep up with blood tests or other matters.

As for all students, activities connected to well-being, joy and new energy – those described as 'good for me' – were important for health. These were activities like going hunting, going to the movie or reading a book. The intentions behind the activities were personal. Toril was a female student using an electric wheelchair due to movement restrictions. She had a personal assistant both at home and at the university. In an interview, she described how she loved making things:

> Making things is relaxing, in the same way as a computer game. It's like: look what I have done! Computer games are so futile. When you crochet, you actually produce something. In a way it's a mental pastime, at the same time as you produce something. I am not that good at not doing anything. That is not for me. Crocheting is a good thing.

Katrine had rheumatoid arthritis and did similar activities. She invited girlfriends for hobby evenings. This made her sit in quiet surroundings, and she got the accommodation she needed. Eli, who had attention-deficit hyperactivity disorder (ADHD), had decided to keep Sundays free of studies. She did handicrafts, and described it as fun making nice things and being by herself, as this was just what she needed on a regular basis. Others talked about physical activities, such as walking in the forest or the mountains. Common reasons to prioritise the activities they talked about was that the activities were joyful, they put stress at a distance, and they gave the students new energy. For some, the activity involved positive feedback. Activities which Helga, a female student with epilepsy, were doing with some others had some of the same effects. In an interview, she said:

> You get a social boost. The people in the choir are so nice. . . and they are so cheerful. They are so happy . . . Yes, there have been periods when I just sat there in front of the television. Just sat there and did nothing. I don't want to do that now. I would like to do something!

Helga also emphasised activities she did at home which gave her relaxation and satisfaction, such as making a cake or a nice meal, or changing the bedlinen.

These three projects included activities that the students thought were important, and which can be seen as natural parts of being a student. However, the time it took to carry out these activities presented a challenge, and this made everyday life tough to handle. Therefore, the participants also talked about strategies to deal with these challenges, such as structure and routines, prioritising, planning and reducing the progression of their studies to a level that was actually possible to achieve.

Barriers to participation

Despite accommodations and individual strategies to handle challenges linked to time use, the students encountered environmental restrictions. In order to be able to participate in learning and socialising, accessibility of the learning environment, housing, transport, welfare services and financing of studies and living had to be in place.

Capacity

The projects described show how *capacity restrictions* influence different parts of everyday life activities, resulting in extended time use even with the accommodation in place. There were also other restrictions which affected their everyday life.

Even if there are political agreements in Norway for increasing the number of disabled students attending university by removing barriers (Lov om forbud mot diskriminering på grunn av nedsatt funksjonsevne, 2008; Lov om universiteter og høgskoler, 2005), the participants in this study encountered restrictions which made their everyday life more challenging than that of other students.

On campus, there were barriers such as stairs, heavy doors, long distances between buildings, a lack of signs in lifts and on the information board, inaccessible websites, and meeting rooms with no or limited space for a wheelchair. Adaptive literature, such as audiobooks, was reserved for blind and extensively visually impaired students. Students with a less extensive visual impairment or dyslexia also experienced reading much easier using an audiobook. They were permitted to borrow audiobooks, but only literature that was already produced for blind students.

For some students, restrictions were removed if the lecturer used a microphone or the student could record the lecture. Lecturers showing a negative attitude to the use of this equipment, or who refused to give the students copies of lecture notes or other support, demonstrated how new restrictions could arise when different opinions or attitudes about teaching and learning were encountered.

Despite the importance of friendship and of developing a social network, the students experienced limited opportunities for social participation due to capacity restrictions and time use in general. Socialising for students in general mostly happens spontaneously, and the students with disability needed time to plan to meet with fellow students. In addition, there were restrictions in getting to the meeting places, getting in and out of the meeting places, and getting around in the buildings. Therefore, socialising was not prioritised because it demanded too much from them in time and energy.

Coupling

Coupling restrictions come into being when people meet. Students with disabilities who were in need of services from different providers were at risk of not getting the promised support they needed. Students needing transport to get to the university were dependent on its ability to arrive on time. Similarly, for students receiving home help, the service provider had to show up when the student was at home. If the time schedule was tight, the students were at risk of being late for lectures or group work with other students, or of not getting the necessary help at home. Planning and dealing with these issues were also time-consuming. In reducing coupling restrictions, personal assistance was of great importance for students needing extensive services.

Authority

Local authorities and the government can remove or build *authority restrictions* for students with disability. Financial support is one example. In Norway, educational funding is given according to study progression in order to motivate students to study full time. This means that a student studying full time gets a maximum loan, and this support reduces according to actual study progression and income. In this study, a few students had the right to rehabilitation benefits from the Work and Welfare Administration to cover daily expenses during their education. For the other students, educational funding was of special importance because they were at risk of slower study progression, and they were in a situation where paid work in their free time and holidays was hard. As such, funding was not adjusted to the life situation of disabled students.

Summary

The time-geographic method activities performed by an individual are contextually integrated (Ellegård, 1999). For young adults with disabilities who encounter difficulties with participation, a time-geographic approach is a useful tool for highlighting the obstacles they face. The everyday context constitutes the sequence of all activities performed by a person within a certain time period; the social context indicates when a person is together with other people; the geographical context shows where people perform activities and their movement during the day. The project context shows how different performed activities are connected by their objectives. During most of what an individual does, she or he will sometimes experience restrictions which indicate what is possible and not possible for that person to do.

Despite restrictions on campus and in other parts of their everyday life, these students expressed a will to study in accessible surroundings, and they made the necessary personal adjustments.

In addition, attitudinal and social elements, such as how disability is seen and understood or how people with disability are expected to participate or not, influence the way students with disabilities participate in desirable life situations. Despite strategies to increase participation for all, individuals with disabilities encounter participation barriers (Frank et al., 2008). Time use in daily routines can, to a limited degree, be supported by universal design and anti-discrimination strategies. Universal design (Nussbaumer, 2012) and individual strategies are of extreme importance, but not enough to secure participation. For many, individual adaptation will still be needed in homes, in education, in work and in leisure time to ensure participation in attractive situations (Pemberton & Cox, 2015).

References

Aamodt, P.O., Hovdhaugen, E., & Opheim, V. (2006). *Evaluering av Kvalitetsreformen. Delrapport 6. Den nye studiehverdagen* (Evaluation of the Quality Reform of Higher Education). Oslo – Bergen: Norges forskningsråd, Rokkansenteret, NIFU STEP.

Alsaker, S., Jakobsen, K., Magnus, E., Bendixen, H.J., Kroksmark, U., & Nordell, K. (2006). Everyday Occupations of Occupational Therapy and Physiotherapy Students in Scandinavia. *Journal of Occupational Science*, 13, 17–26.

Ellegård, K. (1999). A Time-Geographical Approach to the Study of Everyday Life of Individuals – A Challenge of Complexity. *GeoJournal*, 48(3), 167–175.

Frank, G., Block, P., & Zemke, R. (2008). Anthropology, Occupational Therapy, and Disability Studies: Collaborations and Prospects. *Practicing Anthropology*, 30(3), 2–5.

Hägerstrand, T. (1985). Time-geography: Focus on the Corporeality of Man, Society, and Environment. In: *The Science and Praxis of Complexity*. Tokyo: The United Nations University, 193–216.

Hammel, J., Magasi, S., Heinemann, A., Whiteneck, G., Bogner, J., & Rodriguez, E. (2008). What Does Participation Mean? An Insider Perspective from People with Disability. *Disability Rehabilitation*, 30(19), 1445–1460.

Hammel, K.W. (2009). Self-Care, Productivity and Leisure or Dimensions of Occupational Experience? Rethinking Occupational "Categories". *Canadian Journal of Occupational Therapy*, 71, 107–114.

Hasselkus, B. (2006). The World of Everyday Occupation: Real People, Real lives. *American Journal of Occupational Therapy*, 60, 627–640.

Hasselkus, B. (2011). *The Meaning of Everyday Occupation* (2nd ed). Thorofare, NJ: Slack.

Holstein, J.F., & Gubrium, J.A. (1995). *The New Language of Qualitative Method*. Oxford: Oxford University Press.

Kroksmark, U., & Nordell, K. (2001). Adolescence: The Age of Opportunities and Obstacles for Students with Low Vision in Sweden. *Journal of Visual Impairment & Blindness*, 95(4), 213–225.

Kroksmark, U., & Nordell, K. (2013). Aday – Life Context Evaluation. http://www.aday.se/

Krueger, R.A. (2009). *Focus Groups: A Practical Guide for Applied Research*. London: Sage Publications.

Lov om forbud mot diskriminering på grunn av nedsatt funksjonsevne (2008). *The Act on Accessibility and Discrimination*. Oslo: Barne- og likestillingsdepartementet.

Lov om universiteter og høgskoler (2005). *The Higher Education Act*. Oslo: Kunnskapsdepartementet.

Magnus, E. (2009). *Student, som alle andre. En studie av hverdagslivet til studenter med nedsatt funksjonsevne* (Student, Like Everybody Else. A Study of the Everyday Life of Students with Impairments). PhD. Trondheim: NTNU.

McCracken, G. (1988). *The Long Interview*. (Vol. 13) London: SAGE Publications.

Meyer, A. (1922/1977). The Philosophy of Occupation Therapy. *Archives of Occupational Therapy*, 1(1), 1–10.

Nilsson-Lindström, M. (2003). *Studenter med funktionshinder och deras erfarenheter av utbildning vid Lunds universitet* (Students with Disabilities and Their Experiences in Studying at Lund University). Lund: Utvärderingsenheten, Lunds universitet.

Nordell, K. (2002). *Women's Health – About Awareness, Possibilities and Power*. Thesis, summary. Gothenburg: Department of Human and Economic Geography. University of Gothenburg.

Nussbaumer, L.L. (2012). *Inclusive Design: A Universal Need*. New York, London: Fairchild.

Pemberton, S., & Cox, D. L. (2015). Synchronisation: Co-Ordinating Time and Occupation. *Journal of Occupational Science*, 22(3), 291–303.

Rønning, E., & Våge, O. F. (2002). *Tidsbruksundersøkelsen 2000/2001*. Oslo – Kongsvinger: Statistisk sentralbyrå.

Shakespeare, T. (2006). *Disability Rights and Wrongs*. London: Routledge.

Stockholms universitet (2006). *Studier och funktionshinder. Enkätundersökning genomförd 2005 bland studenter med funktionshinder vid Stockholms universitet* (Studies and Disability Questionnaire Carried out in 2005 among Students with Impairments at Stockholm University). Stockholm: Studentbyrån, Handikappservice.

UN (2006). *Convention on the Rights of Persons with Disabilities*. www.un.org/disabilities/documents/convention/convoptprot-e.pdf (18th of March 2016)

Wilcock, A.A. (2010). Population Health: An Occupational Rational. In M. E. Scaffa, S. Maggie Reitz, Michael A. Pizzi (Eds.), *Occupational Therapy in the Promotion of Health and Wellness* (pp. 110–119). Philadelphia: F.A. Davis Company.

Wilcock, A. A., & Hocking, C. (2015). *An Occupational Perspective on Health*. Thorofare, NJ: Slack Incorporated.

WHO (2001). *International Classification of Functioning, Disability and Health (ICF)*. Geneva: WHO.

17 Participation and inclusion

Mental health service users' lived experience – an international study

Elizabeth McKay, Deirdre Mahon, Grainne Donellan, Kirsti Haracz, Sarah Sheldon and Susan Ryan

Introduction

In the UK, progress has been made in terms of awareness of the barriers to participation and social inclusion that is experienced by people with severe and enduring mental health problems (Office of the Deputy Prime Minister, 2004). Yet it is unclear whether mental health service users in other countries report similar or differing experiences of social inclusion and/or exclusion. Rudman et al. (2008: p. 142) argued that an international perspective was needed to 'add new ideas to existing theories, raise awareness of the assumptions underpinning existing concepts, and help guard against assumptions of universality'. If there were any, the particular in each country needed to be emphasised.

This three-centre international study examined, compared and contrasted the experiences of mental health service users with enduring problems in regional areas of Ireland, Canada and Australia, focusing on the factors that influenced their experience of participation and social inclusion in their respective communities. This was a two-phase, mixed-methodology study utilising the International Classification of Functioning, Disability and Health (ICF) as a framework for enquiry for practice and research. In the first phase, a questionnaire was developed from the ICF components of Activities and Participation to examine enduring mental health users' experiences. The second, qualitative, phase, reported here, captured participants' experiences through interviews about these issues.

Literature review

Social inclusion has received considerable attention in recent years. This is evidenced by the implementation of recent legislative and policy developments in various countries that aim to increase community participation for those experiencing enduring mental ill-health (Australian Government National Action Plan on Mental Health, 2006–2011; Department of Health and Children, 2006; Mental Health Commission of Canada, 2012). Such policy developments have significantly raised expectations that mental health services should address and promote *social inclusion* and participation. Participation is defined as 'a person's involvement in a life situation or role in society' (World Health Organisation [WHO], 2001: p. 4), and engagement in activities that provide meaning and purpose (Lloyd et al., 2007). Any difficulties in participating in everyday activities significantly increase the experience of social exclusion.

People with enduring mental health difficulties are among the most excluded in society (Harrison and Sellers, 2008; Office of the Deputy Prime Minister, 2004). Simply put, social exclusion limits a person's opportunities for participation in social, cultural and economic life (Lloyd et al., 2006; Repper and Perkins, 2003; Russell and Lloyd, 2004; Sayce, 2001; Stickley and Shaw, 2006). Poverty is not the only factor leading to social exclusion. Limited 'access to valuable contacts within a social network' (Morgan et al. 2007: p. 479), stigma and prejudice, even outright rejection, are also relevant to many with enduring mental health problems (Parr et al., 2004; Stickley, 2005).

According to Morgan et al. (2007), there is no simple definition of *social inclusion* existing, but only assumptions for its promotion. Nonetheless, Repper and Perkins (2003) suggest *social inclusion* can only be achieved by addressing the stigma of mental ill-health and valuing the contribution that all individuals make to society as citizens, employees and neighbours (Stickley, 2005). Mueller et al. (2007) highlighted that people who experience stigma and discrimination may withdraw from society and isolate themselves socially. Furthermore, these negative experiences and social exclusion can lead to people experiencing deterioration in their physical and mental health, and developing a limited self-image and reduced self-esteem (Bryant et al., 2004; Erdner et al, 2005; Lloyd et al., 2008b).

There have been no cross-society comparisons, apart from one study of patterns of daily occupations among people with mental health problems who live in Japan and the US (Haertl and Minato, 2006). So, in order to make these comparisons, an accepted international framework was needed, and the ICF was chosen. To date, the use of the ICF in mental health settings has been limited (Daremo and Haglund 2008; Stucki et al., 2002). Major themes were mapped from an existing study by Shaw et al. (2007) onto the Activity, Participation and Environmental components of the ICF. The results provided strong support for the use of the ICF, as it was effective in identifying even the subtle societal barriers to participation. They found that the greatest numbers of facilitators within the Activity and Participation components were clustered in Communication and Major Life Areas, whereas the greatest number of barriers were found in Communication, Major Life Areas and Mobility. These findings were a step towards evaluating and validating the use of the ICF in practice. Nonetheless, it has been suggested that the Participation construct in the ICF is restrictive. It does not consider the subjective experience of the meaning of participation for individuals themselves (Hemmingsson and Jonsson, 2005).

With the growing trend for community mental health services to focus on promoting social inclusion (Repper and Perkins, 2003), there is therefore a need to explore the more recent experiences of participation and exclusion among people living with enduring mental health problems, and to compare and contrast their experiences in different societies.

In light of the above, this qualitative study aimed to address this need and to explore service users' perspectives by enhancing understanding of the complexities of social inclusion and participation in the three locations across three continents and countries: Ireland (Limerick), Canada (London, Ontario) and Australia (Newcastle), and to consider implications for practice, research and policy.

Method

Interviews were used to gain more nuanced experiences of **social inclusion** from the service users' lived experience. Interviews are a way of uncovering and exploring the meanings that underpin people's lives, routines, behaviours and feelings (Forchuk et al., 2006). Therefore, semi-structured interview questions broadly based on the two ICF components Environment and Participation (see Table 17.1 below) were conducted to elicit personal subjective data.

Ethics

Ethical Approval for this study was granted from the three countries involved. Informed written consent was sought and identities protected by only referring to the participants' nationalities.

Inclusion criteria

Participants were aged between 18 and 65 years; had a range of diagnoses, including schizophrenia, bipolar disorder, depression and Obsessive Compulsive Disorder; and had attended day centres in the three regions. All lived in the community, either at home or in supported or hostel accommodation. Participants in an acute stage of illness were excluded.

Table 17.1 Interview topics

Environment	Participation
Physical barriers	Experiences of social inclusion
Access to activities	Mobility
Transport	Participation in self-care and domestic life
Support and relationships with people	Participation in education and work
Attitudes of others	Interpersonal Interactions
Services and policies that impact on participation in everyday life	

Data collection

In Ireland, Donnelly and Mahon conducted the interviews in 2009. In Canada, all data were collected by the Principal Investigator (McKay) in 2009. In Australia, interviews were conducted by Sheldon in 2010.

In each country, one community service in the local area was targeted for recruitment. Purposive sampling was used. Possible participants who met the inclusion criteria in each geographical area were informed of the research through professional team members. Posters were also displayed in centres. Once possible participants were identified, the researchers approached these service users to establish their interest, first, in participating in the Phase One questionnaire. Following the Phase One data collection, the same participants were then asked if they would be willing to be interviewed at a later date for Phase Two. If interest was expressed, new informed written consent forms were signed and collected at the time of interview. Participation was voluntary, and all responses were kept anonymous and confidential. The four interviewers utilised the same interview protocol. In all locations, interviews were conducted in the day centres/services. The interviews were digitally recorded and subsequently transcribed verbatim. The average interview was 24 minutes in duration.

Data analysis

The interview captured a dialogue between researcher and interviewee, allowing for questions to be clarified and adapted (Green and Thorogood, 2004). These descriptions of participants' experiences of participation, social inclusion and exclusion enabled links to be established between theory and their lived reality. Following transcription, manual coding techniques were used, and subsequently the first themes were entered into the qualitative software N-Vivo8 (QSR International, 2009). Analysis of the data was approached from a constructionist perspective, creating a thematic analysis approach to identify recurrent themes (Braun and Clarke, 2006). The data captured the person–environment relationship and the barriers and facilitators that participants deemed to have contributed to their **social inclusion** and exclusion experiences. Themes were identified in each location group and subsequently cross-checked in order to ensure that interpretation of data was credible. The Irish findings were used as a framework onto which the Canadian data initially, and then the Australian data, were overlaid. Additional categories/themes were identified with cross-checking by the Principal Investigator (PI). Finally, peer checking was conducted by a colleague from the PI's location. This process is reported to ensure trustworthiness and credibility of findings (Finlay and Ballinger, 2006).

Findings

A total of 30 people (20 men and 10 women) participated. The age range of the participants was 18–65 years, although the majority (19) were 45 years and above. There were 11 Irish participants (7 men and 4 women); 10 Canadian participants (6 men and 4 women); and 9 Australian participants (7 men and 2 women).

Table 17.2 Themes and related ICF categories

Theme		ICF category
'My mental health affects my relationships with others': experiences of support, rejection and loss in personal and professional relationships	1	Interpersonal Interactions and Relationships
'There is a public ignorance regarding mental health': varied experiences of prejudice, rejection and social isolation	2	Attitudes
'Some training and support to build back up the confidence': key sources of social inclusion	3	Services, Systems and Policies
'I go see the movies a lot': but inclusive participation choices are limited	4	Support and Relationships
'I have a voice in what's going on which is how things should be going': experiences of agency and control in mental health services	5	Community, Social and Civic Life, Environment

From the data analysis, five main themes emerged placing the participants' voices to the fore. Each theme reflected the main issues discussed by the partici-pants according to the five ICF categories as shown in Table 17.2.

'*My mental health affects my relationships with others*': experiences of sup-port, rejection and loss in personal and professional relationships.

ICF (1) – Interpersonal Interactions and Relationships

Participants felt that their mental health profoundly impacted on their interac-tions and relationships with others. Most stated that family and friends were a source of significant support, although some highlighted they were treated differ-ently since the onset of mental health problems. Several participants perceived that, although supportive, family members did not always have a clear understanding of their condition and its effects on their participation in daily life. One Irish partici-pant linked a lack of understanding to the breakdown in his relationship with his children who refused to maintain contact with him. He said, '*my marriage broke down over it [mental health condition]; she divorced me over my mood swings*'.

Others made reference to some form of relationship breakdown within the fam-ily. One Canadian participant, commenting on his wife, stated, '*I'm not the same person that I was, I know it, she knows it, she misses what I was*'.

Making friendships outside the mental health services appeared to be difficult for half of the participants, leading to feelings of social isolation and loneliness. An Australian participant described his experience: 'the worst part for me . . . that I find it really tricky to make new friendships'. A similar experience was reported by a Canadian participant: for years I didn't go anywhere, I didn't know anybody, I didn't do anything, I was too sick to work, I was too sick to maintain relationships – I didn't want one anyway'.

For the most part, participants' interactions with health professionals were positive, and many described them as being caring and helpful. A Canadian participant appreciated their input. He said:

> These professionals have spotted many things where I needed areas of improvement. They taught me how to control my symptoms – first of all, [to] recognise them and [then] what to do when that happens and [to] keep them under control.

However, some participants experienced negative interactions with staff. For example, an Irish participant stated:

> One particular psychiatrist did all the talking. He never asked me if there was anything I would like to talk about. He talked at me, and ended up with, 'is that alright?' He would have been put out if one had said 'no!'

This negative interaction with staff aspect was not reflected by the Australian participants.

'*There is public ignorance regarding mental illness*': varied experiences of prejudice, rejection and social isolation.

ICF (2) – Attitudes

A lack of public understanding about mental health was a widely held view expressed by the majority. For example, an Irish participant stated: 'they don't understand, it's an ignorance'. Links were made between this ignorance and subsequent stigmatising attitudes and discriminatory behaviours by society. An Australian and a Canadian participant, respectively, said:

> People treat you differently if you tell them – some people just look at you like you are a malingerer, if you do mention it . . . I don't mention it very often.

> Sometimes at social events – right away they see your mannerisms, the way you dress, you don't have much money. In wider society, if you don't meet the status quo; you are kind of shunned a bit.

As a result of these feelings, it emerged that over half the participants were reluctant to reveal their mental health condition or past history.

A further effect of stigma was described by an Australian as avoiding certain situations resulting in an exclusionary lifestyle:

> I keep to myself totally; I don't invite them [the neighbours] in. I am just frightened if they get to know too much about me, you know the word will get around, that he is strange, or something like that.

Some discussed how the negative experiences or attitudes they received from other people resulted in lowering their self-esteem, confidence and self-value. An Australian participant said: 'It's not a stigma from the outside, mine is sort of internalised'.

The participants said they experienced 'being different'. This was also emphasised by those who highlighted differences in relation to their sexual orientation, their weight and physical ill-health. However, more positively, there was an awareness that some things had changed over time as a result of improved public education, the media and the mental health service users themselves.

The role the media has played in changing societal attitudes was emphasised: 'people are pouring out their souls and it's breaking down huge barriers and stereotypes in society' (Irish participant). A Canadian participant highlighted the influence that service users themselves play in educating people. She said, 'I don't keep my illness a secret I try to educate more people about my illness so that they are more understanding about everybody'.

Discrimination was an issue that was frequently discussed; significantly, for half of the participants, no discriminatory experiences were encountered at either the workplace or at leisure facilities. However, others reported discrimination at previous points in their lives. One Irish participant reported name-calling and verbal abuse like 'they started chanting 'weirdo' which was very embarrassing'.

Despite the prevalence of stigma in participants' lives, the majority described themselves as feeling socially included within their own immediate communities of people. A Canadian participant summed this up:

> But for the most part my friends are wonderful, most of my friends have psychiatric illnesses as well. It's easy to talk to people in that group because they understand and they are forgiving and they know what it's like.

In summary, stigma and discrimination were still experienced to some extent by participants in all three countries, and the internalisation of these processes led to reduced self-esteem, self-isolation and limited participation.

'*Some training and support to build back up the confidence*': key sources of social inclusion.

ICF (3) – Services, Systems and Policies

The overall consensus among all three countries' participants was that issues relating to entry into education, housing, transport, services and systems were not problematic and acted as facilitators to participation and inclusion.

The majority of participants were satisfied with their ability to access or return to education. 'I've achieved all I want with education' (Irish participant). A Canadian participant added: 'Education would be [accessible] – but I don't want to do it.'

All participants were satisfied with their housing situation at the time of the interviews, and either lived with family members or in supported accommodation. For those who did wish to move to independent living, they described being met with significant support. An Irish participant stated:

> It's a six month programme; they cover lots of independent living skills. It's hard to get decent accommodation; they make sure you get decent accommodation before you leave the service.

That said, several participants were worried about future housing should there be changes in their circumstances or finances.

Participants agreed that free public transport supported their participation in daily activities, and they used the variety of transport available in their regional areas.

Most participants, however, raised access to employment as a key barrier to social inclusion. Although most were not in any paid employment at the time of interview, they acknowledged that the reasons they were not working were due to both internal and external barriers. Internal barriers included feeling unable to cope with having to interact with colleagues and work-related stress.

In relation to accessing paid employment, this was experienced as difficult for those who wished to return to work or participate in the workforce. Some of the participants, as a strategy, actively highlighted that they withheld their mental health history from possible employers and others.

> I made out a second resume – one saying I worked out here, it was a lie but it was the only way I could get round it. Well I know . . . it looks pretty stupid someone with a college education looking for a job in Subway or a sandwich shop. Maybe I could just get something small to start off with till I'm back in the work force. I went to Quiznos, Tacobells, Tim Hortons and Zellers. I went to all places around my neighbourhood . . . and not a response from any of them. A lot of these places had 'help wanted' signs out and I couldn't get a job.
>
> (Canadian participant)

Many would like to have part-time paid work; however, the recession made this even more difficult, as employment opportunities were limited. Some were volunteers in a range of settings and valued doing things with others. Several wished to gain voluntary experience, seeing this as perhaps a step nearer to paid work. However, the lack of paid employment remains a significant issue and limits their social inclusion.

'*I go see the movies a lot*': but inclusive participation choices are limited.

ICF (4) – Support and Relationships

Most participants referred to the importance of involving themselves in leisure activities and support outside of their mental health service. Examples of participation in a range of activities were evidenced, although limitations were acknowledged. Participation was facilitated with people with whom they had trusted relationships, who were from small social networks, and often with whom they shared mental health problems and felt they belonged. They went to places that were easily available to them, affordable, and had ease of access; and to those places which reflected their pastimes/interests – some from their childhood, others they had developed – such as attending recitals, or going for a meal or to the cinema in their community. They did not report any difficulties with accessing such facilities, although financial constraints were highlighted as an issue. Participants emphasised the need for acceptance, understanding and supportive relationships with good friends in order to maximise their experiences:

> They understand what I'm going through and so they don't pressure me. . ..
> If I say 'No' now, they understand that I am not doing so well at the moment.
> (Australian participant)

> That's right, I do church – it's a meeting place. There's a book club. At the church, I take the notes, I'm the secretary. . .. I enjoy it.
> (Canadian participant)

Environments, specifically climate, were also an issue, particularly for Canadian and Australian participants. The climate in their countries was sometimes at the extreme and impacted on their participation in activities, as it stopped them going out. However, the unique place of shopping malls in enabling social participation in both these locations was highlighted, as the weather extremes were regulated in these environments and they were places to go and meet others.

'*I have a voice in what's going on which is how things should be going*': experiences of agency and control in mental health services.

ICF (5) – Community, Social and Civic Life – Environments

Participants identified that they now had a voice in their life decisions. They believed that this was a positive development and was different from their past experience:

> I'm now totally in control. Before I was in their (the professional's) hands and I did trust them but then I just got lost. Now it's like – there's a programme. This programme and the doctor is a total good match and my clinicians are a really good match.
> (Canadian participant)

Importantly, most participants highlighted their role in maintaining their mental health to maximise their participation in their social life, for example structuring their day, engaging in daily activities, and participating in relevant activity or social groups. Participants in all the countries drew special attention to the importance that routine, structure and participation in meaningful activities played in keeping them in contact with their wider community. They were aware this fostered their inclusion in society. Significant recognition was given to attending the mental health services, such as day centres or community groups, for example the Young Men's Christian Association (YMCA), and taking part in the courses, classes and groups on offer. 'I'm happy coming here and my days are filled up with lots of different things to take part in' (Irish participant). 'Coming here keeps me occupied and gives me a reason to get up in the morning' (Australian participant).

All highlighted how their involvement in their mental health service activities created positive social experiences for them. They felt this participation assisted them to engage further in their community, now or at a later date.

> Coming here, the groups that were offered here that I came to were the best that I ever did, because I came and there was people like me . . . and it was just great to know that I wasn't the only person in the world, which we knew, but, you just had not met them.
>
> (Australian participant)

People and the relationships they established in these services were very influential for an individual's ongoing participation. In contrast, the consequences of having no daily routine were indicated:

> If I didn't have programmes to attend, I'd have a huge amount of time on my hands, which would play straight into the hands of the OCD [Obsessive Compulsive Disorder]. That time would be filled with obsessive thoughts . . . the key is to keep occupied . . . routine is good.
>
> (Irish participant)

Similar sentiments were reflected by an Australian participant:

> I cannot stress enough how important it is to have something to do. Not having something to do makes things worse. If you are not having stuff to do you will sleep in, you will wake up at mid-day, you will throw your sleep schedule out of whack. . . .. But, like the whole thing about it, sort of getting to planning for and going there . . . it was a good thing!

An important factor raised by many participants for participating in civic and social life was that of taking their medications and acknowledging that their past choices about taking them regularly had affected their mental well-being. The importance of regular medication in helping them to carry out tasks of daily living independently was clear to all. Also, it was felt that it contributed to participants' having more positive and meaningful relationships with others. An Irish participant stated: 'I'm on my medication now so I'm sort of leading a more normal life and I get on better with people now because of it'. This was also echoed by a Canadian participant: 'Part of my participation in my recovery is staying on the meds, that's a major part of my progress'.

Taking control of their own decisions regarding participating was key for participants: 'It gave me such a boost and I really started to get a lot better after [attending] those two groups I came to here' (Australian participant).

Overall, this theme suggests that, for these participants, it was easier to participate in social activities within the community mental health context in which they belonged or in local community groups where they were known. Being with people who understood, or who were in a similar position – and significantly, who were not stigmatising – was important. However, this suggestion also implies that wider social inclusion was limited and experienced as hard, beyond the participants' 'safe' social networks, and that this limited social inclusion was happening only up to a point. This indicates that it is harder to be accepted and included in 'mainstream' society or environments.

Discussion

This international study explored participants' experiences of social inclusion in communities in three developed countries. The findings emphasised many similarities and few discrepancies across these groups, illustrating that the construct of 'universality' (Rudman et al., 2008: p. 142) could be valid in these particular instances, e.g. developed countries; provincial cities; comparable governmental policies being created; and similarities in the focus of interventions, professionals' education and the health services. Nevertheless, subtle nuances from these contexts and differences between individuals have still to be taken into consideration. The voices of the participants gave meaning and feelings to the findings that may raise professional and public awareness and give new ideas for practice.

The participants from all three countries highlighted their 'mixed' experiences of feeling socially included in the mainstream population. Their voices reiterated the results of previous studies, yet added subtleties of texture that could enhance existing practice and future research. Certain aspects in the findings that supported their participation were family understanding, friendships and belonging up to a point; choices and support in the mental health settings; and transport and educational opportunities. Limited finances reduced their opportunities, e.g. for leisure activities. Nonetheless, major barriers were still the experiences of ignorance, stigma and discrimination from the population and consequent fear and loneliness for the service users. Some of these barriers led to problems in gaining meaningful work, whether voluntary or paid employment.

For most of the participants, family relationships or supportive friendships were the key to their ongoing ability to experience social inclusion positively. Two participants told of a lack of understanding from their immediate families about their actual ongoing condition and how this was the cause of further tension.

This reiterated Murray-Swank et al's (2007) conclusions about worsening mental health effects which had negative outcomes for assisting in improving their *social inclusion* with their family and others.

Some participants had realised that they were not the same as before and that both they and their spouses were aware of these changes in their behaviours and personalities (Champlin, 2009). Participants spoke of how family members approached them in another manner than they would have done prior to the onset of their condition. As Topor et al. (2006: p. 19) stated, 'memories of the individual's earlier life begin to fade'.

Friendships that helped the participants to feel like they belonged and were more socially included were extremely important. According to Hall-Lande et al. (2007), the significance of friendships in the lives of this vulnerable population was paramount. They argued that close and supportive friendships resulted in higher levels of acceptance, increased social competence, higher levels of motivation and increased levels of self-worth for the individuals. These points were emphasised by several participants who found comfort in the friendships they had made in their mental health services, because these friends had similar problems and they understood their reactions and responses (Bryant et al., 2010; McKay, 2010). The next step would be for close friends such as these to venture together into **inclusive** activities within the mainstream facilities in their communities.

In contrast, participants also spoke of the strain on ordinary friendships as well as the strains within the family. They said they found it difficult to make friends outside of the service or they had lost the friends they had before they became unwell. Topor et al. (2006) found that friendships were broken off, either by the friends themselves or by the person, as a result of the mental health difficulty. Several participants spoke of their loneliness, and others spoke of their fear of making new friendships.

The majority of participants reported a general lack of understanding of mental health by the public, family members and close friends, and termed it 'public ignorance'. In contrast, one Canadian participant spoke of her belief in disclosure about her condition, saying that she believed this was a form of public education. Many avoided social settings and opportunities in their communities to be socially included. However, the area that was most affected was in seeking and maintaining employment, as the majority here were not in paid employment.

With regards to employment, more than half of the participants omitted personal details from CVs and wondered about how to explain time gaps in their work experience. Alterations in facts then caused additional distress if these were revealed. There was a strong connection made by the participants here between reluctance to disclose information about their mental health and a perceived lack of public/employer understanding or systems to support re-employment. Work was seen as positive and a path to increased participation in the wider community. Therefore, strategies need to be put in place in order to change societal attitudes and promote awareness of mental health in the workplace.

Lack of paid employment limits the social inclusion of many people, with the majority finding it problematic to obtain and retain employment (Crowther et al., 2001; Davis and Rinaldi, 2004; Henry and Lucca, 2004; Letts et al., 2003; Russell and Lloyd, 2004; Stickley and Shaw, 2006). The significance of gaining a valued social role through employment cannot be underestimated as this confers a positive identity, a way to participate in the wider community, a sense of responsibility, a reward, a value, and thus improved self-esteem (Commonwealth of Australia, 2009; Evans and Repper, 2001; Stickley, 2005).

Optimistically, participants from all countries talked about how public attitudes were beginning to change and the role that all types of media played in this reformation. Opportunities via social media to share experiences, join existing blogs or create new ones, and viewing YouTube on the web are escalating worldwide. These will widen the public's awareness and knowledge further and help in some way to break down barriers.

On the other hand, no amount of support will be effective without the underpinning services, systems and policies being in place. All countries were working on and implementing policies to provide a legislative framework as a foundation. In this study, the questions derived from the ICF components of Environment and Participation did not probe the participants about these relatively new higher-level policy issues. The participants' responses focused more on the services and systems they were exposed to and used.

Support, in whatever system or service, appears to be the key to further social inclusion and the deterrent to discrimination. All the participants said they were satisfied with, and some praised, their mental health staff and services, and that they did not experience discrimination currently, although it had happened in the past. In 2003, Pinfold et al. (2003a, 2003b) highlighted widespread discrimination as being the predominant problem for people with mental health issues, saying it had a deleterious effect on their confidence and well-being. This discrimination caused many of the participants to seek out more passive leisure pursuits that reduce social interaction, such as going to the movies. It is therefore in the more active leisure areas that support is needed to increase participation.

It was clear that all participants valued their mental health services and felt that they were given choices and had a voice in their decisions. Additionally, most participants acknowledged the need for maintaining their engagement with services and meaningful activities in order to remain well and maximise their participation in society. As McKay and Robinson (2011) suggest, such participation provides opportunities for the development of a sense of meaning, increased self-esteem, skill acquisition and improved sense of identity.

Limitations of the study

Nevertheless, there are limitations with this study, as with most research. As 'users' of mental health services, the participants were not representative of people with mental health problems living and working independently in the community. The majority (20/30) of the participants were men, and this would have brought a particular perspective on *social inclusion* and further integration into the mainstream community, although this focus was not followed up. It could also be argued that those who did agree to be interviewed were likely to have been more forthcoming in offering their opinions. Additionally, the group was drawn from older generations, and another study with younger participants might give more information about being socially included in mainstream education and employment.

This three-country study also used four interviewers to collect the data. Although initial preparation was organised as part of the research protocol, each interviewer did not have the same research experience. Nonetheless, having a large international team to analyse the data was an advantage to the credibility of the study.

Conclusion

This research provides evidence and informs multidisciplinary professionals on best practice in promoting participation and social inclusion, and the need for graded/supported participation in the mainstream community. Additionally, the importance of listening and understanding their client voices when designing individual programmes is paramount.

It can be concluded from the findings that people have been victims of societal ignorance. Associations were made between stigmatising attitudes and a lack of public understanding of mental health. Such ignorance had detrimental effects on individuals and their relationships with others. Internalisation of negative attitudes has led to exacerbation of participants' symptoms with subsequent effects of family strain and relationship breakdown.

It is evident that individuals here were not presented with the same life opportunities as their counterparts due to their mental health. The opportunities to obtain work and form close friendships were hindered by discriminatory attitudes and led to feelings of frustration, inadequacy and loneliness. Both negative and positive portrayals of mental health were attributed to the media, and it was concluded that the media must persist in breaking down negative stereotypes.

The ICF has proved to be a useful framework for exploring social inclusion and exclusion in terms of environmental components and their unique relationship with activities and participation. Because of the uniformity of language in these categories, all elements were included in this research, providing a comprehensive insight into people's experiences of social inclusion.

To conclude, the findings are somewhat contradictory. Although participants felt socially included, it should be acknowledged that they still had the support of the services they were involved with and access to multidisciplinary team members. They were socially included within their particular environments but not in mainstream society.

References

Blank, A.A., Harries, P., & Reynolds, F. (2015). 'Without occupation you don't exist': Occupational engagement and mental illness. *Journal of Occupational Science*, 22(2), 197–209.

Braun, V., & Clarke, V. (2006). Using thematic analysis in psychology. *Qualitative Research in Psychology*, 3(2), 77–101.

Bryant, W., Craik, C., & McKay, E.A. (2004). Living in a glasshouse: Exploring occupational alienation. *Canadian Journal of Occupational Therapy*, 71(5), 282–363.

Bryant, W., Vacher, G., Beresford, P., & McKay, E.A. (2010). The modernisation of mental health day services: Participatory action research exploring social networking. *Mental Health Review Journal*, 15(3), 11–21.

Champlin, B.E. (2009). Being there for another with serious mental illness. *Qualitative Health Research*, 19(11), 1525–1535.

Commonwealth of Australia. (2009). Fourth National Mental Health Plan: An agenda for collaborative government action in mental health 2009–2014, retrieved from: https://www.health.gov.au/internet/main/publishing.nsf/Content/9A5A0E8BDFC55D3BCA25 7BF0001C1B1C/$File/plan09v2.pdf [accessed 4 January 2017].

Crowther, E.R., Marshall, M., Bond, R.G., & Huxley, P. (2001). Helping people with severe mental illness to obtain work: Systematic review. *British Medical Journal*, 322, 204–208.

Daremo, A., & Haglund, L. (2008). Activity and participation in psychiatric institutional care. *Scandinavian Journal of Occupational Therapy*, 15(3), 131–142.

Davis, M., & Rinaldi, M. (2004). Using an evidence-based approach to enable people with mental health problems to gain and to retain employment, education and voluntary work, *British Journal of Occupational Therapy*, 67(7), 319–322.

Department of Health and Children (2006). *A Vision for Change: Report of the Expert Group on Mental Health Policy*, Dublin: Stationery Office.

Erdner, A., Magnusson, A., Nystrom, M., & Lutzen, K. (2005). Social and existential alienation experienced by people with long-term mental illness. *Scandinavian Journal of Caring Sciences*, 19(4), 373–380.

Evans, J., & Repper, J. (2001). Employment, social inclusion and mental health. *Journal of Psychiatric and Mental Health Nursing*, 7, 15–24.

Finlay, L., & Ballinger, C., eds. (2006). *Qualitative Research for Allied Health Professionals: Challenging Choices*, West Sussex: Whurr Publishers Ltd.

Forchuk, C., Nelson, G., & Brent-Hall, G. (2006). It's important to be proud of the place you live in: Housing problems and preferences of psychiatric survivors. *Perspectives in Psychiatric Care*, 42(1), 42–51.

Green, J., & Thorogood, N. (2004). *Qualitative Methods for Health Research*, London: Sage.

Haertl, K., & Minato, M. (2006). Daily occupations of persons with mental illness: Themes from Japan and America. *Occupational Therapy in Mental Health*, 22(1), 9–32.

Hall-Lande, J., Eisenberg, M.E., Christenson, S.L., & Neumark-Sztainer, D. (2007). Social isolation, psychological, health, and protective factors in adolescence. *Adolescence*, 42(166), 265–286.

Harrison, D., & Sellers, A. (2008). Occupation for mental health and social inclusion. *British Journal of Occupational Therapy*, 71(5), 216–218.

Hemmingsson, H., & Jonsson, H. (2005). The issue is – An occupational perspective on the concept of participation in the international classification of functioning, disability and health – Some critical remarks. *American Journal of Occupational Therapy*, 59, 569–576.

Henry, D.A., & Lucca, M.A. (2004). Facilitators and barriers to employment: The perspectives of people with psychiatric disabilities and employment service providers. *Work*, 22, 169–182.

Letts, L., Rigby, P., & Stewart, D. (2003). *Using Environments to Enable Occupational Performance*, Thorofare, NJ: Slack Incorporated.

Lloyd, C., King, R., McCarthy, M., & Scanlan, M. (2007). The association between leisure motivation and recovery: A pilot study. *Australian Occupational Therapy Journal*, 54, 33–41.

Lloyd, C., Samson, T., & Deane, F. (2006). Community participation and social inclusion: How practitioners can make a difference. *Australian e-Journal for the Advancement of Mental Health*, 5(3), 1–10, retrieved from: www.auseinet.com/journal/vol5iss3/lloyd.pdf [accessed 24 October 2008].

Lloyd, C., Waghorn, G., & Williams, P.L. (2008). Conceptualising recovery in mental health rehabilitation. *British Journal of Occupational Therapy*, 71(8), 321–328.

McKay, E.A. (2010). Rip that book up I've changed: Unveiling the experiences of women living with and surviving enduring mental illness. *British Journal of Occupational Therapy*, 73(3), 96–105.

McKay, E.A., & Robinson, K (2011). Creating occupational engagement to maximise recovery in mental health: The place of occupation analysis. In McKenzie, L., & O'Toole, G., eds., *Occupation Analysis in Practice*, Wiley-Blackwell, Oxford, 217–231.

Mental Health Commission of Canada (2012). *Changing Directions Changing Lives: The Mental Health Strategy for Canada*, Calgary, AB: Mental Health Commission Canada.

Morgan, C., Burns, T., Fitzpatrick, R., Pinfold, V., & Priebe, S. (2007). Social exclusion and mental health. *British Journal of Psychiatry*, 191, 477–483.

Mueller, B., Nort, C., Lauber, C. Rueesch, P., Meyer, P.C., & Roessler, W. (2007). Changes in social network diversity and perceived social support after psychiatric hospitalisation: Results from a longitudinal study. *International Journal of Social Psychiatry*, 53(6), 564–575.

Murray-Swank, A., Glynn, S., Cohen, A.N., Sherman, M., Medoff, D.P., Fang, L., Drapalski, A., & Dixon, L.B. (2007). Family contact, experience of family relationships, and views about family involvement in treatment among VA consumers with serious mental illness. *Journal of Rehabilitation Research and Development*, 44, 801–812.

Office of the Deputy Prime Minister (2004). *Mental health and social exclusion*. Wetherby, OPDM publications. Summary report, retrieved from: www.nfao.org/Useful . . . /MH_Social_Exclusion_report_summary.pdf.

Parr, H., Philo, C., & Burns, N. (2004). Social geographies of rural mental health: Experiencing inclusions and exclusions. *Transactions of the Institute of British Geographers*, 29, 401–419.

Pinfold, V., Huxley, P., Thornicroft, G., Farmer, P., Toulmin, H., & Graham, T. (2003a). Reducing psychiatric stigma and discrimination. *Social Psychiatry Psychiatric Epidemiology*, 38, 337–344.

Pinfold, V., Toulmin, H., Thornicroft, G., Huxley, P., Farmer, P., & Graham, T. (2003b). Reducing psychiatric stigma and discrimination: evaluation of educational interventions in UK secondary schools. *British Journal of Psychiatry*, 182, 342–346.

QSR International (2009). NVivo 9, retrieved from http://www.qsrinternational.com/ [accessed 15 November 2016].

Repper, J., & Perkins, R. (2003). *Social Inclusion and Recovery: A Model for Mental Health Practice*, Edinburgh: Balliere Tindall.

Rudman, D.L., Dennhardt, S., Fok, D., Huot, S., Molke, D., Park, A., & Zur, B. (2008). A vision for occupational science: Reflecting on our disciplinary culture. *Journal of Occupational Science*, 15(1), 136–146.

Russell, A., & Lloyd, C. (2004). Partnerships in mental health: Addressing barriers to social inclusion. *International Journal of Therapy & Rehabilitation*, 11(6), 267–274.

Sayce, L. (2001). Social inclusion and mental health. *Psychiatric Bulletin*, 25(4), 121–123.

Shaw, L., Leyshon, R., & Liu, M. (2007). Validating the potential of the international classification of functioning, disability and health to identify barriers to and facilitators of consumer participation. *Canadian Journal of Occupational Therapy*, 74, 255–266.

Stickley, T. (2005). Developing a social inclusion strategy for people with ongoing mental health problems. *Mental Health Practice*, 8(6), 12–15.

Stickley, T., & Shaw, R. (2006). Evaluating social inclusion. *Mental Health Practice*, 9(10), 14–20.

Stucki, G., Cieza, A., Ewert, T., Anjsek, N., Chatterji, S., & Ustun, T. (2002). Application of the international classification of functioning, disability and health (ICF) in clinical practice. *Disability and Rehabilitation*, 24(5), 281–282.

Topor, A., Borg, M., Mezzina, R., Sells, D., Marin, I., & Davidson, L. (2006). Others: The role of family, friends, and professionals in the recovery process. *American Journal of Psychiatric Rehabilitation*, 9(1), 17–37.

World Health Organisation (2001). *The International Classification of Functioning: Disability and Health (ICF)*. Geneva: World Health Organisation.

Epilogue

*Staffan Josephsson, Arne H. Eide
and Kjersti Vik*

In the introduction to this book, the intention of describing and discussing participation as a phenomenon and as a conceptual frame of reference is stated. Further, it is asserted that participation will be discussed in relation to its usefulness in research on the user/patient–provider interface. Finally, the objective is defined of addressing how issues of participation are intertwined with daily and social life, with examples from practice; and the various meanings of the concept, depending on when, how and by whom it is used, highlighted and discussed. Before closing, we will reflect on how the different contributions have met these ambitions.

The material and arguments presented in the various chapters of this book clearly confirm the diversity in use and conceptualisation of participation. This is, of course, significant when the ambition is to discuss participation as a phenomenon and as a conceptual frame of reference. The review of the term in the introduction identified a complex web of different understandings, depending on professional background and scientific discipline. This diversity in understanding and use of the concept can also be seen in the different chapters. For example, when comparing Leiulfrud's introduction to the International Classification of Functioning, Disability and Health (ICF) model (Chapter 2), and its use of the word 'participation', with Horghagen and Hocking's activist framing of the concept (Chapter 11), one might begin to wonder whether their different use of the concept refers to a diversity in the basic phenomena of interest. Are we talking about the same thing, or is participation a kind of 'elastic concept' that can even serve as an umbrella for the relevant issues at stake for people living with illness or chronic conditions and staff working with these persons?

However, we could also reverse this observation and argue that when shifting the focus of interest from traditional professional realms such as medicine to the everyday, it is to be expected that multifaceted and complex understandings will follow. The expansion of participation, as it is discussed within health and welfare services, into 'engagement in daily life' (ICF) and 'everyday life' lies at the heart of all the chapters in this book. With the broadening of the role of services to enable, prepare and stimulate users/patients to participate in everyday mainstream society, there is also a need to critically discuss what this means and implies for practice. We hope the book will be a useful contribution to this discussion.

One way in which the book addresses these matters is by drawing from the debate around how accurately the conceptualisations of participation within the ICF framework fit the everyday needs of people living with chronic conditions. One critical point concerns the classification of people, with the risk of labelling, stigma and abuse of the classification in priority settings. Is the professionalisation of the everyday really the right way to go? (Dahl 2002; Hammel 2004; Hurst 2003). Another point is that the subjective experience of participation is not sufficiently taken into account in the ICF (Hemmingsson & Jonsson 2005; Udea & Okawa, 2003). Imrie (2004) also points to the lack of a theoretical foundation of the ICF, stating that it is based on a 'political/professional compromise' rather than theory. Further, there are already related terms, such as autonomy, in use, and the relationship between participation and autonomy is not clear (Cardol, de Jong & Ward, 2002; Grimby 2002). The term 'activity' is another related concept that needs further clarification in terms of its relationship to and distinction from participation (Eide et al. 2008; Jette, Haley, & Kooyookijan, 2003; Jette, Tao, & Haley, 2007; Nordendfelt, 2003). In the chapters of this book, these issues are addressed, helping to further the current understanding of the term and possible future developments. When reading the arguments presented throughout the chapters, two central threads stand out. First, there seems to be a movement and development of the term participation towards a relational concept. Second, we see the interpretation of participation in terms of the active user rather than the passive receiver of care.

Towards a relational understanding of participation

Both Imrie (2004) and Shakespeare (2006) argue that the ICF and its use of the term participation represent the development of a relational understanding of determinants of disease and disability. This shift is not without complications. The knowledge derived from medicine, and the labelling tradition mostly identifying health and lack of health as concerning discrete components within the individual, are challenged with a situated understanding. It could be said that the use of participation has caused a shift in health, and services supporting health, from underlying discrete components to the situated web of social processes in everyday life that people are involved in on a daily basis. This move has important consequences for how service and healthcare function. In Chapter 7, Witsø and Vik address how different service users and providers might interpret and deal with problems that are at stake differently. Redzovic and Eide (Chapter 5) add to this complexity by discussing the impact of both cultural context and individual cultural preferences on the understanding of participation. Elstad and Johanssen argue in Chapter 13 how participation requires reciprocal relationships, a challenge for traditional service providers and healthcare. All the different chapters serve as a tentative and emerging map of challenges and opportunities following the move to a relational understanding of participation.

One core challenge is, of course, how and if a more relational social and situated understanding of participation can and should be measured. In Chapter 16,

Magnus, Kroksmark and Nordell present a time-geographical method as relevant in assessing participation. Even if the method is not chiefly presented as an assessment, they do touch upon the complex issue of measurement of participation. If participation is situated socially, can it then be measured on an individual level? What constitutes the unit of analysis in the emergent relational understanding of participation? The contribution from Dashner et al. (Chapter 4) represents a different tradition in participation research, and does in fact demonstrate the viability and usefulness of measuring participation at the individual level in combination with contextual variables. Rather than viewing different scientific traditions as contradictory, it may thus be useful to agree on the challenges posed by the shift to a relational understanding of participation.

From receiver of care to active user

Another key issue emerging from the analysis of participation in this book is the role of the users of health and social services. What does the shift towards participation mean for people using social and healthcare services? In Chapter 6, Beresford informatively portrays the groundings of a participatory approach within social and healthcare services. However, in several of the other chapters, the authors complicate the picture. Is it the case that professionals tend to see the voice of the user as a stable resource just waiting to be taken into account? How does such a simplistic understanding comply with more complex understandings of the everyday, such as the one presented by Alsaker, Josephsson and Dickie in Chapter 15? What about ambiguity and inconsistency? What about unequal power relations, not only between service users and providers, but also among users?

However, maybe the most urgent aspect of the move from receiver towards active participating user is the handling of the complex borders between taking personal responsibility for health and needs, and the relevant right to seek help when challenges emerge. Such questions exemplify how the shift to participation leads to new discussions and the need for a lively debate. To what extent the conceptual shifts discussed in this book will impact on the highly professionalised health and welfare services is a very relevant question. Understanding users as active participants could push forward changes in professional practice and healthcare provision, making them more tuned into current societal and individual needs for social inclusion, and reducing marginalisation.

It will be a mission for coming generations of discussants not only to engage in debates about participation, but also include new participants and forms of participation in the development of concepts that can be used to support future health and social services.

Finally, we would like to say that we hope this book has succeeded in portraying some of the consequences and discussions emerging from the shift of focus from disease as an individual impairment to participation as a shared situated phenomenon. Many of them have been touched upon, but there are numerous others. And maybe that is one of the core lessons that can be learned from this book. When moving to participation as a core concept within service delivery and the everyday life of persons in need of service, there will be a continuous need for discussion and contestation on what participation is and how it can be promoted, and more voices need to be invited into the dialogue. It is our hope that the voices in this book will be heard in such dialogues.

References

Cardol M, de Jong B, Ward C D (2002) On autonomy and participation in rehabilitation. *Disability and Rehabilitation*, 24, 18, 970–974.

Dahl T H (2002) International classification of functioning, disability and health: An introduction and discussion of its potential impact on rehabilitation services and research. *Journal of Rehabilitation Medicine*, 34, 201–204.

Eide A H, Jelsma J, Loeb M E, Maart S, Ka' Toni M (2008) Exploring ICF components in a survey among Xhosa speakers in Eastern & Western Cape, South Africa. *Disability and Rehabilitation*, 30, 11, 819–829.

Grimby G (2002) On autonomy and participation in rehabilitation. *Disability and Rehabilitation*, 24, 18.

Hammel K W (2004) Deviating from the norm: A sceptical interrogation of the classificatory practices of ICF. *British Journal of Occupational Therapy*, 67, 9, 408–411.

Hemmingsson H, Jonsson H (2005) An occupational perspective on the concept of participation in the international classification of functioning, disability and health – Some critical remarks. *American Journal of Occupational Therapy*, 59, 5, 569–576.

Hurst R (2003) The international disability rights movement and the ICF. *Disability and Rehabilitation*, 25, 11–12, 572–576.

Imrie R (2004) Demystifying disability: A review of the international classification of functioning, disability and health. *Sociology of Health and Illness*, 26, 3, 287–305.

Jette A M, Haley S M, Kooyookijan J T (2003) Are the ICF activity and participation dimensions distinct? *Rehabilitation Medicine*, 35, 145–149.

Jette A M, Tao W, Haley S M (2007) Blending activity and participation sub-domains of the ICF. *Disability and Rehabilitation*, 29, 22, 1742–1750.

Nordenfelt L (2003) Action theory, disability and ICF. *Disability & Rehabilitation*, 25, 18, 1075–1079.

Shakespeare T. (2006) *Disability Rights and Wrongs*. Routledge: London and New York.

Udea S, Okawa Y (2003) The subjective dimension of functioning and disability: What is it and what is it for? *Disability and Rehabilitation*, 25, 11–12, 596–601.

Index

Milton Keynes UK
Ingram Content Group UK Ltd.
UKHW040105071024
449327UK00019B/822